Multidisciplinary Approaches to Breathing Pattern Disorders

For Churchill Livingstone:

Editoral Director, Health Professions: Mary Law
Head of Project Management: Ewan Halley
Project Development Manager: Katrina Mather
Design Direction: George Ajayi/Judith Wright

Multidisciplinary Approaches to Breathing Pattern Disorders

Foreword by

Leon Chaitow ND DO
Registered Osteopathic Practitioner and Senior Lecturer,
University of Westminster, London, UK

Dinah Bradley DipPhys NZRP MNZSP
Private Consultant Respiratory Physiotherapist,
Breathing Works, Remuera, Auckland, New Zealand

Christopher Gilbert PhD
Psychologist, Chronic Pain Management Program,
Kaiser Permanente Medical Center, San Francisco,
California, USA

Foreword by

Ronald Ley
Research Professor, University of Albany,
State University of New York, New York, USA

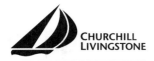

EDINBURGH LONDON NEW YORK OXFORD PHILADELPHIA ST LOUIS SYDNEY TORONTO 2002

CHURCHILL LIVINGSTONE
An imprint of Elsevier Science Limited

First published 2002
Reprinted 2002

ISBN 0 443 07053 9

British Library Cataloguing in Publication Data
A catalogue record for this book is available from the British Library.

Library of Congress Cataloging in Publication Data
A catalog record for this book is available from the Library of Congress.

Note
Medical knowledge is constantly changing. As new information becomes available, changes in treatment, procedures, equipment and the use of drugs become necessary. The authors and the publishers have taken care to ensure that the information given in this text is accurate and up to date. However, readers are strongly advised to confirm that the information, especially with regard to drug usage, complies with the latest legislation and standards of practice.

Neither the publisher nor the authors will be liable for any loss or damage of any nature occasioned to or suffered by any person acting or refraining from acting as a result of reliance on the material contained in this publication.

Before treating breathing pattern disorders it is important for practitioners and therapists to ensure that a valid diagnosis exists in case more serious pathology is also a factor. Differential diagnosis by a suitably qualified and licensed healthcare provider offers a degree of safety to both the patient and the practitioner/therapist, especially when patients have self-referred. No claims are made in this book to teach medical diagnoses other than to offer guidelines, and to encourage interprofessional liaison (with the patient's permission), between the practitioner/therapist and the patient's primary health care provider/general practitioner/specialist. It is important for practitioners/therapists to check their regional professional medical standards requirements in order to establish appropriate patient/therapist protocols.

ELSEVIER SCIENCE
your source for books, journals and multimedia in the health sciences
www.elsevierhealth.com

The publisher's policy is to use paper manufactured from sustainable forests

Printed in China
C/02

Contents

Foreword

Breathing is a complicated dynamic process with some crucial parameters that were until recently difficult to measure non-invasively. It may be for this reason that respiration has taken so long to come to the attention of scientists who study psychophysiology and clinicians who treat psychophysiological disorders. Although the International Society for the Advancement of Respiratory Psychophysiology, an organization whose membership includes both scientists and clinicians, was founded less than a decade ago, there is a considerably longer history of individual scientists and clinicians, sometimes in informal groups but usually in individual efforts, who have pondered the complications of breathing in a quest for knowledge and a quest for applications designed to help those who suffer respiratory diseases or suffer disorders associated with dysfunctional breathing.

Although my training in experimental psychology included the rudiments of neurophysiology and the physiological substratum of sensation and emotions, my first encounter with what would come to be known as respiratory psychophysiology was in 1971 at the Temple University School of Medicine on the occasion of a demonstration by Joseph Wolpe of the anxiolytic effects of single inhalations of large concentrations of carbon dioxide mixed with oxygen (65% CO_2 with 35% O_2). The procedure required that the patient put an inhalation mask to the face and take a full capacity inhalation of the CO_2—O_2 mixture. Although the patient was told what the resulting sensation would be, the sharp respiratory response driven by the CO_2 inhalation (rapid cycles of full capacity ventilation) elicited a wide-eyed mouth-agape expression of startle, and rendered the patient momentarily incapable of speech. After a very brief period of recovery (about one minute), the patient regained control of breathing and speech; the muscles of the face relaxed, the stiffened posture of the upper torso relaxed, and the patient reported a pleasant sense of relaxation and release from anxiety. Why?

While the effects of CO_2 inhalation on breathing were clearly a consequence of the CO_2-sensitive chemoreceptors that drive respiration, why should the dissipation of CO_2 following a single inhalation of a colorless and odorless combination of CO_2 and O_2 have such rapid and profound effects on muscle tension and mood? I was intrigued, as was Herb Walker, a clinical professor of psychiatry at the New York University School of Medicine. Together, with Wolpe's approval and encouragement, we conducted an experiment in Wolpe's lab. The study, published in 1973, documented the anxiolytic effects of the CO_2 inhalation, provided data on changes in heart rate and blood pressure, and ultimately (1994) led to a satisfactory theoretical explanation of the anxiolytic effects in terms of Dick Solomon's opponent-process theory of emotion. Most important, for the purpose of this foreword, Wolpe's demonstration and the ensuing experiment conducted with Walker left me with a newfound interest in the study of breathing.

My new interest led me to the works of Claude Lum and to others who had written seminal papers on hyperventilation and its production of a broad range of psychosomatic complaints. With metabolism relatively constant (i.e. insignificant variance from moment to moment), an increase in ventilation (the volume of air breathed from respiratory cycle to respiratory cycle) will increase the rate of flow of CO_2 from tissue cells to the point of diffusion of CO_2 from the pulmonary artery to the alveoli of the lungs. If this rate of flow is too fast, the concentration of CO_2 in blood will be too lean, acid level of blood will drop, the crucial ratio of base to acid will increase, and the unbalanced pH will be alkalotic. If the rate of flow of CO_2 is too slow, its concentration in blood will be too rich, acid level will rise, the crucial ratio of base to acid will decrease, and the unbalanced pH will be acidic. In healthy individuals under non-stressful conditions, the self-regulatory mechanisms of breathing will automatically calculate the amount of O_2 needed for metabolism and increase or decrease the volume of air breathed per unit of time so that the rate of flow of CO_2 from cells to lungs will be just right, neither too fast nor too slow, and a stable level of balanced pH will be maintained. And what a delicate balance it is.

Disease aside, the delicate balance is upset when problems of everyday living arise. Breathing is exquisitely sensitive to stress. Apneusis, apnea, and hyperventilation occur in different stages of the respiratory response to stress, depending on the qualitative and quantitative nature of the stress. While apneusis and apnea are limited to relatively brief periods by physiological barriers that can not be overridden, hyperventilation is not. Additional complications result from the fact that breathing is the only vital function under voluntary as well as involuntary control. Although voluntary control is limited by physiological mechanisms, the breathing behavior within these limits can be modified by learning. The conditionability of breathing behavior has a negative and a positive side. The negative side is that unhealthy dysfunctional habits of breathing can be acquired. The positive side is that bad habits can be extinguished and replaced with good habits.

Leon Chaitow, Dinah Bradley, and Christopher Gilbert have written a thorough and highly readable book that provides detailed information on the relevant physiological and psychological processes that underlie breathing. The unique backgrounds that each of the authors bring to the study of breathing and the treatment of its disorders provide a vast amount of information that is nicely synthesized in their vivid description of breathing pattern disorders and their detailed explanation of how these patterns of breathing disorders can be remedied. This book marks a singular advancement in clinical respiratory psychophysiology.

Albany, NY 2002 Ronald Ley

Preface

Many bodily functions are essential to survival, but breathing is our lifeline, linking us with the world from birth to death. Just as we eat food, extract nourishment from it, and excrete the leavings, we must take in air, extract oxygen, and exhale carbon dioxide as if each breath were a separate meal. Precise regulation of respiration is crucial to health, but many things can go wrong. Breathing is subject to major interference and disruption, in large part because of thinking, feeling, and experience, and also as a result of biomechanical and biochemical factors.

This book concentrates on problems in the breathing process as seen and treated by our three professional disciplines: osteopathy, physiotherapy, and psychology. The first and third basically anchor the ends of a body–mind continuum, while the middle one spans the gap. Yet each of us uses techniques from the entire continuum. Most readers will go first to the chapters that confirm and enlarge upon what they already know. But that will not be as challenging as exploring the other chapters; much as we have tried to define things and avoid jargon, some of the terms and concepts will be foreign at first. But to the curious reader, some meta-variables should emerge.

There are principles in the operation of an organism that cut across mind–body borders. Writing this book, reading each other's material, we often felt that we were using the same concepts to talk about very different subject matter. We write about rigidity in the muscles of the thorax, and about rigidity as expressed in fearful attitudes; both affect breathing. We describe hyperventilation as compensating for blood acidity and also as compensating for feelings of helplessness. Flexibility is as important for a muscle as for social behavior; both can influence breathing. Protection, preparation, compensation, adaptation: these happen at many levels from the cellular to the behavioral to the attitudinal. Traces of an old trauma can disrupt free breathing through bracing of abdominal muscles; is this psychological, physiological, or some dimension of life which finally unites the two?

It is difficult, if not impossible, to separate psychological from physiological features in normal and unbalanced breathing. Emotion can alter, and be altered by, changes in the pH of the blood. Patterns of use, such as habitual upper-chest breathing, which are directly linked to such chemical modifications, ultimately modify the very structures that perform the functions involved in respiration. These structural musculoskeletal changes eventually become major obstacles to the resumption of normal patterns of breathing.

The concepts and methods of psychotherapy, physiotherapy and osteopathy, although different, are united in recognizing the potency of self-regulating homeostatic systems and mechanisms on which the maintenance and recovery of health depend. Making sense of the interacting biochemical, emotional and biomechanical etiological features of breathing pattern disorders is the clinician's struggle. As efforts are made to reduce the individual's adaptive load and/or to enhance the ability to handle that load, the wide perspectives and practical solutions that the authors bring to this task offer a set of clinical choices from which an integrated therapeutic and rehabilitation approach can be constructed to meet the unique needs of each patient.

The widespread commercialization of health and the ability of people to avail themselves of detailed information on health issues via the internet have helped create a subculture of apprehension in many people. The bewildering collection of seemingly unrelated symptoms experienced by those suffering from chronic breathing pattern dysfunction leads to increasing levels of fear and anxiety and loss of quality of life.

Whether hyperventilation syndrome/breathing pattern dysfunctions (HVS/BPDs) are primarily psychiatric or physical disorders has been the subject of lively debate among clinicians in all disciplines. Various avenues of research have gained ascendancy at different times, emphasizing the dualistic approach to health in modern medicine – that is, that mental and physical disorders are separate, coexisting issues. Continuing research into human stress and relaxation responses, however, has brought HVS/BPDs back under scrutiny in the last couple of decades.

Another factor in the reappraisal of HVS/BPDs as a primary health problem is tighter health funding. Misdiagnosis is expensive; patients may be repeatedly sent for costly, sometimes risky or invasive, investigations, only to be told 'nothing is wrong' in spite of recurring symptoms. Anxiety levels further increase as patients continue to experience very real symptoms.

Our goal in this book is to redress the lack of awareness of these disabling and distressing disorders. We have all gained from working together on this text. Our aim has been that those reading our three different approaches will gain much as well – not only to enhance their own clinical skills but also to stimulate research and bring these ubiquitous disorders the recognition they deserve.

Leon Chaitow
Dinah Bradley
Chris Gilbert

Acknowledgments

To British physicians Claude Lum and Peter Nixon many thanks for, and appreciation of, their elegant writtings and outstanding research on breathing pattern disorder. To Beverly Timmons, warmest appreciation for master-minding and holding together ISARP (International Society for the Advancement of Respiratory Psychophysiology), where new research and ideas are presented annually. My appreciation and thanks to David Scott MB ChB B Med Sci FRCP(Lond) FRACP for invaluable help with tables and medical text and for constructive advice; John Henley MB ChB FRACP for continuing professional support; the Respiratory Medicine and Physiotherapy Department at Green Lane Hospital for recognizing the value to patients of this work; special thanks to physiotherapists Annette Jackman and Pam Young.

I want to thank Leon Chaitow and Chris Gilbert for the opportunity to work with them both on this book and for the sharing of ideas and information, especially Leon for putting the mix together and having the drive to get us, from our three disciplines, together from such distant parts of the world. Inevitably, embarking on a project such as this has made demands on family and friends. I want to give special appreciation to my sons, Jake and Keir, and my practice partner at B r e a t h i n g Works Tania Clifton-Smith.

Dinah Bradley

I wish to thank these leaders and original thinkers in the area of hyperventilation: Robert Fried, Claude Lum, Ronald Ley, Beverly Timmons and Peter Nixon. These were my main guides for combining psychological and behavioral observations with the intricacies of respiratory physiology. Herbert Fensterheim, Bernard Landis, Ashley Conway, David Mars, and many others, including my co-authors, enlarged my understanding of this endlessly intriguing topic.

Chris Gilbert

I join my co-authors in their acknowledgments, and wish to add the many osteopathic and other clinicians and researchers whose ideas and methods broadened my horizons as to how to recognize and handle (literally) the biomechanical and other dysfunctional tendencies associated with problems such as breathing pattern disorders, particularly Karel Lewit, Vladimir Janda, Craig Liebenson, Fred Mitchell Sr, Laurence Jones, Irvin Korr, Michael Kuchera, Phil Latey, David Simons, Janet Travell, and all the others quoted and referenced in this book. My particular and special thanks to Dinah Bradley and Chris Gilbert for their enthusiastic collaboration on this interdisciplinary project.

Leon Chaitow

Glossary/Abbreviations

A alveolar (e.g. PA_{O_2})

a arterial (e.g. Pa_{O_2})

Ach acetylcholine

AHI Aviation Health Institute

ALTEs apparent life-threatening events

anaerobic threshold highest oxygen consumption during exercise, above which sustained lactic acidosis occurs

ASI Anxiety Sensitivity Index

ARTT asymmetry/range of motion alteration/tissue texture alteration/tenderness

ASIS anterior superior iliac spine, an anatomical location

ATP adenosine triphosphate

BPD breathing pattern disorder

BBT Buteyko breathing technique

BUL, BUM backward upward laterally, backward upward medially

C cervical (as in C7, or seventh cervical vertebra)

CAL chronic airway limitation (e.g. COAD)

Catecholamines collective term for compounds with a sympathomimetic action (e.g. adrenaline)

CCP common compensatory pattern

CHD coronary heart disease

CNS central nervous system

CO_2 carbon dioxide

COAD chronic obstructive airways disease

CPAP continuous positive airways pressure

CT cervicothoracic

CXR chest X-ray

ECG electrocardiogram

EIA exercise induced asthma

EMG electromyography

end-tidal CO_2 measure of CO_2 in exhaled air

ET CO_2 end-tidal CO_2 (normal 4–6%)

FVC forced vital capacity

FEV_1 forced expiratory volume in one second

Hb (hemoglobin) respiratory pigment in red blood cells, combines reversibly with O_2 (normal: men: 14.0–18.0 g/100 ml; women: 11.5–15.5 g/100 ml)

HVPT hyperventilation provocation test

HVT high velocity thrust, a manipulative method (also known as HVLA – high velocity low amplitude – thrust)

hyperventilation CO_2 removal in excess of CO_2 production, producing $Pa_{CO_2} < 4.6$ kPa or 35 mmHg

hypoventilation CO_2 production in excess of CO_2 removal producing $Pa_{CO_2} > 6.0$ kPa or 45 mmHG

IgE immunoglobulin E, an antibody involved in allergic reactions

IMT inspiratory muscle training

INIT integrated neuromuscular inhibition technique (a combination of different soft tissue approaches used to deactivate trigger points)

kPa kilopascal

L lumbar (as in L1, or first lumbar vertebra)

LS lumbosacral

MV resting minute volume

NANC nonadrenergic noncholinergic

NMT neuromuscular technique(s), a treatment method, or neuromuscular therapy, a therapeutic approach

µg microgram

mmHg millimeters of mercury

MET muscle energy techniques, a treatment method

MFR myofascial release, a treatment method

MPI myofascial pain index (evaluation of the average current poundage required to evoke pain in an individual, on applied pressure, using a series of test points)

MWM mobilization with movement, a therapeutic approach

NAGs neutral apophyseal glides (treatment method)

OMT osteopathic manipulative therapy (or treatment)

OA occipito-atlantal

OSA obstructive sleep apnea

PEFR peak expiratory flow rate

PLB pursed-lips breathing

Pao$_2$ partial pressure of oxygen in the blood

Paco$_2$ partial pressure of carbon dioxide in the blood

PETco$_2$ measure of end-tidal CO_2 from exhaled air

pH relative alkalinity or acidity of body fluids

PIR post-isometric relaxation (an effect achieved in application of MET)

PRT positional release techniques

PSG polysomnograph

QL quadratus lumborum

QOL quality of life

REM rapid eye movement

RI reciprocal inhibition (an effect achieved in application of MET)

RRAF Ruddy's reciprocal antagonist facilitation (a version of MET)

RSA respiratory sinus arrhythmia

RV residual value

SaO$_2$ saturation of hemoglobin with oxygen from arterial sampling

SCS strain/counterstrain (an osteopathic treatment method)

SI(J) sacroiliac (joint)

SCM sternocleidomastoid (muscle)

SNAGs sustained neutral apophyseal glides (treatment method)

SpO$_2$ noninvasive estimation of arterial oxyhemoglobin by pulse oximetry

SIDS sudden infant death syndrome

TFL tensor fasciae latae (muscle)

TL thoracolumbar

TMJ temporomandibular joint

torr mmHg

T thoracic (as in T1, or first thoracic vertebra)

TCM Traditional Chinese Medicine

TLC total lung capacity

UPPP ulvulopalatopharyngoplasty

VC vital capacity

Vt tidal volume

1

The structure and function of breathing

Leon Chaitow
Dinah Bradley

THE STRUCTURE–FUNCTION CONTINUUM

Nowhere in the body is the axiom of structure governing function more apparent than in its relation to respiration. This is also a region in which prolonged modifications of function – such as the inappropriate breathing pattern displayed during hyperventilation – inevitably induce structural changes, for example involving accessory breathing muscles as well as the thoracic articulations. Ultimately, the self-perpetuating cycle of functional change creating structural modification leading to reinforced dysfunctional tendencies can become complete, from whichever direction dysfunction arrives, for example: structural adaptations can prevent normal breathing function, and abnormal breathing function ensures continued structural adaptational stresses leading to decompensation.

Restoration of normal function requires restoration of adequate mobility to the structural component and, self-evidently, maintenance of any degree of restored biomechanical integrity requires that function (how the individual breathes) should be normalized through re-education and training.

MULTIPLE INFLUENCES: BIOMECHANICAL, BIOCHEMICAL, AND PSYCHOLOGICAL

The area of respiration is one in which the interaction between biochemical, biomechanical, and psychosocial features is dramatically evident

1

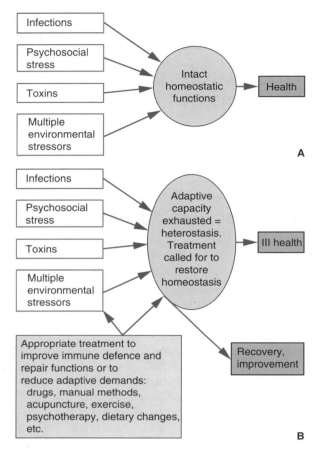

Figure 1.1 A Homeostasis. **B** Heterostasis. (Reproduced with kind permission from Chaitow 1999.)

(Fig. 1.1A, 1.1B). Inappropriate breathing can result directly from structural, biomechanical causes, such as a restricted thoracic spine or rib immobility or shortness of key respiratory muscles.

Causes of breathing dysfunction can also have a more biochemical etiology, possibly involving an allergy or infection which triggers narrowing of breathing passages and subsequent asthmatic-type responses. Acidosis resulting from conditions such as kidney failure will also directly alter breathing function as the body attempts to reduce acid levels via elimination of CO_2 through the means of hyperventilation.

The link between psychological distress and breathing makes this another primary cause of many manifestations of dysfunctional respiration. Indeed, it is hard to imagine examining a person suffering from anxiety or depression without breathing dysfunction being noted.

Other catalysts which may impact on breathing function include environmental factors (altitude, humidity, etc.). Even factors such as where an individual is born may contribute to subsequent breathing imbalances: 'People who are born at high altitude have a diminished ventilatory response to hypoxia that is only slowly corrected by subsequent residence at sea level. Conversely, those born at sea level who move to high altitudes retain their hypoxic response intact for a long time. Apparently therefore ventilatory response is determined very early in life' (West 2000).

How we breathe and how we feel are intimately conjoined in a two-way loop. Feeling anxious produces a distinctive pattern of upper-chest breathing which modifies blood chemistry, leading to a chain reaction of effects, inducing anxiety, and so reinforcing the pattern which produced the dysfunctional pattern of breathing in the first place.

Even when an altered pattern of breathing is the result of emotional distress, it will eventually produce the structural, biomechanical changes which are described below. This suggests that when attempting to restore normal breathing – by means of re-education and exercise for example – both the psychological initiating factors and the structural compensation patterns need to be addressed. (The psychological effects of breathing dysfunction are covered in greater detail in Chapter 5.)

Homeostasis and heterostasis

The body is a self-healing mechanism. Broken bones mend and cuts usually heal, and most health disturbances – from infections to digestive upsets – get better with or without treatment (often faster without!), and, in a healthy state, there exists a constant process for normalization and health promotion. This is called homeostasis.

However, the homeostatic functions (which include the immune system) can become overwhelmed by too many tasks and demands as a result of any, or all, of a selection of negative impacts, including nutritional deficiencies, accumulated toxins (environmental pollution, either as food or inhaled, in medication, previous or current use of drugs, etc.), emotional stress, recurrent or current infections, allergies, modified functional ability due to age, or inborn factors, or acquired habits involving poor posture, breathing imbalances and/or sleep disturbances, and so on and on … (Fig. 1.2).

At a certain point in time the adaptive homeo-static mechanisms break down, and frank illness – disease – appears. At this time the situation has modified from homeostasis to *heterostasis*, and at this time the body needs help – treatment. Treatment can take a number of forms, which are usually classifiable as involving one of three broad strategies:

1. Reducing the load impacting the body by taking away as many of the undesirable adaptive factors as possible (by avoiding allergens, improving posture and breathing, learning stress coping tactics, improving diet, using supplements if called for, helping normalize sleep and circulatory function, introducing a detoxification program if needed, dealing with infections) and generally trying to keep

the pressure off the defense mechanisms while the body focuses on its current repair needs.
2. Enhancing, improving, modulating the defense and repair processes by a variety of means, sometimes via specific intervention and sometimes involving non-specific, constitutional methods.
3. Treating the symptoms while making sure that nothing is being done to add further to the burden of the defense mechanisms.

Not all available therapeutic measures need to be employed, because once the load on the adaptation and repair processes has reduced sufficiently, a degree of normal homeostatic self-regulating function is automatically restored, and the healing process commences.

Therapy as a stress factor

A corollary to the perspective of therapy being aimed at the 'removal of obstacles to self-healing'

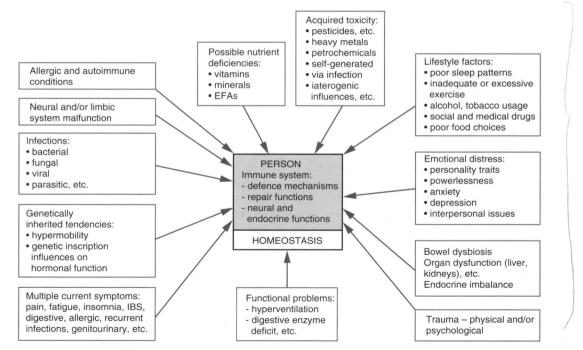

When homeostatic adaptive capacity is exhausted treatment calls for:
1. Restoration of immune competence, enhancement of defence capabilities, support of repair functions
2. Reduction of as many of the multiple interacting stressors impacting the individual as possible
3. Attention to symptoms (ideally without creating new problems).

Figure 1.2 Multiple stressors in fibromyalgia. (Reproduced with kind permission from Chaitow 1999.)

is that, since almost any form of 'treatment' involves further adaptive demands, therapeutic interventions need to be tailored to the ability of the individual to respond to the treatment. Excessive adaptive demands made of an individual, already in a state of adaptive exhaustion, are bound to make matters worse.

A clinical rule of thumb adopted by one of the authors (LC) is that the more ill a patient is, the more symptoms are displayed, and the weaker is the evidence of vitality, the lighter, gentler, and more 'constitutional' (whole person) the intervention needs to be. (See Ch. 4 for discussion of adaptation exhaustion, and Zink's protocols.) Whereas a robust, vital individual might well respond positively to several simultaneous therapeutic demands, for example a change in diet together with medication, bodywork, and rehabilitation exercises, someone who is more frail and less vital might well collapse under such an adaptive therapeutic assault. For the frail patient, a single modification or therapeutic change might be called for, with ample time allowed to adapt to the change (whether this involves exercise, posture, diet, bodywork, medication, psychological intervention, or anything else).

In any given case it is necessary to focus attention on what seems to be the likeliest and easiest targets (perhaps using a team approach in which more than one therapist/therapy is being utilized) which will achieve this desirable end. In one person this may call for rehabilitation exercises accompanied by psychotherapy/counseling; in another, dietary modification and stress reduction could be merited; while in another, enhancement of immune function and structural mobilization using bodywork and exercise may be considered the most appropriate interventions. The 'art' of health care demands the employment of safe and appropriate interventions to suit the particular needs of each individual.

OBJECTIVES AND METHODS

The focus of this book is on normal versus abnormal respiratory patterns (function), and how best to restore normality once an altered pattern has been established. This commonly requires the removal of causative factors, if identifiable, and, if possible, the rehabilitation of habitual, acquired dysfunctional breathing patterns, and, in order to achieve this most efficiently, some degree of structural mobilization to restore the machinery of breathing towards normality.

If rehabilitation is attempted without taking account of etiological features or maintaining features – restricted rib articulations, shortened thoracic musculature, etc. – results will be less than optimal.

An example of extreme breathing pattern alteration is hyperventilation. Hyperventilation and its effects occupy a major part of the book. It will also be necessary to explore the widespread gray area in which normal patterning is clearly absent, even though patent hyperventilation is not demonstrable.

A perspective needs to be held in which function and structure are kept in mind as dual, interdependent features. The thoracic cage can be thought of as a cylindrical structure housing most major organs – lungs, heart, liver, spleen, pancreas, kidneys. The functions associated with the thorax (or with muscles attached to it) include respiration, visceral activity, stabilization, and movement (and therefore posture) of the head, neck, ribs, spinal structures, and upper extremity.

The causes of dysfunctional breathing patterns will be seen to possibly involve etiological features which may in nature be largely biomechanical (for example post-surgical or postural factors), biochemical (including allergic or infection factors), or psychosocial (chronic emotional states such as anxiety and anger). Etiology may also involve combinations of these factors, or established pathology may be the cause. In many instances, altered breathing patterns, whatever their origins, are maintained by nothing more sinister than pure habit (Lum 1994).

Where pathology provides the background to altered breathing patterns, the aim of this book is not to explore these disease states (e.g. asthma, cardiovascular disease) in any detail except insofar as they impact on breathing patterning (for example where airway obstruction causes normal nasal inhalation to alter to mouth breathing). The changes which concern this text are largely functional in nature rather than pathological, although the impact on the physiology of the individual of an altered breathing pattern such as hyperventilation can be profound, possibly resulting in severe health problems ranging from anxiety and panic attacks to fatigue and chronic pain.

It is axiomatic that in order to make sense of abnormal respiration, it is essential to have a reasonable understanding of normality. As a foundation for what follows, this chapter will outline the basic characteristics of normal breathing. The biochemical and alveolar processes involved in respiration (as distinct from the biomechanical process of breathing) will be covered in later chapters.

NORMAL BREATHING

RESPIRATORY BENEFITS

Optimal respiratory function offers a variety of benefits to the body:

- It allows an exchange of gases involving
  — the acquisition of oxygen (O_2)
  — the elimination of carbon dioxide (CO_2).
- The efficient exchange of these gases enhances cellular function and so facilitates normal performance of the brain, organs, and tissues of the body.
- It permits normal speech.
- It is intimately involved in human non-verbal expression (sighing, etc.).
- It assists in fluid movement (lymph, blood).
- It helps maintain spinal mobility through regular, mobilizing, thoracic cage movement.
- It enhances digestive function via rhythmic positive and negative pressure fluctuations, when diaphragmatic function is normal.

Any modification of breathing function from the optimal is capable of producing negative effects on these functions.

THE UPPER AIRWAY (Figs 1.3–1.10)

To enter the air sacs of the lungs, air journeys through a series of passages: nose, nasopharynx, oropharynx, laryngeal pharynx, larynx, trachea, bronchi, and bronchioles. Disease and dysfunction can affect any of these segments and cause abnormal breathing patterns, and it is important to recognize and treat any such conditions before attempting to correct abnormal patterns such as hyperventilation.

The nose

The nose is an intriguing characteristic facial feature, taking on a variety of shapes and sizes, and changing with age. It is a complex structure with a number of vital functions:

- Air enters each narrow nostril (the external *naris*), streaming into a tall *cave*.
- Further turbulence is created by three curved bony plates (termed *conchae*) on the outer wall. These increase the mucosal surface area.
- Bristling hairs (*vibrissae*) inside the nostril trap large floating debris, while fine dust is arrested by a forest of fine hairs and a film of mucus floating on the nasal mucosa.
- In this fashion, the air is filtered, warmed, and humidified before leaving the nose via large apertures (*choanae*) above the hard palate.
- The mucosa has a rich blood supply providing heat and fluid, and is thickest over the tips of the conchae.
- During (for instance) a cold, the mucous membrane can swell, blocking the passage of air.
- Air in the upper reaches of the tall cave can enter *attics* (cool air sinuses) through narrow openings (*ostia*). Here, warming and further filtering takes place.
- These sinuses are named the *frontal* behind the forehead, the *maxillary* behind the cheek, and the *ethmoid* and *sphenoid* under the bridge of the nose.
- The dust-laden mucus can work forward toward the nostrils, where it dries and can be removed.
- There is a backward flow as well, and this collection can be swallowed or coughed out.

Box 1.1 gives details of the osseous and muscular components of the nasal apparatus, and Chapter 6 describes palpation/treatment exercises relating to them.

Box 1.1 Key facial and cranial structures associated with the nasal function

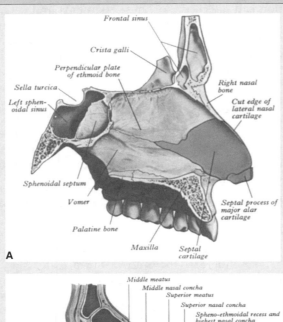

A

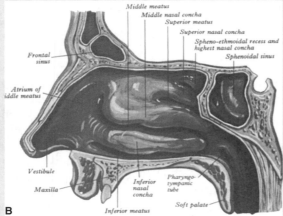

B

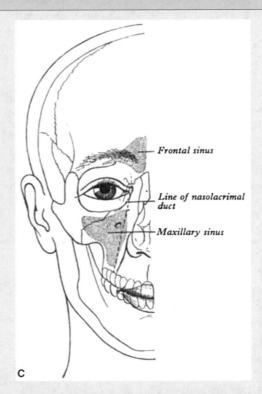

C

Figure 1.3 A The right side of the septum of the nose, showing its constituent bones and cartilages. **B** The lateral wall of the right half of the nasal cavity: internal aspect. **C** An outline of the bones of the face, showing the positions of the frontal and maxillary sinuses. (Reproduced with kind permission from Gray 1989.)

Sphenoid (see Fig. 1.4)
- The body of the sphenoid – a hollow structure enclosing an air sinus – is situated at the centre of the cranium
- Two 'great' wings, the lateral surfaces of which form the temples, are the only aspect of this bone palpable from outside the head
- The anterior surfaces of the great wings form part of the eye socket
- The anterior surfaces of the two lesser wings form part of the eye socket
- Two pterygoid processes hang down from the great wings and are palpable intraorally posteromedial to the eighth upper tooth
- The pterygoid plates form part of the pterygoid processes and are important muscular attachment sites

- The sella turcica ('Turkish saddle') houses the pituitary gland
- The sphenobasilar junction with the occiput is a synchondrosis which fuses in adult life

Articulations relevant to respiration
- Anteriorly with the ethmoid
- Inferiorly with the palatine bones
- Inferiorly with the vomer
- Anterolaterally with the zygomata

Relevant muscular attachments
- The temporalis muscle attaches to the great wing and the frontal, parietal, and temporal bones, crossing important sutures such as the coronal, squamous, and frontosphenoidal

Box 1.1 (Continued)

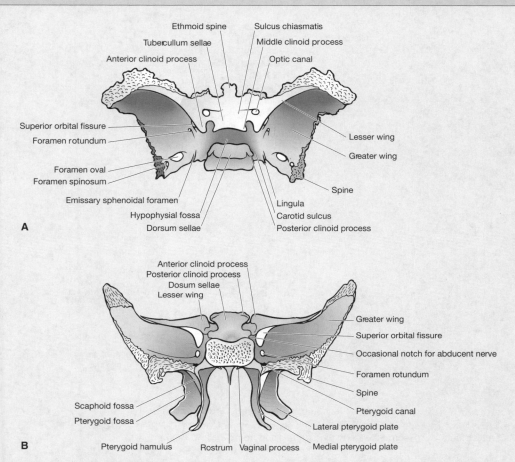

Ethmoid spine
Sulcus chiasmatis
Tuberculum sellae
Middle clinoid process
Anterior clinoid process
Optic canal
Superior orbital fissure
Foramen rotundum
Lesser wing
Greater wing
Foramen oval
Foramen spinosum
Spine
Emissary sphenoidal foramen
Lingula
Hypophysial fossa
Carotid sulcus
Dorsum sellae
Posterior clinoid process

A

Anterior clinoid process
Posterior clinoid process
Dosum sellae
Lesser wing
Greater wing
Superior orbital fissure
Occasional notch for abducent nerve
Foramen rotundum
Spine
Scaphoid fossa
Pterygoid canal
Pterygoid fossa
Lateral pterygoid plate
Pterygoid hamulus   Rostrum   Vaginal process   Medial pterygoid plate

B

Figure 1.4 A Superior aspect of the sphenoid bone and its major features. **B** Posterior aspect of the sphenoid bone and its major features. (Reproduced with kind permission from Chaitow 1998.)

- Specifically, the attachments of temporalis are to the temporal bone, the zygomatic arch, the mandible, and the lateral and medial pterygoid plates of the sphenoid
- Attaching to the internal pterygoid plate are buccinator as well as a number of small palate-related muscles
- Medial pterygoid attaches to lateral pterygoid plate and palatine bones, running to the medial ramus and angle of the mandible
- Lateral pterygoid attaches to the great wing of the sphenoid, the lateral pterygoid plate, and the anterior neck of the mandible

Neural associations
The first six cranial nerves have direct associations with the sphenoid, with the 2nd (optic), 3rd (part of oculomotor), 4th (trochlear), 5th (nasociliary, frontal, lacrimal, mandibular,

and maxillary branches of trigeminus), and 6th (abducens) all passing through the bone into the eye socket (the 1st, the olfactory nerve, runs superior to the lesser wings).

Ethmoid (see Fig. 1.5)
A tissue paper thin construction comprising a central horizontal plate (cribriform) which contains tiny openings for the passage of neural structures, surrounded by shell-shaped air sinuses forming a honeycomb framework to each side of the plate, which is crowned by: a thin crest (crista galli) formed by the dragging attachment of the falx cerebri; thin, bony, plate-like structures which form the medial eye socket; additional projections and plates, one forming part of the nasal septum, with the perpendicular plate being a virtual continuation of the vomer (see below).

Box 1.1 (Continued)

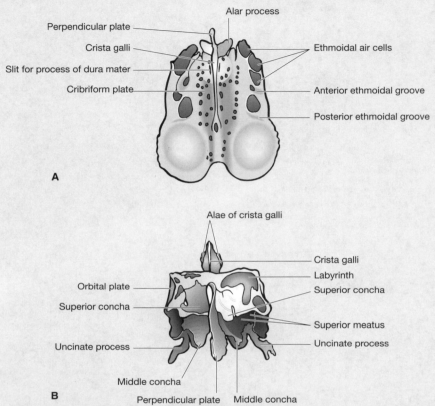

Figure 1.5 A Superior aspect of the ethmoid bone showing major features. **B** Posterior aspect of the ethmoid bone showing major features. (Reproduced with kind permission from Chaitow 1998.)

Articulations
There are interdigitated sutures with the sphenoid and non-digitated sutures with the vomer, nasal bones, palatines, maxillae, and frontal bone.

Reciprocal tension membrane relationships
• The falx cerebri attaches directly to the crista galli
• The inferior border connects with the nasal cartilage

Other associations and influences
Air passing through the shell-like ethmoid air cells is warmed before reaching the lungs and the alternation of pressures as air enters and leaves the ethmoid results in minor degrees of motion between it and its neighboring structures. Because in life its tissue paper like delicacy has a spongy consistency, it must be presumed that the structure acts as a local shock absorber.

The first cranial (olfactory) nerve lies superior to the cribriform plate and from this derive numerous neural penetrations of it which innervate mucous membranes which provide the olfactory sense.

Treatment protocols for the ethmoid will be found in Chapter 6.

Vomer
This is a plough-shaped sandwich of thin, bony tissue which houses a cartilaginous membrane, which forms the nasal cartilage. It is a junction point between the ethmoid and the maxillae, and the maxillae and the sphenoid.

Articulations
• Superiorly, it articulates with the sphenoid at a tongue-and-groove joint of spectacular beauty, as the vomer forms two wing-shaped expansions which dovetail with the receptacle offered by the inferior aspect of the centre of the sphenoid
• On the inferior aspect of the sphenoid the vomer also has minor articulation contacts with the palatine bones at the rostrum
• There is a direct, plain (not interdigitated) suture with the ethmoid at its anterosuperior aspect, the vomer

Box 1.1 (Continued)

being a virtual continuation of the ethmoid's perpendicular plate
- The inferior aspect of the vomer articulates with the maxillae and the palatines
- There is a cartilaginous articulation with the nasal septum

Muscular attachments
There are no direct muscular attachments.

Associations and influences
As with the ethmoid, this is a pliable, shock-absorbing structure which conforms and deforms, depending on the demands made on it by surrounding structures. The mucous membrane covering the vomer assists in warming air in nasal breathing.

Treatment protocols for the vomer will be found in Chapter 6.

Zygomata
Each zygoma has:
- A central broad curved malar surface
- A concave 'corner' which makes up most of the lateral, and half of the inferior, border of the orbit
- An anteroinferior border which articulates with the maxilla
- A superior jutting frontal process which articulates superiorly via interdigitations with the temporal portion of the frontal bone and posteriorly with the greater wing of the sphenoid
- A posteromedial border which articulates via interdigitations with the greater wing above and the orbital surface of the maxilla below

Articulations
The zygoma articulates:
- With the temporals via the zygomatic bone where it meets the zygomatic process at the zygomaticotemporal suture
- With the frontal bone at the frontozygomatic suture
- With the maxillae at the zygomaticomaxillary suture
- With the sphenoid at the zygomatic margin

Muscular attachments
- Masseter attaches from the zygomatic arch both superficially and deep, running superficially to the lower lateral ramus of the mandible and deep to the coronoid process and upper ramus of the mandible
- Zygomaticus minor and major extend from the zygomatic bone to the upper lip and to the angle of the mouth (involved in raising the upper lip and in laughing)
- Orbicularis oculi is a broad, flat muscle which forms part of the eyelids, surrounds the eye and runs into the cheeks and temporal region. Parts are continuous with occipitofrontalis. It is the sphincter muscle of the eyelids, causing blinking and, in full contraction, drawing the skin of the forehead, temple, and cheek toward the medial corner of the eye

- Levator labii superioris arises from the frontal portion of the maxilla and runs obliquely laterally and inferior to insert partly in the greater alar cartilage and partly into the upper lip. Its actions are to raise and evert the upper lip and dilate the nostrils

Associations and influences
The zygomata offer protection to the temporal region and the eye and, like the ethmoid and vomer, act as shock absorbers which spread the shock of blows to the face. The zygomaticofacial and zygomaticotemporal foramina offer passage to branches of the 5th cranial nerve (maxillary branch of trigeminal).

Treatment protocols for the zygomata will be found in Chapter 6.

Maxilla (see Fig. 1.6)
This extremely complex bone is made up of:
- The body which houses an air sinus
- A superior concave orbital surface which forms part of the floor of the eye socket
- An infraorbital foramen and canal which offers passage to part of the 5th cranial (trigeminal) nerve and to the infraorbital artery
- An anterior spine to which the nasal septum attaches
- An aperture (maxillary hiatus) on the medial wall of the air sinus which is largely covered by the palatines posteriorly and the inferior conchae anteriorly
- A jutting superior projection which articulates by interdigitation with the frontal bone
- A notch (ethmoid notch) on the medial surface of this projection which articulates with the middle conchae
- A lateral zygomatic process which articulates with the zygoma at the dentate suture
- An inferiorly situated palatine process which forms most of the hard palate (anterior portion)
- An inferiorly situated central suture for articulation with its pair, the intermaxillary suture
- A suture which runs transversely across the palate where the maxillary palate and the palatine bone articulates (maxillopalatine suture)
- A central (incisive) canal, placed inferiorly and anteriorly, for passage of the nasopalatine nerve
- The alveolar ridge, an anterior/inferior construction for housing the teeth

Articulations
As described above, the maxillae articulate at numerous complex sutures with each other, as well as with the teeth they house, the ethmoid and vomer, the palatines and the zygomata, the inferior conchae and the nasal bones, the frontal bone and the mandible (by tooth contact), and sometimes with the sphenoid.

Muscular attachments
- Medial pterygoid runs from the palatine bones and the medial surface of the lateral pterygoid plate of the sphenoid and the tuberosity of the maxilla to the

Box 1.1 (Continued)

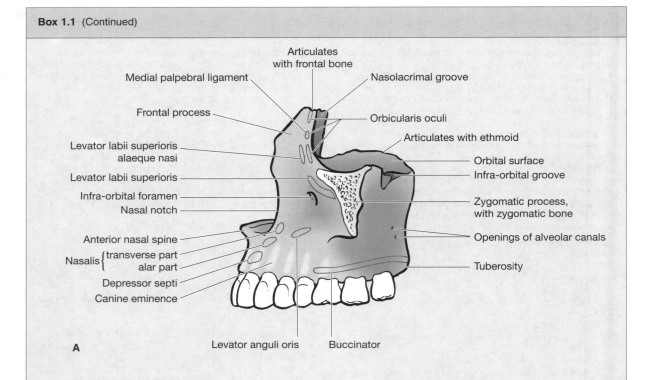

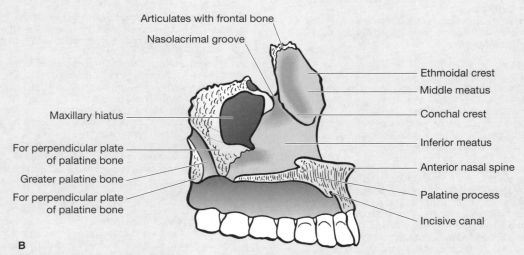

Figure 1.6 A Left maxilla, lateral aspect, showing major features, articulations, and muscular attachment sites. **B** Left maxilla, medial aspect, showing major features and articulations. (Reproduced with kind permission from Chaitow 1998.)

ramus and angle of the mandible to which it attaches via a tendon. The action is to close the jaw, elevating the mandible. Hypertonic states will interfere with sphenoid function, with the maxilla, and with normal motion of the palatines. It is commonly involved in temporomandibular problems.

- Masseter attaches from the zygomatic arch both superficially and deep, running superficially to the lower

Box 1.1 (Continued)

lateral ramus of the mandible and deep to the coronoid process and upper ramus of the mandible

- Buccinator is a thin four-sided muscle which forms part of the cheek, occupying the space between the maxilla and the mandible. It attaches to the alveolar processes of the maxilla and the mandible, opposite the three molar teeth. Its fibers converge toward the angle of the mouth and the lips. Its action is to compress the cheeks against the teeth during chewing and it is involved in the act of blowing ('buccinator' means trumpeter)
- Of lesser importance but also attaching to the maxillae are various muscles, many of which have to do with facial expression and with mouth movement in eating, such as orbicularis oris, depressor anguli oris, levator labii superioris, levator labii superioris alaeque nasi, levator anguli oris, nasalis, depressor septi nasi, risorius
- There are also strong influences from the muscles of the tongue, although these do not directly attach to the maxillae

Associations and influences
Because of the involvement of both the teeth and the air sinuses, the causes of pain in this region are not easy to diagnose. These connections (teeth and sinuses), as well as the neural structures which pass through the bone, plus its multiple associations with other bones and its vulnerability to trauma, make it one of the key areas for therapeutic attention where problems associated with the area are concerned.

Treatment protocols for the maxillae will be found in Chapter 6.

Palatines
This complex, extremely thin, hook-shaped structure includes:
- A perpendicular plate which forms part of the wall for the maxillary sinus
- A horizontal plate which makes up the posterior aspect of the hard palate as well as the floor of the nose
- A pterygoid process which articulates with the sphenoid
- An ethmoidal crest which articulates with the middle conchae of the ethmoid
- A ridge which articulates with the inferior conchae
- An orbital process which articulates with the maxilla, ethmoid, and sphenoid
- A sphenoid process which articulates with the vomer and the inferior aspect of the sphenoid

- A nasal crest which is a continuation of the suture which links the two palatines (median palatine suture)
- A sulcus which houses the greater palatine nerve and the descending palatine artery

Articulations
- The conchal crest for articulation with the inferior nasal concha
- The ethmoidal crest for articulation with the middle nasal concha
- The maxillary surface has a roughened and irregular surface for articulation with the maxillae
- The anterior border has an articulation with the inferior nasal concha
- The posterior border is serrated for articulation with the medial pterygoid plate of the sphenoid
- The superior border has an anterior orbital process, which articulates with the maxilla and the sphenoid concha, and a sphenoidal process posteriorly, which articulates with the sphenoidal concha and the medial pterygoid plate, as well as the vomer
- The median palatine suture joins the two palatines

Muscular attachments
The medial pterygoid is the only important muscular attachment. It attaches to the lateral pterygoid plate and palatine bones running to the medial ramus and angle of the mandible.

Associations and influences
- These delicate shock-absorbing structures with their multiple sutural articulations spread force in many directions when any is exerted on them
- They are capable of deformation and stress transmission and their imbalances and deformities usually reflect what has happened to the structures with which they are articulating
- Great care needs to be exercised in any direct contact on the palatines (especially cephalad pressure) because of their extreme fragility and proximity to the sphenoid in particular, as well as to the nerves and blood vessels which pass through them (see cautionary note below).

⚠ **CAUTION:** No guidelines are presented in this text for treatment involving the palatines due to reported iatrogenic effects resulting from inappropriate degrees of pressure being applied (McPartland 1996).

Diaphragmatic and intercostal breathing

Breathing through the nose involves overcoming a resistance, and this favours the slow, rhythmic, diaphragmatic breathing of sleep, rest, and quiet activity. As exercise increases the nostrils at first widen, but when larger volumes of air are required the person resorts to mouth breathing, where there is much less resistance to flow. This breathing involves the intercostal and anterior neck muscles and is termed 'intercostal breathing'.

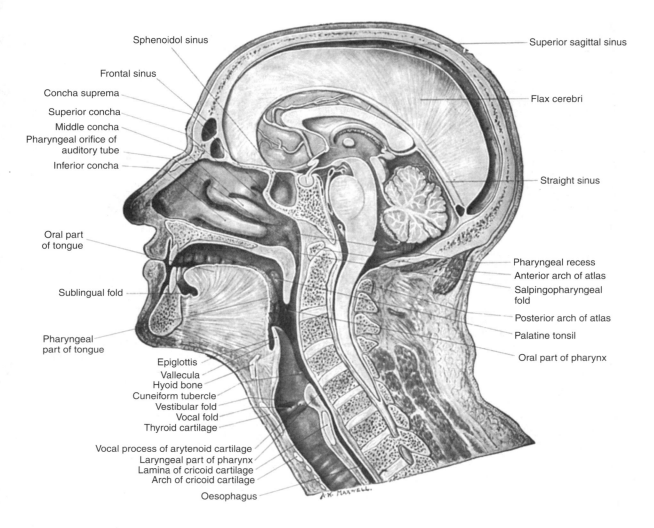

Figure 1.7 Sagittal section through the nose, mouth, pharynx, and larynx. Where it divides the skull and the brain, the section passes slightly to the left of the median plane, but below the base of the skull it passes slightly to the right of the median plane. (Reproduced with kind permission from Gray 1989.)

Sense of smell

The sense of smell, the second function, is served by an olfactory membrane lining the roof of the ethmoid sinuses. Protruding among supporting cells are tiny buttons, each with three to four fine hairs lying in a special secretion. Turbulence ensures that the scent of roses, for example, or the odor of a meal cooking, persists, enabling the cilia to sense the stimulus and activate the receptor cell below. An impulse is sent along the nerve fiber to the brain for deciphering, recognition, and initiating the appropriate response – for example irritating substances can cause violent sneezing which expels the offensive material. In humans there is a further mechanism elsewhere in the nose for the recognition of powerful and dangerous substances such as smoke and noxious chemicals which evoke violent alarm, coughing, and avoidance behavior. The sense of smell is much more sophisticated and sensitive in the dog, which has a much larger area of olfactory membrane than man.

Protective function

A third function of the nose is as a defence against both viral and bacterial infections, protecting the lungs and the rest of the body against these organisms. The first reaction to invasion is a vascular engorgement, bringing phagocytes into the nasal mucosa to engulf the invading organisms. The blood also brings cells which stimulate and secrete antibodies against the invaders. The debris of phagocytes with their contents is carried via the lymphatics to small satellite lymph nodes. In many cases the infection is limited to a cold in the nose, a tonsillitis, or a pharyngitis.

Tear duct drain into the nose

The nasopharynx has a curved, sloping roof. Its floor is made up of a bony hard palate in the front and a soft palate behind. The soft palate ends in the uvula. In swallowing and vomiting, the soft palate and uvula rise to cut off the nasal cavity. On each side wall is the opening of the eustachian tube, draining the middle ear and equalizing the pressure with the external atmosphere. In childhood the opening is surrounded by the adenoids, a collection of lymphoid tissue.

The oropharynx

The oropharynx lies between the tip of the uvula above, and, below, the epiglottis, a cartilaginous flap at the back of the tongue. The mouth opens into the oropharynx (Fig. 1.7). On each lateral wall is a recess, housing the tonsil, which can vary in size. Tonsils are large in childhood, when recurrent infection and inflammation favor increased size. On the medial surface of each tonsil are 12–15 orifices of the narrow tonsilar crypts lined with stratified squamous epithelium with invading lymphocytes. Behind these are germinal centers, generating lymphocytes. The

tonsils are part of the defense system of the upper airway.

The laryngeal pharynx lies between the epiglottis above, and the cricoid cartilage of the larynx below, merging with the larynx in front and the esophagus behind.

Swallowing

In the first, voluntary, stage of swallowing the front of the tongue is raised to press against the hard palate, pushing back the bolus of food to the soft palate, which descends to grip the bolus. With the rising of the back of the tongue, the food bolus is propelled into the oropharynx. Here the involuntary second stage ensues. The soft palate rises to close off the nasopharynx. The epiglottis is bent back to close off the entry to the larynx and the food bolus slips down into the esophagus, partly by gravity and partly by the action of the constricture muscles of the pharynx.

The larynx

The larynx is the next segment in the air passages, joining the pharynx with the trachea. In its wall are nine cartilaginous plates with connecting muscles. The cavity has an upper pair of vestibular folds and a lower set, termed the vocal chords, which can be more tightly brought together. The whole structure forms a mechanism to produce speech by opposing the vocal folds to varying degrees. Alternatively the folds may be completely closed off to protect the airway from fluid and food or to enable the lungs to build up pressure to cough out sputum.

Air proceeds to the trachea, dividing into right and left bronchi and on through diminishing orders of bronchi and bronchioles to the terminal air sacs where gaseous exchange takes place.

PATHOLOGICAL STATES AFFECTING THE AIRWAYS

Chronic obstruction of the nose and oropharynx can arise from a deviated nasal septum, exuberant distorted conchae, enlarged adenoids, hay fever, cluster headaches, nasopharyngeal tumors, or Wegener's granulomatosis. Obstruction increases the resistance to airflow, necessitating intercostal breathing and a switch to mouth breathing. The patient should be referred back to a general practitioner, or to an ear, nose, and throat surgeon, or perhaps an allergist. In obese people, redundancy and laxity of the mucosal folds can give rise to laryngeal obstruction and cause sleep apnea or the obstructive sleep syndrome. Tumors of the vocal chords can cause laryngeal obstruction. In acromegaly, where there is a pituitary tumor overproducing growth hormone, the vestibular folds enlarge and tend to obstruct breathing. A previous tracheotomy can give rise to a tracheal stenosis. Chronic, inadequately-treated asthma causes spasm of the bronchioles, producing an expiratory wheeze and breathlessness. Lung tumors are another cause of breathlessness, while emphysema and heart disease are more common causes.

The therapist who concentrates on psychological causes and on correcting abnormal breathing patterns in these patients is unlikely to succeed, since the major factor is not psychological but physical, is often life-threatening, and requires precise diagnosis and treatment. Such patients should be referred to an appropriate specialist – a general physician or an expert in respiratory diseases.

NORMAL POSTURE AND OTHER STRUCTURAL CONSIDERATIONS

It is a truism worth repeating that in order to appreciate dysfunction, a clear picture of what lies within normal functional ranges is needed. For normal breathing to occur, a compliant, elastic, functional state of the thoracic structures, both osseous and soft tissue, is a requirement. If restrictions are present which reduce the ability of the rib cage to appropriately deform in response to muscular activity and altered pressure gradients during the breathing cycle, compensating adaptations are inevitable, always at the expense of optimal function.

In manual medicine it is vital that practitioners and therapists have the opportunity to evaluate and palpate normal individuals with pliable musculature, mobile joint structures, and sound

respiratory function so that dysfunction can be more easily identified. Apart from standard functional examination, it is also important that practitioners and therapists acquire the ability to assess by observation and touch, relearning skills familiar to former generations of 'low-tech' health care providers. Assessment approaches will be outlined in Chapters 6 and 7.

Is there such a thing as an optimal breathing pattern?

If structural modifications result from, and reinforce, functional imbalances (see Ch. 4 in particular) in respiration as in other functions, it is of some importance to establish whether an optimal, ideal, state is a potential clinical reality.

Since breathing function is, to a large extent, dependent for its efficiency on the postural and structural integrity of the body, the question can be rephrased: 'Is there an optimal postural state?' (Fig. 1.8).

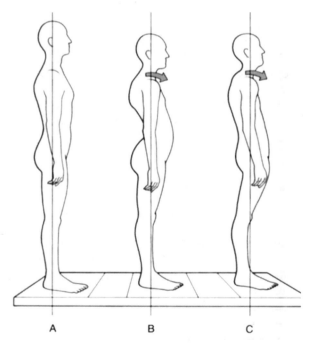

Figure 1.8 Balanced posture (**A**) compared with two patterns of musculoskeletal imbalance which involve fascial and general tissue and joint adaptations. (Reproduced with kind permission from Chaitow 1996a.)

Is there an ideal posture?

Kuchera & Kuchera (1997) describe what they consider an ideal posture:

Optimal posture is a balanced configuration of the body with respect to gravity. It depends on normal arches of the feet, vertical alignment of the ankles, and horizontal orientation (in the coronal plane) of the sacral base. The presence of an optimum posture suggests that there is perfect distribution of the body mass around the centre of gravity. The compressive force on the spinal disks is balanced by ligamentous tension: there is minimal energy expenditure from postural muscles. Structural and functional stressors on the body, however, may prevent achievement of optimum posture. In this case homeostatic mechanisms provide for 'compensation' in an effort to provide maximum postural function within the existing structure of the individual. Compensation is the counterbalancing of any defect of structure or function.

This succinct description of postural reality highlights the fact that there is hardly ever an example of an optimal postural state, and, by implication, of optimal respiratory function. However, there can be a well-compensated mechanism (postural or respiratory) which, despite asymmetry and compensations, functions as close to optimally as possible. This is clearly an acceptable 'ideal' and approaches the reality normally observed in most symptom-free people. Where dysfunction is apparent, or symptoms are evident, a degree of adaptive overload will have occurred.

If postural features are a part of such a scenario it is necessary to take account of emotional states, occupational and leisure influences, proprioceptive and other neural inputs, inborn characteristics (for example an anatomical short leg), as well as habitual patterns of use (for example upper-chest breathing), along with clinical evidence of joint and soft tissue restrictions and imbalances. It is also necessary to be able to evaluate and assess patterns of use which indicate just how close to, or far from, an optimal postural or respiratory state the individual is. Examples of useful structural and functional assessment methods will be found in Chapters 4, 5, 6, and 7.

Further structural considerations

As described above, the cylindrical thoracic cage houses most major organs – the lungs, the heart, the liver, the spleen, the pancreas, and the kidneys. It has a number of functions associated with it (or with its muscular attachments), including visceral support and influence, stabilization, and movement (and therefore posture) of the head, neck, ribs, spinal structures, and upper extremity.

Since the volume of the lungs is determined by changes in the vertical, transverse, and anteroposterior diameters of the thoracic cavity, the ability to produce movements which increase any of these three diameters (without reducing the others) should increase respiratory capacity, under normal circumstances (i.e. if the pleura are intact).

Inhalation and exhalation involve expansion and contraction of the lungs themselves, and this takes place:

- By means of a movement of the diaphragm, which lengthens and shortens the vertical diameter of the thoracic cavity. This is the normal means of breathing at rest. This diameter can be further increased when the upper ribs are raised during forced respiration, where the normal elastic recoil of the respiratory system is insufficient to meet demands. This brings into play the accessory breathing muscles, acting rather like a reserve tank, including sternocleidomastoid, the scalenes, and the external intercostals.

- By means of movement of the ribs into elevation and depression which alters the diameters of the thoracic cavity, vertical dimension is increased by the actions of diaphragm and scalenes. Transverse dimension is increased with the elevation and rotation of the lower ribs ('bucket handle' rib action) involving the diaphragm, external intercostals, levatores costarum. Elevation of the sternum is provided by upwards pressure due to spreading of the ribs ('pump handle' rib action), and the action of sternocleidomastoid and the scalenes.

what about cxVBs?

Kapandji's model

Kapandji (1974), in his discussion of respiration, has described a respiratory model. A crude model can be created by replacing the bottom of a flask with a membrane (representing the diaphragm), and providing a stopper with a tube set into it (to represent the trachea) and a balloon within the flask at the end of the tube (representing the lungs within the rib cage). By pulling down on the membrane (the diaphragm on inhalation), the internal pressure of the flask (thoracic cavity) falls below that of the atmosphere, and a volume of air of equal amount to that being displaced by the membrane rushes into the balloon, inflating it. The balloon relaxes when the lower membrane is released, elastically recoiling to its previous position as the air escapes through the tube.

The human respiratory system works in a similar manner, while at the same time being much more complex and highly coordinated:

- During inhalation, the diaphragm displaces caudally, pulling its central tendon down, thus increasing vertical space within the thorax.
- As the diaphragm descends, it is resisted by the abdominal viscera.
- At this point, the central tendon becomes fixed against the pressure of the abdominal cavity, while the other end of the diaphragm's fibers pull the lower ribs cephalad, so displacing them laterally.
- As the lower ribs are elevated and simultaneously moved laterally, the sternum moves anteriorly and superiorly.
- Thus, by the action of the diaphragm alone, the vertical, transverse, and anteroposterior diameters of the thoracic cavity are increased.
- If a greater volume of breath is needed, other accessory muscles must be recruited to assist.
- Abdominal muscle tone provides correct positioning of the abdominal viscera so that appropriate central tendon resistance can occur. If the viscera are displaced, or abdominal tone is weak and resistance is reduced, lower rib elevation may be impeded and volume of air intake will be reduced.

STRUCTURAL FEATURES OF BREATHING

The biomechanical structures which comprise the mechanism with which we breathe include the sternum, ribs, thoracic vertebrae, intervertebral discs, costal joints, muscles, and ligaments. Structural and functional aspects of all of these are summarized below (see also Figs 1.9–1.12).

Put simply, the efficiency of breathing/respiration depends upon the production of a pumping action carried out by neuromuscular and skeletal exertion. The effectiveness of the pumping mechanism may be enhanced or retarded by the relative patency, interrelationships, and efficiency of this complex collection of structures and their activities:

Is this well documented?

- On inhalation, air enters the nasal cavity or mouth and passes via the trachea to the bronchi, which separate to form four lobar bronchi and subsequently subdivide into ever narrower bronchi until 'At the 11th subdivision, the airway is called a bronchiole' (Naifeh 1994).
- Normal nasal function in respiration includes filtration of the air as well as warming and humidifying it as it passes towards the trachea. This function is lost if there is obstruction of the airways involved, or in chronic mouth breathers. Quiet inhalation function should be effortless if all the mechanical characteristics of the structures involved are optimal and airways are patent. Altered compliance (the expansibility potential of the lungs and thoracic cage), tissue resistance (how elastic, fibrotic, mobile the structures are), and airway resistance all increase the amount of effort required to inhale.
- The structure of the trachea and bronchi includes supporting rings which are made up of varying proportions of cartilage – for rigidity – and elastic muscle. While the wider and more cephalad trachea has a larger proportion of cartilage, the narrower and more caudad bronchioles are almost entirely elastic.
- Gas exchange takes place in the alveoli (air sacs) which are situated toward the end of the

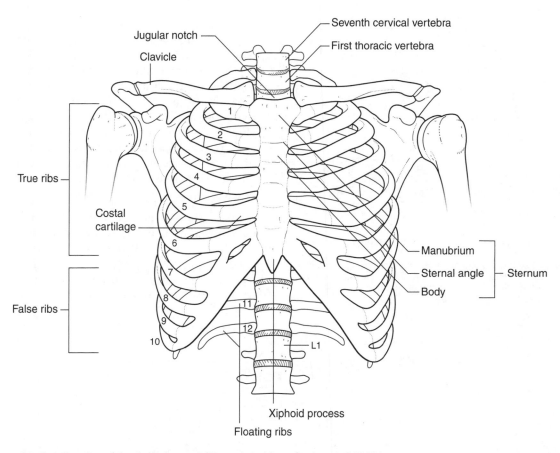

Figure 1.9 Anterior view of the thoracic cage. (Reproduced from Seeley et al 1995.)

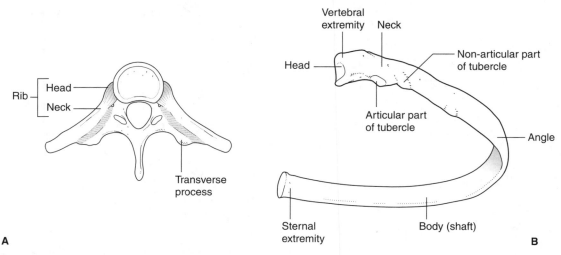

Figure 1.10 The rib and its vertebral articulation. **A** Articulation with the thoracic vertebra. **B** Posterior view of the rib. (Reproduced from Beachey 1998.)

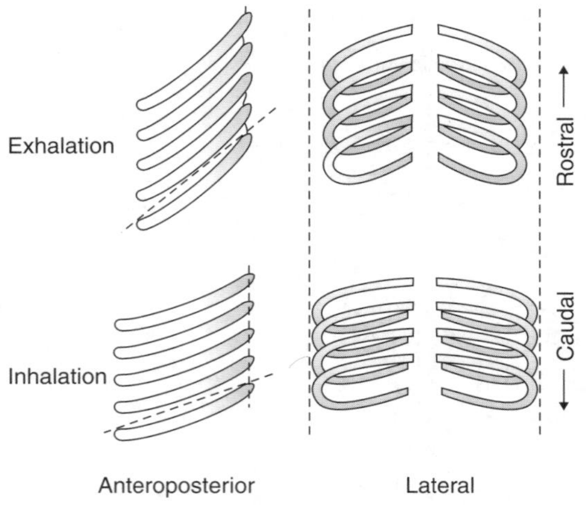

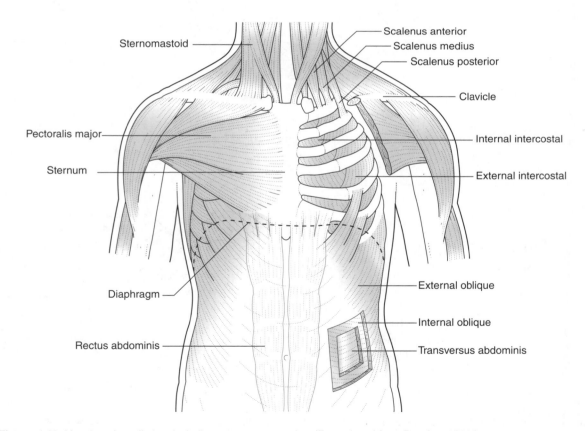

Figure 1.11 Chest wall dimension changes during breathing. The left column illustrates the pump-handle movement of the ribs. The right column illustrates the bucket-handle movement. (Reproduced from Beachey 1998.)

bronchioles, mainly in the alveolar ducts (Fig. 1.13). These air sacs have fine membraneous walls surrounded by equally thin-walled capillaries which allow gas exchange to occur. In order for the lungs to expand and contract, the thoracic cavity lengthens and shortens due to the rise and fall of the diaphragm as the ribs elevate and depress to produce an increase and decrease in the anteroposterior diameter of the rib cage. Any restrictions imposed by joint or soft tissue dysfunction will retard the efficiency of this pumping process.

Some of the thoracic activities described are under muscular control, whereas others result from elastic recoil: 'When the chest wall is opened during surgery the lungs have a continual elastic tendency to collapse, pulling away from the chest wall, whereas the chest wall tends

Figure 1.12 Muscles of ventilation, including accessory muscles. (Reproduced from Beachey 1998.)

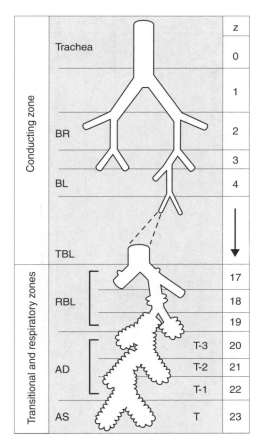

Figure 1.13 Branching of the conducting and terminal airways. Alveoli first appear in the respiratory bronchioles marking the beginning of the respiratory or gas exchange zone. *BR* bronchus, *BL* bronchiole, *TBL* terminal bronchiole, *RBL* respiratory bronchiole, *AD* alveolar duct, *AS* alveolar space, and *Z* order of airway division. (Reproduced from Beachey 1998.)

to recoil outwards. These movements, in opposite directions, are responsible for the development of negative pleural pressure when the respiratory system functions in the intact state' (D'Alonzo & Krachman (1997)). In quiet breathing, at the end of exhalation, with the lungs partially inflated, an elastic recoil occurs which contracts and starts to empty the lungs. This passive elastic recoil which empties the lungs in quiet breathing should not involve any muscular activity. If more air is required than can be introduced by quiet breathing, accessory breathing muscles come into play. And with such deeper

breathing, where muscular activity is used to overcome airway resistance, elastic recoil must also be overcome during inhalation. During exhalation from deeper breathing, the tendency for the thorax to increase its volume also has to be overcome by muscular effort.

If the accessory breathing muscles become shortened or fibrotic they negatively influence the efficiency of these processes.

LUNG VOLUMES AND CAPACITIES

- Total lung capacity (TLC) is the amount of air the lung can contain at the height of maximum inspiratory effort. All other lung volumes are natural subdivisions of TLC.
- Residual volume (RV) is the amount of air remaining within the lung after maximum exhalation. Inhaled at birth, it is not exhaled until death because the rib cage prevents total lung collapse. The volumes and capacities within these two limits are described in Figure 1.14.
- Lung volumes are measured in a variety of ways. From simple hand-held peak expiratory flow (PEF) meters used by patients with asthma to record air flow resistance to sophisticated laboratory equipment to establish both static and exercise lung capacities, volumes, and pressures, accurate information can be gained as to lung health or otherwise. For instance, vital capacity (VC) may be greatly reduced by limited expansion (restrictive disease) or by an abnormally large tidal volume (chronic obstructive airways disease or during asthma attacks). During vigorous exercise, tidal volume (Vt) may increase to half the VC to maintain adequate alveolar ventilation. Limitation of exercise capacity is often the first sign of early lung disease that limits VC (Berne & Levy 1998, p. 530).

Respiratory function (breathing) therefore demonstrably depends on the efficiency with which the structures constituting the pump mechanisms operate. At its simplest, for this pump to function optimally, the thoracic spine and the

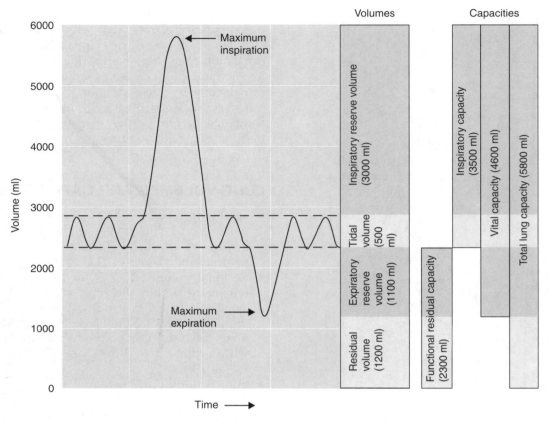

Figure 1.14 Lung volumes and capacities as displayed by a time versus volume spirogram. Values are approximate. The tidal volume is measured under resting conditions. (Reproduced from Beachey 1998.)

attaching ribs, together with their anterior sternal connections and all the soft tissues, muscles, ligaments, tendons, and fascia, need to be structurally intact, with an uncompromised neural supply.

Without an efficient pump mechanism all other respiratory functions will be suboptimal. Clearly, a host of dysfunctional patterns can result from altered airway characteristics, abnormal status of the lungs, and/or from emotional and other influences. However, even if allergy or infection is causal in altering the breathing pattern, the process of breathing can be enhanced by relatively unglamorous nuts-and-bolts features such as the normalization of rib restrictions or shortened upper fixator muscles (see Ch. 6 for further discussion).

The major structural components of the process of breathing are briefly outlined in the observations below. These notes discuss the fascia, the joints of the thoracic cage – including spinal and rib structures – and the musculature and other soft tissues of the region. Functional influences on these structures (e.g. gait and posture) are evaluated insofar as they impact on the efficiency of the respiratory process.

FASCIA AND RESPIRATORY FUNCTION

● Page (1952) describes the fascial linkage as follows:

The cervical fascia extends from the base of the skull to the mediastinum and forms compartments enclosing oesophagus, trachea, carotid vessels and provides support for the pharynx, larynx and thyroid gland. There is direct continuity of fascia from the apex of the diaphragm to the base of the skull. Extending through the fibrous pericardium upward through the deep cervical fascia and the continuity extends not only to the outer surface of the sphenoid, occipital and temporal bones but proceeds further through the foramina in the base of the skull around the vessels and nerves to join the dura.

An obvious corollary to this vivid description of the continuity of the fascia is that distortion or stress affecting any one part of the structure will have repercussions on other parts of the same structure. For example, if the position of the cervical spine in relation to the thorax alters (as in a habitual forward-head position), or if the position of the diaphragm alters relative to its normal position (as in a slumped posture), the functional efficiency of the breathing mechanisms may be compromised.

- Rolfer Tom Myers (1997) has described what he terms the 'deep front line' – fascial connections linking the osseous and soft tissue structures which highlight clearly how modifications in posture involving spinal and/or other attachment structures will directly modify the fascia which envelops, supports, and gives coherence to the soft tissues of the breathing mechanism:
  - the anterior longitudinal ligament, diaphragm, pericardium, mediastinum, parietal pleura, fascia prevertebralis and the scalene fascia connect the lumbar spine (bodies and transverse processes) to the cervical transverse processes and via longus capitis to the basilar portion of the occiput
  - other links in this chain involve a connection between the posterior manubrium and the hyoid bone, via the subhyoid muscles and the fascia pretrachealis, between the hyoid and the cranium/mandible, involving the suprahyoid muscle as well as the muscles of the jaw linking the mandible to the face and cranium.
- Barral (1991) details additional fascial features of the respiratory mechanism, pointing out that there are five lung lobes (segments), three

on the right and two on the left, wrapped in a membranous fascial structure, the pleura, which separates the lungs from the inner thoracic wall, and attaches to the thoracic structures superiorly at the hilum and inferiorly to the diaphragm. Barrell highlights the importance of this connection: 'The pleura is probably the structure most affected by the twenty-four thousand daily diaphragmatic movements, particularly in its superior attachments.' (Ideally, breathing rates are between 10 and 14 per minute; therefore, the normal 24-hour total would range from 14 000 to 20 000.) The suspensory attachment of the pleura (and pericardium), to the skeleton, is via a connective tissue dome comprising a variety of myofascial tissues and ligaments which attach to the spine and deep cervical aponeurosis close to the cervicothoracic junction. Barrell (1991) points out that while the mobile pleura require a point of stability, 'it is somewhat paradoxical that the cervical spine is much more mobile than the thorax, but at the same time serves as a superior fixed point for the pleural system.' Barrell observes that on dissection of degenerated lower cervical structures it is common to find associated excessive thickening and fibrotic change to the pleuropulmonary attachments: 'in view of the relationships between the pleural attachments and neurovascular system, it is easy to imagine the disorders which can arise in this strategic area, and their effects on nearby organs.'

In considering function and dysfunction of the respiratory system, fascial continuity should be kept in mind, since evidence of a local dysfunctional state (say of a particular muscle, spinal segment, rib, or group of ribs) can be seen to be capable of influencing (and being influenced by) distant parts of the same mechanism, as well as other areas of the body, via identifiable fascial connections.

THORACIC SPINE AND RIBS

The posterior aspect of the thorax is represented by a mobile functional unit, the thoracic spinal column, through which the sympathetic nerve supply emerges:

- The degree of movement in all directions (flexion, extension, sideflexion, and rotation) allowed by the relatively rigid structure of the thorax is less than that available in the cervical or lumbar spines, being deliberately limited in order to protect the vital organs housed within the thoracic cavity.
- In most individuals the thoracic spine has a kyphotic (forward-bending) profile which varies in degree from individual to individual.
- The thoracic spinous processes are especially prominent, and therefore easily palpated.
- The transverse processes from T1 to T10 carry costotransverse joints for articulation with the ribs.

The thoracic facet joints, which glide on each other and restrict and largely determine the range of spinal movement, have typical plane-type synovial features, including an articular capsule.

Facet orientation

Hruby and colleagues (1997) describe a useful method for remembering the structure and orientation of the facet joints (of particular value when using mobilization methods, see Ch. 6):

The superior facets of each thoracic vertebrae are slightly convex and face posteriorly (backward), somewhat superiorly (up), and laterally. Their angle of declination averages 60° relative to the transverse plane and 20° relative to the coronal plane. Remember the facet facing by the mnemonic. 'BUL' (backward, upward, and lateral). This is in contrast to the cervical and lumbar regions where the superior facets face backwards, upwards, and medially ('BUM'). Thus, the superior facets [of the entire spine] are BUM, BUL, BUM, from cervical, to thoracic to lumbar.

Discs

The disc structure of the thoracic spine is similar to that of the cervical and lumbar spine. The notable difference is the relative broadness of the posterior longitudinal ligament which, together with the restricted range of motion potential of the region, makes herniation of thoracic discs an infrequent occurrence. Degenerative changes due to osteoporosis and aging, as well as trauma, are relatively common in this region and may impact directly on respiratory function as a result of restricted mobility of the thoracic structures.

Structural features of the ribs
(see Fig. 1.9, above)

The ribs are composed of a segment of bone and a costal cartilage. The costal cartilages attach to the costochondral joint of most ribs (see variations below), depressions in the bony segment of the ribs.

Ribs 11 and 12 do not articulate with the sternum ('floating ribs'), whereas all other ribs do so, in various ways, either by means of their own cartilaginous synovial joints (i.e. ribs 1–7, which are 'true ribs') or by means of a merged cartilaginous structure (ribs 8–10, which are 'false ribs').

The head of each rib articulates with its thoracic vertebrae at the costovertebral joint. Ribs 2–9 also articulate with the vertebrae above and below by means of a demifacet. Ribs 1, 11, and 12 articulate with their own vertebrae by means of a unifacet.

Typical ribs (3–9) comprise a head, neck, tubercle, angles, and shafts and connect directly, or via cartilaginous structures, to the sternum.

The posterior rib articulations allow rotation during breathing, while the anterior cartilaginous elements store the torsional energy produced by this rotation. The ribs behave like tension rods and elastically recoil to their previous position when the muscles relax. These elastic elements reduce with age and may also be lessened by intercostal muscular tension.

Rib articulations, thoracic vertebral positions, and myofascial elements must all be functional for normal breathing to occur. Dysfunctional elements may reduce the range of mobility, and, therefore, lung capacity.

Atypical ribs

Atypical ribs and their key features include:

- Rib 1, which is broad, short and flat, is the most curved. The subclavian artery and cervical plexus are anatomically vulnerable to compression if the 1st rib becomes compromised in relation to the anterior and/or middle scalenes, or the clavicle.

● Rib 2 carries a tubercle which attaches to the proximal portion of serratus anterior.
● Ribs 11 and 12 are atypical due to their failure to articulate anteriorly with the sternum or costal cartilages.

Rib dysfunction and appropriate treatments are discussed in Chapter 6.

Intercostal musculature

Stone (1999) amplifies the generally understood role of the intercostal muscles and their functions: 'For many years the intercostals were attributed with a very complex biomechanical effect, such that the internal intercostals were considered expiratory muscles and the external intercostals inspiratory muscles' (Kapandji 1974). Stone continues by explaining that the processes involved are far more complicated and that they relate to air and fluid movement within the thoracic cavity: 'During inspiration and expiration there are cascades of action within the intercostal muscles, which start at one end of the rib cage and progress to the other to produce the required changes in rib cage shape.'

De Troyer & Estenne (1988) showed that during inhalation the external intercostals are activated from superior to inferior, while during forced exhalation the internal intercostals are activated from inferior to superior. The implication is that, on inhalation, stabilization of the upper ribs is required, involving scalenes (De Troyer 1994) to allow the sequential intercostal contraction wave to progress inferiorly. In contrast, during forced exhalation the lower ribs require stabilization – by quadratus lumborum – to allow the superiorly directed wave to occur. Muscular imbalances (shortness, weakness, etc.) could therefore inpact on normal breathing function. (Assessment and treatment of muscular imbalances are discussed in Chapters 6 and 7.)

Structural features of the sternum
(see Fig. 1.9, above)

There are three key subdivisions of the sternum:

1. The manubrium (or head) which articulates with the clavicles at the sternoclavicular joints. The superior surface of the manubrium (jugular notch) lies directly anterior to the 2nd thoracic vertebra. The manubrium is joined to the body of the sternum by means of a fibrocartilaginous symphysis, the sternal angle (angle of Louis), which lies directly anterior to the 4th thoracic vertebra (Fig. 1.15).
2. The body of the sternum provides the attachment sites for the ribs, with the 2nd rib attaching at the sternal angle. This makes the angle an important landmark when counting ribs.
3. The xyphoid process is the 'tail' of the sternum, joining it at the xyphisternal symphysis (which fuses in most people during the fifth decade of life), usually anterior to the 9th thoracic vertebra.

Posterior thorax

In regional terms, the thoracic spine is usually divided into (White & Panjabi 1978): upper (T1–4), middle (T5–8), lower (T9–12):

● The total range of thoracic flexion and extension combined (between T1 and T12) is approximately 60° (Liebenson 1996)
● The total range of thoracic rotation is approximately 40°
● Total range of lateral flexion of the thoracic spine is approximately 50°.

Palpation landmarks

A useful way of identifying the thoracic vertebrae involves the so-called 'rule of threes'. This 'rule' is simply an approximate generalization, but it positions the palpating fingers in the estimated positions for locating individual thoracic vertebrae (Hruby et al 1997):

● The spinous processes of T1–3 project directly posteriorly so that the tip of each spinous process is in the same plane as the transverse process of the same vertebra

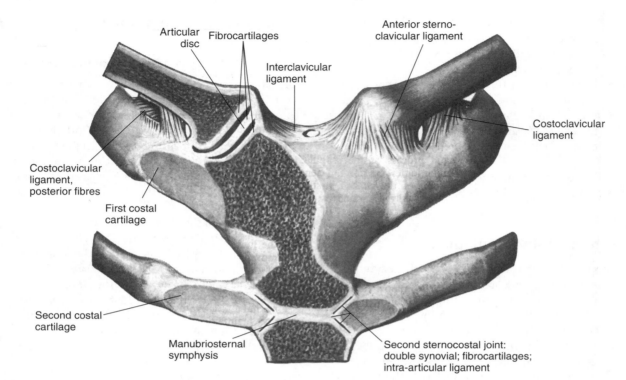

Figure 1.15 Manubrium sternum. (Reproduced with kind permission from Gray 1995.)

- The spinous processes of T4–6 project caudally so that the tip of each spinous process is in a plane that is approximately halfway between the transverse processes of its own vertebra and those of the vertebra immediately below
- The spinous processes of T7–9 project more acutely caudally so that the tip of each spinous process is in the same plane as the transverse processes of the vertebra immediately below
- T10 spinous process is similar to T7–9 (same plane as the transverse processes of the vertebra immediately below)
- T11 spinous process is similar to T4–6 (in a plane that is approximately halfway between the transverse processes of its own vertebra and those of the vertebra immediately below)
- T12 spinous process is similar to T1–3 (in the same plane as the transverse process of the same vertebra).

Box 1.2 describes some research into respiratory synkinesis and Box 1.3 describes the segmental coupling that takes place during compound spinal movements.

NEURAL REGULATION OF BREATHING

Respiratory centres in the most primitive part of the brain, the brainstem, unconsciously influence and adjust alveolar ventilation to maintain arterial blood oxygen and carbon dioxide pressures ($P\text{CO}_2$) at relatively constant levels in order to sustain life under varying conditions and requirements.

There are three main groups:

1. The **dorsal respiratory group** is located in the distal portion of the medulla. It receives input

---

Box 1.2   Respiratory synkinesis

Numerous adaptive combinations are possible in the thoracic spine, partly as a result of the compound influences and potentials of the muscles attaching to each segment. There seems to be a potential for compensatory patterning at all thoracic spinal levels. Lewit (1999) describes some research by Gaymans (1980) into *respiratory synkinesis*. This explains the apparent alternating inhibitory and mobilizing effects on spinal segments during inhalation and exhalation which appear to follow a predictable pattern in the cervical and thoracic spine during side-flexion. For example:

- On inhalation, resistance increases to side-flexion in the *even* segments (occiput–atlas, C2 etc. T2, T4, etc.) while in the *odd* segments there is a mobilizing effect (i.e. they are more free)
- On exhalation, resistance increases to side-flexion in the *odd* segments (C1, C3, etc., T3, T5, etc.) while in the *even* segments there is a mobilizing effect (i.e. they are more free)
- The area involving C7 and T1 seems 'neutral' and uninvolved in this phenomenon
- At the cervicocranial junction, the restrictive and mobilizing effects to inhalation and exhalation respectively seem to involve not just side-bending but all directions of motion
- The 'mobilizing influences' of inhalation as described above, diminish in the lower thoracic region.

The clinical value of this knowledge would be apparent during mobilization of segments in which side-flexion is a component of the restriction. In the thoracic region in particular there would be value in encouraging the appropriate phase of respiration when applying specific segmental mobilization techniques.

Box 1.3   Segmental coupling

Biomechanical coupling of segments occurs during compound movements of the spine. During side-flexion an automatic rotation occurs due to the planes of the facets. In the thoracic spine this coupling process is less predictable than in the cervical region, where from C3 downwards type 2 coupling (also known as 'non-neutral') is the norm (i.e. side-bending and rotation occur to the same side).

Hruby and colleagues (1997) state:

Upper thoracic coupling is typically neutral/type 2 [i.e. side-bending and rotation take place towards the same side] and generally occurs as low as T4 ... [whereas] ... middle thoracic coupling is commonly a mix of neutral/type 1 and non-neutral/type 2 movements, that may rotate to either the formed convexity [type 1] or concavity [type 2]. Lower thoracic coupling is more apt to accompany lumbar neutral/type 1 mechanics.

---

from peripheral chemoreceptors and other types of receptors via the vagus and glosso-pharyngeal nerves. These impulses generate inspiratory movements and are responsible for the *basic rhythm of breathing.*

2. The **pneumotaxic centre** in the superior part of the pons transmits inhibitory signals to the dorsal respiratory centre, controlling the *filling phase of breathing*.
3. The **ventral respiratory group**, located in the medulla, causes either inspiration or expiration. It is inactive in quiet breathing but is important in stimulating abdominal expiratory muscles during levels of high respiratory demand.

The *Hering-Breuer reflex* prevents overinflation of the lungs and is initiated by nerve receptors in the walls of the bronchi and bronchioles sending messages to the dorsal respiratory centre, via the vagus nerves. It 'switches off' excessive inflation during inspiration, and also excessive deflation during exhalation.

Chemical control of breathing

The central role of respiration is to maintain balanced concentrations of oxygen (O_2) and carbon dioxide (CO_2) in the tissues. Increased levels of CO_2 act on the central chemosensitive areas of the respiratory centres themselves, increasing inspiratory and expiratory signals to the respiratory muscles. O_2, on the other hand, acts on peripheral chemoreceptors located in the carotid body (in the bifurcation of the common carotid arteries) via the glossopharyngeal nerves, and the aortic body (on the aortic arch) which sends the appropriate messages via the vagus nerves to the dorsal respiratory centre.

Voluntary control of breathing

Automatic breathing can be overridden by higher cortical conscious input (directly, via the spinal neurons which drive the respiratory muscles) in response to, for instance, fear or sudden surprise. Speaking requires voluntary control to interrupt the normal rhythmicity of breathing, as does singing and playing a wind instrument. There is evidence that the cerebral cortex and thalamus also supply part of the drive for normal respiratory rhythm during wakefulness (cerebral influences on the medullary centres are withdrawn during sleep). Breathing pattern disorders (BPDs) and hyperventilation syndromes (HVSs) probably originate from some of these higher centres (Timmons 1994, p. 35).

THE AUTONOMIC NERVOUS SYSTEM
(Table 1.1)

This system enables the automatic unconscious maintenance of the internal environment of the body in ideal efficiency, and adjusts to the various demands of the external environment, be it sleep with repair and growth, quiet, or extreme physical activity and stress. The nerves innervate the smooth muscle of the alimentary canal causing propulsion of food, while the nerves to exocrine glands initiate secretion of digestive juices. The system is also concerned with the emptying of the bladder and with sexual activity.

Innervation of smooth muscle in the walls of the arterioles varies their caliber, permitting the maintenance of blood pressure and the switching up and down of various parts of the circulation according to whether digestion, growth and repair, heat conservation or loss, or strong muscular activity are required. The maintenance of an adequate circulation also depends on the heart rate, the strength of the cardiac muscle contraction thereby varying the cardiac output.

The hypothalamus in the brainstem has a key role in coordinating the diverse functions of the autonomic nervous system, as well as controlling the release of hormones from the pituitary gland, to which it is connected by a stalk carrying the releasing factors. Some pituitary hormones directly control the biochemical processes of the body. On the other hand, the pituitary trophic hor-

Table 1.1 Comparison of the autonomic and somatic motor nervous systems (from Beachey 1998)

Features	Somatic motor nervous system	Autonomic nervous system
Target tissues	Skeletal muscle	Smooth muscle, cardiac muscle, and glands
Regulation	Control of all conscious and unconscious movements of skeletal muscle	Unconscious regulation, although influenced by conscious mental functions
Response to stimulation	Skeletal muscle contracts	Target tissues are stimulated or inhibited
Neuron arrangement	One neuron extends from the central nervous system (CNS) to skeletal muscle	Two neurons in series; the preganglionic neuron extends from the CNS to an autonomic ganglion, and the postganglionic neuron extends from the autonomic ganglion to the target tissue
Neuron cell body location	Neuron cell bodies are in motor nuclei of the cranial nerves and in the ventral horn of the spinal cord	Preganglionic neuron cell bodies are in autonomic nuclei of the cranial nerves and in the lateral horn of the spinal cord; postganglionic neuron cell bodies are in autonomic ganglia
Number of synapses	One synapse between the somatic motor neuron and the skeletal muscle	Two synapses; first in the autonomic ganglia, second at the target tissue
Axon sheaths	Myelinated	Preganglionic axons myelinated, postganglionic axons unmyelinated
Neurotransmitter substance	Acetylcholine	Acetylcholine released by preganglionic neurons; either acetylcholine or norepinephrine released by postganglionic neurons
Receptor molecules	Receptor molecules for acetylcholine are nicotinic	In autonomic ganglia, receptor molecules for acetylcholine are nicotinic; in target tissues, receptor molecules for acetylcholine are muscarinic, whereas receptor molecules for norepinephrine are either α- or β-adrenergic

mones control the activity of target endocrine glands, such as the thyroid and adrenals, in secreting their own hormones, which in turn control other metabolic processes. The hypothalamus has connections with the preganglionic neurons further down the brainstem and the spinal cord.

The system has a set of receptors from which afferent nerve fibers carry impulses to the central nervous system for integration and action. This action is mediated by impulses transmitted down a set of efferent nerves to effector organs which are mainly smooth muscles and glands. Besides the afferent and efferent pathways, there are two divisions:

- The sympathetic, mainly concerned with preparing the body for, and handling stressful situations, adapting to the needs of the external environment
- The parasympathetic, serving visceral functions such as digestion, absorption, and growth (see Tables 1.2 and 1.3).

Sympathetic division (Tables 1.2 and 1.3; Figs. 1.16, 1.17)

- The sympathetic outflow from preganglionic neurons in the spinal cord is carried by way of their axons through the ventral routes of the first thoracic, all the way down to the third or fourth lumbar spinal nerves, some 15–16 pairs. They make up the white rami communicantes to the paravertebral sympathetic ganglionic chain, where they synapse with postganglionic neurons. These in turn send fibers along the arteries to autonomic effectors, be they glands or smooth muscle.
- The sympathetic ganglion chain has at its upper end the superior, middle, and stellate ganglia, housing the postganglionic neurons which supply effectors in the head, neck, and heart.
- The outflow from thoracic segments 1–4 supplies the larynx, trachea, bronchi, and lungs, while thoracic segments 5–12 fire the greater and small splanchnic nerves, enter the celiac and superior mesenteric ganglia. The inferior mesenteric ganglion is supplied by lumbar segments 1–3, 4. Nerve fibers from these three ganglia supply the organs in the abdomen and the genitalia.

Parasympathetic division (Tables 1.2 and 1.3; Fig. 1.16)

- The parasympathetic outflow occurs in two regions: cranial with the preganglionic axons traveling in the oculomotor, facial, glossopharyngeal, and vagus nerves to ganglia situated close to the effector mechanisms; the sacral outflow supplies the pelvic organs through the second to fourth sacral nerves coming together as the pelvic nerve.
- The lungs are entirely governed by autonomic sensory and motor nerves: there is no voluntary motor control over airway smooth muscles.

Table 1.2 Comparison of the sympathetic and parasympathetic divisions (from Beachey 1998)

Feature	Sympathetic division	Parasympathetic division
Location of preganglionic cell body	Lateral horns of spinal cord gray matter (T1–L2)	Brainstem and lateral horns of spinal cord gray matter (S2–S4)
Outflow from central nervous system	Spinal nerves Sympathetic nerves Splanchnic nerves	Cranial nerves Pelvic nerves
Ganglia	Sympathetic chain ganglia along spinal cord for spinal and sympathetic nerves; collateral ganglia for splanchnic nerves	Terminal ganglia near or on effector organ
Number of postganglionic neurons for each preganglionic neuron	Many	Few
Relative length of neurons	Short preganglionic Long postganglionic	Long preganglionic Short postganglionic

Table 1.3 Comparison of the sympathetic and parasympathetic divisions (from Beachey 1998)

Organ	Effect of sympathetic stimulation	Effect of parasympathetic stimulation
Heart		
Muscle	Increased rate and force (b)	Slowed rate (c)
Coronary arteries	Dilated (b), constricted (a)*	Dilated (c)
Systemic blood vessels		
Abdominal	Constricted (a)	None
Skin	Constricted (a)	None
Muscle	Dilated (b), constricted (a)	None
Lungs		
Bronchi	Dilated (b)	Constricted (c)
Liver	Glucose released into blood (b)	None
Skeletal muscles	Breakdown of glycogen to glucose (b)	None
Metabolism	Increased up to 100% (a, b)	None
Glands		
Adrenal	Release of epinephrine and norepinephrine (c)	None
Salivary	Constriction of blood vessels and slight production of a thick, viscous secretion (a)	Dilation of blood vessels and thin, copious secretion (c)
Gastric	Inhibition (a)	Stimulation (c)
Pancreas	Decreased insulin secretion (a)	Increased insulin secretion (c)
Lacrimal	None	Secretion (c)
Sweat		
Merocrine	Copious, watery secretion (c)	None
Apocrine	Thick, organic secretion (c)	None
Gut		
Wall	Decreased tone (b)	Increased motility (c)
Sphincter	Increased tone (a)	Decreased tone (c)
Gallbladder and bile ducts	Relaxed (b)	Contracted (c)
Urinary bladder		
Wall	Relaxed (b)	Contracted (c)
Sphicter	Contracted (a)	Relaxed (c)
Eye		
Ciliary muscle	Relaxed for far vision (b)	Contracted for near vision (c)
Pupil	Dilated (a)	Constricted (c)
Errector pili muscles	Contraction (a)	None
Blood	Increased coagulation (a)	None
Sex organs	Ejaculation (a)	Erection (c)

a Mediated by α-adrenergic receptors; b, mediated by β-adrenergic receptors; c, mediated by cholinergic receptors.
*Sympathetic stimulation of the heart normally increases coronary artery blood flow because of increased cardiac muscle demand for oxygen.

- A further subdivision of the autonomic nervous system is on the basis of the chemical transmission across the synapses.

NANC system

Researches have recognized a 'third' nervous system regulating the airways called the *non-adrenergic noncholinergic* (NANC) system, containing inhibitory and stimulatory fibers; nitric oxide (NO) has been identified as the NANC neurotransmitter (Snyder 1992).

- NANC inhibitory nerves cause calcium ions to enter the neuron, mediating smooth muscle relaxation and bronchodilation
- NANC stimulatory fibers – also called C-fibers – are found in the lung supporting tissue, airways, and pulmonary blood vessels, and appear to be involved in bronchoconstriction following cold air breathing and in exercise-induced asthma (Beachey 1998, p. 30).

Box 1.4 gives an example of autonomic responses following stress/distress.

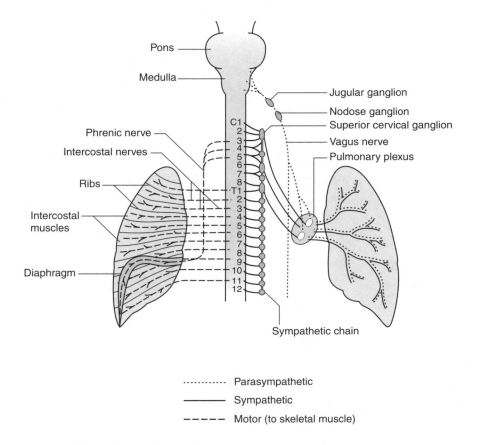

Figure 1.16 Schema of the autonomic innervation (motor and sensory) of the lung and the somatic (motor) nerve supply to the intercostal muscles and diaphragm. (Reproduced from Scanlan et al 1995.)

Box 1.4   An example of autonomic responses

A patient has become alarmed at the sight of blood and the pain from a wound. The immediate reaction to this stress is a strong vagal response, slowing the heart rate. As blood flow slows down in the vertebral arteries supplying the brainstem, a feeling of nausea and faintness supervenes. Pressor receptors in the carotid arteries sense the fall in blood pressure and its threat to the cerebral circulation. From the receptors, impulses travel up the afferents in the glossopharyngeal nerves to the cardiorespiratory center in the medulla. This in turn sends a cascade of efferent impulses down the spinal cord and out along the thoracic spinal nerves. The sympathetic and adrenergic outflow speeds up the heart and constricts the blood vessels of the body. In this way,

normal blood pressure is restored and blood flow to the brain and brainstem increases, thereby preventing a faint. Moreover, there is a discharge in the adrenal medulla releasing epinephrine and norepinephrine which cause a further increase in heart rate and narrowing of the arterioles. These receptors allow the development and use of drugs that either stimulate certain receptors (agonists) or block some receptors (antagonists or blockers). For example, beta-blockers are used in the control of hypertension, favoring the dilation of arterioles and slowing of the heart. A number of beta agonists are useful in asthma, relaxing the bronchospasm of the bronchial musculature set up by allergic responses or infection.

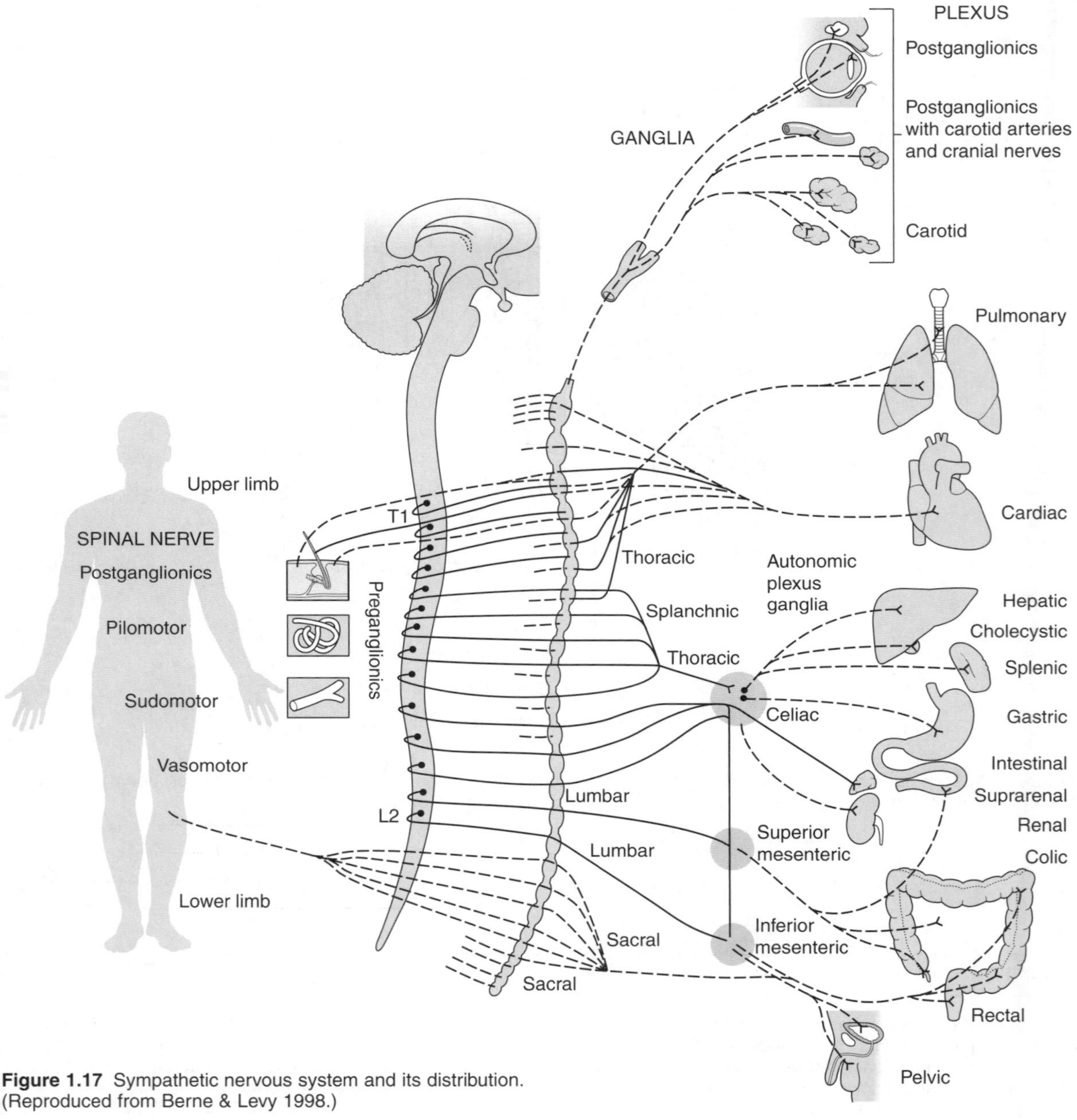

Figure 1.17 Sympathetic nervous system and its distribution. (Reproduced from Berne & Levy 1998.)

THE MUSCLES OF RESPIRATION

The extrinsic thoracic musculature is responsible for positioning the torso, and therefore, also the placement in space of the shoulders, arms, neck, and head. The intrinsic thoracic muscles move the thoracic vertebrae or the rib cage (and possibly the entire upper body) and/or are associated with respiration.

The deeper elements of the thoracic musculature represent a remarkable system by means of which respiration occurs. Some of these muscles also provide rotational components which carry similar, spiraling, lines of oblique tension from the pelvis (external and internal obliques) through the entire torso (external and internal intercostals), almost as if the ribs were 'slipped into' this supportive web of continuous muscular tubes. Rolfer Tom Myers (1997) describes the physical continuity which occurs between these muscles (obliques and intercostals). Above the pelvic crest this myofascial network creates a series of crossover (X-shaped) patterns:

The obliques tuck into the lower edges of the basket of ribs. Between each of the ribs are the internal and external intercostals, which taken all together form a continuation of the same 'X', formed by the obliques. These muscles, commonly taken to be accessory muscles of breathing, are seen in this context to be perhaps more involved in locomotion [and stability], helping to guide and check the torque, swinging through the rib cage during walking and running. (Myers 1997)

Richardson and colleagues (1999) describe research into the behaviour of the abdominal muscles during quiet breathing. They found that the abdominal musculature was activated towards the end of exhalation, and noted that 'Contraction of the abdominal muscles contributes towards the regulation of the length of the diaphragm, end-expiratory lung volume and expiratory airflow'.

With a voluntary increase in exhalation force, all the muscles of the abdomen contract simultaneously. However, when increased exhalation force occurs involuntarily, transversus abdominis is recruited before the other abdominal muscles (rectus abdominis, obliquus externus abdominis), producing enhancement of inspiratory efficiency by increasing the diaphragm's length and permitting an elastic recoil of the thoracic cavity.

Like the erector system of the posterior thorax, the abdominal musculature plays a significant role in positioning the thorax and in rotating the entire upper body. It is also now known to play a key part in spinal stabilization and interseg-

mental stability, particularly transversus abdominis (Hodges 1999). The rectus abdominis, external and internal obliques and transversus abdominis are also involved in respiration due to their role in positioning the abdominal viscera as well as depression of the lower ribs, assisting in forced expiration (especially coughing).

Additional soft tissue influences and connections

- The soft tissue links between the thoracic region and the pelvic region include major structures such as quadratus lumborum, transversus abdominis, and psoas, which merge with the diaphragm and therefore have the potential to influence breathing function.
- The internal and external obliques (usually described as trunk rotators) also merge with the diaphragm and lower ribs and can have marked influences on respiratory function. It is worth reflecting that this works in reverse, and that diaphragmatic and respiratory dysfunction is bound to affect these associated muscles.
- The primary inspiratory muscles are the diaphragm, the more lateral external intercostals, parasternal internal intercostals, scalene group, and levatores costarum, with the diaphragm providing 70–80% of the inhalation force (Simons et al 1998).
- These muscles are supported, or their role is replaced, by the accessory muscles during increased demand (or dysfunctional breathing patterns): sternocleidomastoid (SCM), upper trapezius, pectoralis major and minor, serratus anterior, latissimus dorsi, serratus posterior superior, iliocostalis thoracis, subclavius, and omohyoid (Kapandji 1974, Simons et al 1998).

INSPIRATORY AND EXPIRATORY MUSCLES (Box 1.5)

The muscles associated with breathing function can be grouped as either inspiratory or expiratory, and are either primary in that capacity or provide accessory support. It should be kept in mind that

---

Box 1.5 Muscles of breathing

Muscles of inhalation

Primary
Diaphragm
Parasternal (intercartilaginous) internal intercostals
Upper and more lateral external intercostals
Levatores costarum
Scalenes

Accessory
Sternocleidomastoid
Upper trapezius
Serratus anterior (arms elevated)
Latissimus dorsi (arms elevated)
Serratus posterior superior
Iliocostalis thoracis
Subclavius
Omohyoid

Muscles of exhalation

Primary
Elastic recoil of lungs, diaphragm, pleura and costal cartilages

Accessory
Interosseous internal intercostals
Abdominal muscles
Transversus thoracis
Subcostales
Iliocostalis lumborum
Quadratus lumborum
Serratus posterior inferior
Latissimus dorsi

---

the role that these muscles might play in inhibiting respiratory function (due to trigger points, ischemia, etc.) has not yet been clearly established, and that their overload, due to dysfunctional breathing patterns, is likely to impact on cervical, shoulder, lower back, and other body regions.

Box 1.5 lists the muscles of breathing, both inspiratory and expiratory.

Since expiration is primarily an elastic response of the lungs, pleura, and 'torsion rod' elements of the ribs, all muscles of expiration could be considered to be accessory muscles as they are recruited only during increased demand. They include internal intercostals, abdominal muscles transversus thoracis, and subcostales. With increased demand, iliocostalis lumborum, quadratus lumborum, serratus posterior inferior, and latissimus dorsi may support expiration, including during the high demands of speech, coughing, sneezing,

singing, and other special functions associated with the breath. In addition:

- The intercostal muscles, while participating in inhalation (external intercostals) and exhalation (internal intercostals), are also responsible for enhancing the stability of the chest wall, so preventing its inward movement during inspiration.
- Quadratus lumborum (QL) acts to fix the 12th rib, so offering a firm attachment for the diaphragm. If QL is weak, as it may be in certain individuals, this stability is lost (Norris 1999).
- Bronchial obstruction, pleural inflammation, liver or intestinal encroachment and ensuing pressure against the diaphragm, as well as phrenic nerve paralysis are some of the pathologies which will interfere with diaphragmatic and respiratory efficiency.

Box 1.6 describes some muscle characterization models and the dual roles of some specific muscles.

GAIT INFLUENCES

The major postural muscles of the body (anterior and posterior aspects) are shown in Figure 1.18A and B. Gait involves the spine in general, and the thoracic spinal muscles in particular, and by inference can impact on respiratory function. Gracovetsky (1997) reports: 'In walking, the hip extensors fire as the toe pushes the ground. The muscle power is directly transmitted to the spine and trunk via two distinct but complementary pathways':

- Biceps femoris has its gait action extended by the sacrotuberous ligament, which crosses the superior iliac crest and continues upward as the erector spinae aponeurosis, iliocostalis lumborum, and iliocostalis thoracis (among others), and linking directly with the contralateral latissimus dorsi.
- Gluteus maximus force is transmitted superiorly via the lumbodorsal fascia and latissimus dorsi

In this way, an oblique muscle–tendon–fascial sling is created across the torso, providing a

---

Box 1.6   Muscle characterizations (see also Box 4.1)

Richardson and colleagues (1999) have categorized muscles capable of controlling one joint or one area of the spine as being 'monoarticular'. These could also be referred to as 'local' muscles. They also describe 'multijoint' muscles which are capable of moving several joints at the same time. These muscles are also phylogenetically the oldest. They can be referred to as 'global' muscles. This nomenclature allows clinical disciplines to communicate with other basic science disciplines in order to facilitate research and learning.

Other muscle categorization models include 'postural/phasic' (Janda 1983), and 'mobilizer/stabilizer' (Norris 1999). There are relative advantages in being able to describe and see the way the body works using these models.

Dual roles of specific muscles
Research shows that many of the muscles supporting and moving the thorax and/or the spinal segments (including erector spinae) prepare to accommodate for subsequent movement as soon as arm or shoulder activity is initiated, with deep stabilizing activity from transversus abdominis, for example, occurring miniseconds *before* unilateral rapid arm activity (Hodges & Richardson 1997). Stabilization of the lumbar spine and thorax has been shown to depend, to a large extent, on abdominal muscle activity (Hodges 1999). Transversus abdominis is categorized as a local, stabilizing structure. Richardson and colleagues (1999) note that the direct involvement of this muscle in respiration – where it contributes to forced exhalation – leads to a potential conflict with its role as a spinal stabilizer. They have identified a clear linkage between dysfunction of transversus abdominis and low back pain.

Interestingly the dysfunctional pattern seems to have less to do with strength or endurance capabilities than with motor control. Since the muscle acts to stabilize the spine, dysfunction is bound to contribute to spinal imbalance; however, the impact on respiration is less clear.

Richardson and colleagues also highlight the importance, in postural control, of the diaphragm. In a study which measured activity of both the costal diaphragm and the crural portion of the diaphragm, as well as transversus abdominis, it was found that contraction occurred in all these structures when spinal stabilization was required (in this instance during shoulder flexion). 'The results provide evidence that the diaphragm does contribute to spinal control and may do so by assisting with pressurization and control of displacement of the abdominal contents, allowing transversus abdominus to increase tension in the thoracolumbar fascia or to generate intra-abdominal pressure.' The involvement of the diaphragm in postural stabilization suggests that situations might easily occur where such contradictory demands are evident, where postural stabilizing control is required at the same time that physiological requirements create demands for greater diaphragmatic movement: 'This is an area of ongoing research, but must involve eccentric/concentric phases of activation of the diaphragm' (Richardson et al 1999).

Just what the impact is on respiratory function of transversus abdominis and of the diaphragm when dual stabilizing and respiratory roles occur is an open question; the impact would doubtless be strongly influenced by the relative fitness and health of the individual.

---

mechanism for energy storage, to be utilized in the next phase of the gait cycle. As Lee (1997) points out: 'Together, these two muscles [gluteus maximus and latissimus dorsi] tense the thoracodorsal fascia and facilitate the force closure mechanism through the sacro-iliac joint.'

Gracovetsky (1997) continues: 'As a consequence, firing hip extensors extends and raises the trunk in the sagittal plane. The chemical energy liberated within the muscles is now converted by the rising trunk, into potential energy stored in the gravitational field. When a person is running, so much energy needs to be stored that the necessary rise in the centre of gravity forces the runner to become airborne.'

The intrinsic thoracic muscles are largely responsible for movement of the thoracic spinal column or cage, as well as respiratory function. Though many of these muscles have very short fibers, and therefore may appear relatively unimportant, they are strategically placed to provide, or initiate, precisely directed movement of the thoracic vertebrae and/or ribs. They therefore demand due attention in evaluation of restrictions within these structures.

UPPER THORACIC MUSCLES
(see Fig. 1.18A and B)

When viewing the posterior thorax, the trapezius is immediately obvious as it lies superficially and extensively covers the upper back, shoulder and neck. In addition to trapezius, latissimus dorsi, which superficially covers the lower back, as well

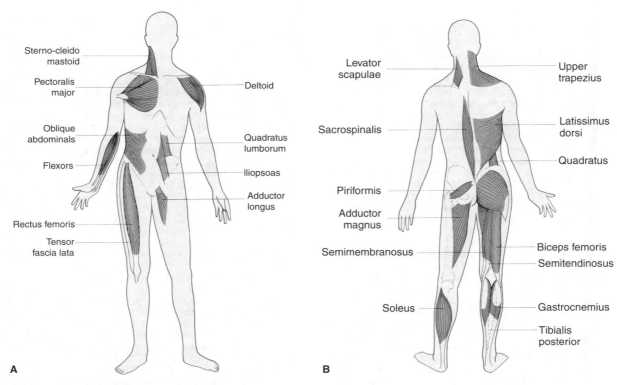

Figure 1.18 A The major postural muscles of the anterior aspect of the body. **B** The major postural muscles of the posterior aspect of the body. (Reproduced with kind permission from Chaitow 1996c.)

as the rhomboids, serratus anterior, and pectoralis major and minor, are of possible clinical significance in breathing imbalance. A complex array of short and long extensors and rotators lies deep to the more superficial trapezius, latissimus dorsi, and rhomboids. Platzer (1992) breaks these two groups into lateral (superficial) and medial (deep) tracts, each having a vertical (intertransverse) and diagonal (transversospinal) component. This subdivision offers a useful mode when assessing rotational dysfunctions, as the superficial rotators are synergistic with the contralateral deep rotators.

Thoracic musculature

- Iliocostalis lumborum extends from the iliac crest, sacrum, thoracolumbar fascia, and spinous processes of T11–L5 to attach to the inferior borders of the angles of the lower 6–9 ribs.
- Iliocostalis thoracis fibers run from the superior borders of the lower 6 ribs to the upper 6 ribs and the transverse process of C7.
- Longissimus thoracis shares a broad thick tendon with iliocostalis lumborum, and fiber attachments to the transverse and accessory processes of the lumbar vertebrae and thoracolumbar fascia, which then attaches to the tips of the transverse processes and between the tubercles and angles of the lower 9–10 ribs.
- The thoracic component of the erector spinae system has numerous attachments onto the ribs.
- Trigger points in these vertical muscular columns refer caudally and cranially across the thorax and lumbar regions, into the gluteal region, and anteriorly into the chest and abdomen.

NOTES ON SPECIFIC MUSCLES

Spinalis thoracis

Attachments. Spinous processes of T11–L2 to the spinous processes of T4–T8 (variable).

Innervation. Dorsal rami of spinal nerves.

Function. Acting unilaterally, flexes the spine laterally; bilaterally, extends the spine.

Synergists. *For lateral flexion*: ipsilateral semispinalis, longissimus and iliocostalis thoracis, iliocostalis lumborum, quadratus lumborum, obliques, and psoas.

Antagonists. *To lateral flexion*: contralateral semispinalis, longissimus and iliocostalis, thoracis, iliocostalis lumborum, quadratus lumborum, obliques, and psoas.

Semispinalis thoracis

Attachments. Transverse processes of T6–T10 to the spinous processes of C6–T4.

Innervation. Dorsal rami of thoracic nerves.

Function. Acting unilaterally, it rotates the spine contralaterally; bilaterally, it extends the spine.

Synergists. *For rotation*: multifidi, rotatores, ipsilateral external obliques and external intercostal, and contralateral internal obliques and internal intercostals. *For extension*: posterior spinal muscles (precise muscles depending upon what level is being extended).

Antagonists. *To rotation*: matching contralateral fibers of semispinalis as well as contralateral multifidi, rotatores, external obliques and external intercostals, and the ipsilateral internal oblique and internal intercostal. *For extension*: spinal flexors (precise muscles depending upon what level is being extended).

Possible signs of dysfunction of spinalis and semispinalis.

Possible impact on breathing function due to association with intercostal musculature
Reduced flexion of spine
Restricted rotation (sometimes painfully)
Pain along spine
Tenderness in laminar groove.

Multifidi

Attachments. From the posterior surface of the sacrum, iliac crest, and the transverse processes of all lumbar, thoracic vertebrae and articular processes of cervicals 4–7, these muscles traverse 2–4 vertebrae and attach superiorly to the spinous processes of all vertebrae apart from the atlas.

Innervation. Dorsal rami of spinal nerves.

Function. When these contract unilaterally they produce ipsilateral flexion and contralateral rotation; bilaterally, they extend the spine.

Synergists. *For rotation*: multifidi, semispinalis muscles, ipsilateral external obliques and external intercostal, and contralateral internal obliques and internal intercostals. *For extension*: posterior spinal muscles (precise muscles depending upon what level is being extended).

Antagonists. *To rotation*: matching contralateral fibers of rotators as well as contralateral multifidi, semispinalis, external obliques, and external intercostals, and the ipsilateral internal oblique and internal intercostal. *For extension*: spinal flexors (precise muscles depending upon what level is being extended).

Possible signs of dysfunction of multifidi.

Possible impact on breathing function due to association with intercostal musculature
Chronic instability of associated vertebral segments
Reduced flexion of spine
Restricted rotation (sometimes painfully)
Pain along spine
Vertebral scapular border pain (referral zone).

Rotatores longus and brevis

Attachments. From the transverse processes of each vertebra to the spinous processes of the second (longus) and first (brevis) vertebra above (ending at C2).

Innervation. Dorsal rami of spinal nerves.

Function. When these contract unilaterally they produce contralateral rotation; bilaterally, they extend the spine.

Synergists. *For rotation*: multifidi, semispinalis muscles, ipsilateral external obliques and external intercostal, and contralateral internal obliques and internal intercostals. *For extension*: posterior spinal muscles (precise muscles depending upon what level is being extended).

Antagonists. *To rotation*: matching contralateral fibers of rotatores as well as contralateral multifidi, semispinalis, external obliques, and external intercostals, and the ipsilateral internal oblique and internal intercostal. *For extension*: spinal flexors (precise muscles depending upon what level is being extended).

Possible signs of dysfunction of rotatores.

Pain and tenderness as associated vertebral segments, tenderness to pressure or tapping applied to the spinous processes of associated vertebrae

Possible impact on breathing function due to association with intercostal musculature.

Spinal musculature: implications for thoracic function

Multifidi and rotatores muscles comprise the deepest layer and are responsible for fine control of the rotation of vertebrae. They exist through the entire length of the spinal column, and the multifidi also broadly attach to the sacrum after becoming appreciably thicker in the lumbar region.

These muscles are often associated with vertebral segments which are difficult to stabilize and should be addressed throughout the spine when scoliosis is presented along with the associated intercostal muscles and pelvic positioning.

Trigger points in rotatores tend to produce rather localized referrals, whereas those in the multifidi refer locally and also to the suboccipital region, medial scapular border, and top of shoulder. These local (for both) and distant (for multifidi) patterns of referral continue to be expressed through the length of the spinal column. In fact, the lower spinal levels of multifidi may even refer to the anterior thorax or abdomen.

Multifidus and the abdominals

Multifidus should co-contract with transversus abdominis to assist in low back stabilization (Richardson & Jull 1995) which suggests that any

chronic weakness (or atrophy) of multifidus is likely to impact strongly on spinal stability – and potentially on breathing function. While shortness and tightness of a muscle are obvious indicators of dysfunction, it is also important when considering muscular imbalances to evaluate for weakness. Actual atrophy of the multifidi has been reported in a variety of low back pain settings. As Liebenson (1996) observes: 'The initial muscular reaction to pain and injury has traditionally been assumed to be an increased tension and stiffness. Data indicates inhibition is at least as significant. Tissue immobilisation occurs secondarily, which leads to joint stiffness and disuse muscle atrophy.'

Serratus posterior superior

Attachments. Spinous processes of C7–T3 attach to the upper borders and external surfaces of ribs 2–5, lateral to their angles.

Innervation. Intercostal nerves (T2–5).

Function. Uncertain role but most likely elevates the ribs (Gray 1995).

Synergists. Diaphragm, levatores costarum brevis, scalenus posterior.

Antagonists. Internal intercostals.

Possible signs of dysfunction of serratus posterior superior.

Pain that seems to be deep to the scapula

Pain may radiate over the posterior deltoid, down the back of the arm and the ulnar portion of the hand, and to the smallest finger

Numbness into the ulnar portion of the hand

Possible impact on breathing function via association with diaphragm and ribs.

Serratus posterior inferior

Attachments. Spinous processes of T11–L3 and the thoracolumbar fascia to the inferior borders of the lower four ribs.

Innervation. Intercostal nerves (T9–12).

Function. Depresses lower four ribs and pulls them posteriorly, not necessarily in respiration (Gray 1989).

Synergists. Internal intercostals.

Antagonists. Diaphragm.

Possible signs of dysfunction in serratus posterior inferior.
Leg length differential
Rib dysfunction in lower four ribs
Lower backache in area of the muscle
Scoliosis.

Levatores costarum longus and brevis (Fig 1.19)

Attachments. *Longus*: tips of transverse processes of T7–T10 to the upper edge and external surface of the tubercle and angle of the second rib below. *Brevis*: tips of transverse processes of C7–T11 to the upper edge and external surface of the tubercle and angle of the next rib below.

Innervation. Dorsal rami of thoracic spinal nerves.

Function. Elevate the ribs: contralateral spinal rotation, ipsilateral flexion, and bilaterally extends the column.

Synergists. *For rib elevation*: serratus posterior superior, external intercostals, diaphragm, scalenes.

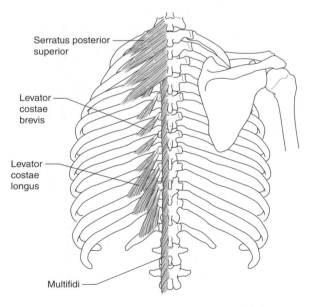

Serratus posterior superior

Levator costae brevis

Levator costae longus

Multifidi

Figure 1.19 Levatores costae elevate and 'spin' ribs during inhalation. (Reproduced with kind permission from Chaitow & Delany 2000.)

Antagonists. Internal intercostals, serratus posterior inferior, elastic elements of thorax.

Possible signs of dysfunction of levatores costarum.
Rib dysfunction
Breathing dysfunctions, especially ribs locked in elevation
Vertebral segmental facilitation
Scoliosis.

Special notes on levatores costarum. The levatores costarum appear innocuous in their small, short passage from the transverse process to the exterior aspect of the ribs. However, this advantageous placement, directly over the costovertebral joint, places them in a powerful position to rotate the ribs during inhalation. Simons and colleagues (1998) state: 'They elevate the rib cage with effective leverage. A small upward movement of the ribs so close to the vertebral column is greatly magnified at the sternum.'

Intercostals (Fig. 1.12)

Attachments. External, internal, and innermost lie in three layers, with the external outermost and attach the inferior border of one rib to the superior border of the rib below it. (See special notes below for direction of fibers.)

Innervation. Corresponding intercostal nerves.

Function. *For respiration. External*: elevates ribs. *Internal*: depresses the ribs. *Innermost*: unclear function but most likely acts with internal fibers (Gray 1995). *For rotation. External*: rotates torso contralaterally. *Internal*: rotates torso ipsilaterally.

Synergists. *For respiration. External*: muscles of inhalation. *Internal and innermost*: muscles of exhalation. *For rotation. External*: ipsilateral multifidi and rotatores, contralateral internal obliques. *Internal*: contralateral external obliques, multifidi, and rotatores.

Antagonists. *For respiration. External*: muscles of exhalation. *Internal and innermost*: muscles of inhalation. *For rotation. External*: contralateral multifidi and rotatores, ipsilateral internal obliques. *Internal*: ipsilateral external obliques, multifidi, and rotatores.

Possible signs of dysfunction in intercostals.
Respiratory dysfunctions, including dysfunctional breathing patterns and asthma
Scoliosis
Rib dysfunctions and intercostal pain
Cardiac arrhythmia.

Special notes on intercostals. Whereas the internal intercostal muscles attach to the ribs and fully to the costal cartilages, the external intercostals attach only to the ribs, ending at the lateral edge of the costal cartilages with the external intercostal membrane expanding the remaining few inches to the sternum.

The external and internal intercostal fibers lie in opposite directions to each other with the external fibers angling inferomedially and the internal fibers coursing inferolaterally when viewed from the front. These fiber directions coincide with the direction of external and internal obliques and provide rotatorial movement of the torso and postural influences in addition to respiratory responsibilities (Simons et al 1998).

The role these muscles play in quiet breathing is uncertain, with some texts suggesting involvement only during forced respiration (Platzer 1992). Simons and colleagues (1998) discuss progressive recruitment depending upon degree of forced respiration. Intercostals may also provide rigidity to the thoracic cage to prevent inward pull of the ribs during inspiration.

The subcostalis muscles (when present) are usually only well developed in the lower internal thoracic region. Their fiber direction is the same as that of internal and innermost intercostals and they span across the internal surface of one or two ribs rather than just the intercostal space. They probably have a similar function to the deeper intercostal muscles (Gray 1995, Platzer 1992, Simons et al 1998).

Interior thorax

Diaphragm

Attachments. Inner surfaces of lower 6 ribs and their costal cartilages, posterior surface of xiphoid process (or sternum), and the body of the upper 1–4 lumbar vertebrae, vertebral discs and the arcuate ligaments, thereby forming a circular attachment around the entire inner surface of the thorax.

Innervation. Phrenic nerves (C3–5) for motor and lower 6–7 intercostal nerves for sensory (Gray 1995, Simons et al 1998).

Function. Principal muscle of inspiration by drawing its central tendon downward to stabilize it against the abdominal viscera, at which time it lifts and spreads the lower ribs.

Synergists. Accessory muscles of inhalation.

Antagonists. Elastic recoil of thoracic cavity and accessory muscles of exhalation

Possible signs of dysfunction in the diaphragm.
Dyspnea or any breathing difficulty (after ruling out more sinister causes)
Dysfunctional breathing patterns
Chronic respiratory problems (asthma, chronic cough, etc.)
'Stitch' in the side on exertion
Chest pain
Hiccup
External compression from tight-waisted clothing.

Special notes on the diaphragm
The diaphragm is a dome-shaped muscle with a central tendon whose fibers radiate peripherally to attach to all the margin of the lower thorax, thereby forming the floor of the thoracic cavity. It attaches higher in the front than in the side or the back. When this muscle contracts, it increases vertical, transverse, and anteroposterior diameter of the internal thorax (Kapandji 1974) and is therefore the most important muscle in inspiration.

A brief summary of some of the diaphragm's key attachments and features indicates the complex nature of this muscle:

- The sternal part of the diaphragm arises from the internal surface of the xiphoid process (this attachment is sometimes absent)
- The costal part arises from the internal aspects of the lower six ribs, 'interdigitating with the transverse abdominis' (Gray 1995)
- The lumbar part arises from two aponeurotic arches (medial and lateral lumbocostal

arches or arcuate ligaments) as well as from the lumbar vertebrae by means of two crura (pillars)

- The lateral crura is formed from a thick fascial covering which arches over the upper aspect of quadratus lumborum, to attach medially to the anterior aspect of the transverse process of L1, and laterally to the inferior margin of the 12th rib
- The medial crura is tendinous in nature and lies in the fascia covering psoas major
- Medially it is continuous with the corresponding medial crura, and also attaches to the body of L1 or L2. Laterally it attaches to the transverse process of L1
- The crura blend with the anterior longitudinal ligament of the spine, with direct connections to the bodies and intervertebral discs of L1, 2 and 3

- The crura ascend and converge to join the central tendon (Fig. 1.20)
- With attachments at the entire circumference of the thorax, ribs, xiphoid, costal cartilage, spine, discs, and major muscles, the various components of the diaphragm form a central tendon with apertures for the vena cava, aorta, thoracic duct, and esophagus
- When all these diaphragmatic connections are considered, the direct influence on respiratory function of the lumbar spine and ribs, as well as psoas and quadratus lumborum, becomes apparent.

Transversus thoracis (Fig. 1.21)

Attachments. Inner surface of the body of sternum and xiphoid process superiolaterally to the lower borders of the 2nd–6th costal cartilages.

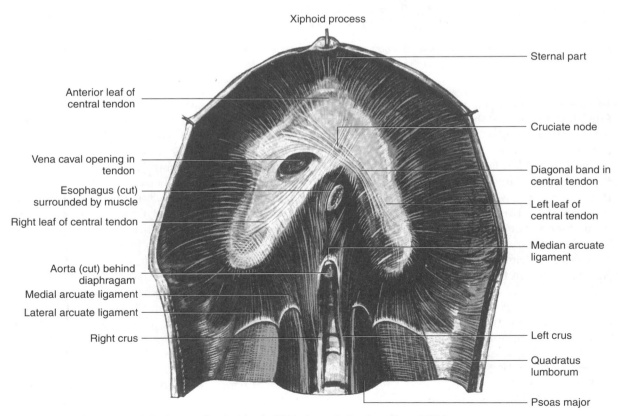

Figure 1.20 Inferior view of diaphragm. (Reproduced with kind permission from Gray 1995.)

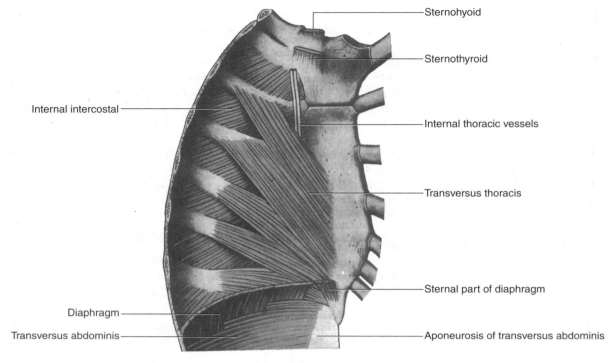

Sternohyoid

Sternothyroid

Internal intercostal

Internal thoracic vessels

Transversus thoracis

Sternal part of diaphragm

Diaphragm

Transversus abdominis

Aponeurosis of transversus abdominis

Figure 1.21 Posterior view of transversus thoracis. (Reproduced with kind permission from Chaitow & DeLany 2000.)

Innervation. Intercostal nerves (2–6).

Function. Depresses the costal cartilages during exhalation, ribs 2–6.

Synergists. Muscles of exhalation.

Antagonists. Muscles of inhalation.

Possible signs of dysfunction of transversus thoracis

Inadequate lifting of the sternum during inhalation, if shortened

Inadequate excursion of upper ribs during exhalation ('elevated ribs'), if lax.

Special notes on transversus thoracis

This muscle (also called the sternocostalis or triangularis sterni) lies entirely on the interior chest and is not available to direct palpation. It varies considerably, not only from person to person, but also from side to side in the same person (Gray 1995), and is sometimes absent (Platzer 1992).

Latey (1996) reports that the transversus thoracis muscle has the ability to generate powerful sensations, with even light contact sometimes producing reflex contractions of the abdomen or chest with feelings of nausea and choking, as well as anxiety, fear, anger, laughter, sadness, weeping, and other emotions. Latey believes that its closeness to the internal thoracic artery is probably significant since, when it is contracted, the muscle can exert direct pressure on the artery. He believes that physiological breathing involves a rhythmical relaxation and contraction of this muscle and that rigidity is often seen where 'control' dampens the emotions which relate to it.

In the following chapter, patterns of dysfunctional breathing will be described. Functional changes always have structural implications, either as part of the etiology, or as a consequence. Keeping in mind the structure while considering functional and dysfunctional behaviour allows for clinical choices and strategies to evolve.

REFERENCES

Barral J-P 1991 The thorax. Eastland Press, Seattle
Beachey W 1998 Respiratory care anatomy and physiology. Mosby, St Louis
Berne RM, Levy M N 1998 Physiology. Mosby, St Louis
Bhagat B D, Young P A, Biggerstall D E 1977 Fundamentals of visceral innervation. Charles C Thomas, Springfield, Ill
Chaitow L 1996a Modern neuromuscular techniques. Churchill Livingstone, Edinburgh
Chaitow L 1996b Positional release techniques. Churchill Livingstone Edinburgh
Chaitow L 1996c Muscle energy techniques. Churchill Livingstone, Edinburgh
Chaitow L 1998 Cranial manipulation. Churchill, Livingstone, Edinburgh
Chaitow L 1999 Fibromyalgia syndrome. Churchill Livingstone, Edinburgh
Chaitow L, Delany J 2000 Clinical application of NMT. Churchill Livingstone, Edinburgh
D'Alonzo G, Krachman S 1997 Respiratory system. In: Ward R (ed) Foundations for osteopathic medicine. Williams and Wilkins, Baltimore
De Troyer A 1994 Do canine scalene and sternomastoid muscles play a role in breathing? Journal of Applied Physiology 76: 242–252
De Troyer A, Estenne M 1988 Functional anatomy of the respiratory muscles. Clinics in Chest Medicine 9: 175–193
Elkiss M, Rentz L 1997 Neurology. In: Ward R (ed) Foundations for osteopathic medicine. Williams and Wilkins, Baltimore
Gaymans F 1980 Die Bedeutung der Atemtypen fur mobilisation der Wirbelsaule. Manuelle Medizin 18: 96
Gracovetsky S 1997 A theory of human gait. In: Vleeming A, Mooney V, Sjniders C, Dorman T, Stoekart R (eds) Movement, stability and low back pain. Churchill Livingstone. Edinburgh
Gray's Anatomy 1989 Edited by P Williams, 37th edn. Churchill Livingstone, Edinburgh
Gray's Anatomy 1995 Edited by P Williams, 38th edn. Churchill Livingstone. Edinburgh
Hodges P 1999 Is there a role for transversus abdominis in lumbo-pelvic stability? Manual Therapy 4(2): 74–86
Hodges P, Richardson C 1997 Feedforward contraction of transversus abdominis is not influenced by direction of arm movement. Experimental Brain Research 114: 362–370
Hruby R, Goodridge J, Jones J 1997 Thoracic region and rib cage. In: Ward R (ed) Foundations for osteopathic medicine. Williams and Wilkins, Baltimore
Janda V 1983 Muscle function testing. Butterworths, London
Kapandji I 1974 The physiology of the joints, 2nd edn. Churchill Livingstone, Edinburgh, Vol 3
Kuchera M, Kuchera W 1997 General postural considerations. In: Ward R (ed) Foundations for osteopathic medicine. Williams and Wilkins, Baltimore
Latey P 1996 Feelings, muscles and movement. Journal of Bodywork and Movement Therapies 1(1): 44–52

Lee D 1997 Treatment of pelvic instability. In: Vleeming A, Mooney V, Dorman T, Snijders C, Stoeckart R (eds) Movement, stability and low back pain. Churchill Livingstone, Edinburgh
Leff A R, Shumacker P T 1993 Respiratory physiology: basics and applications. W B Saunders, Philadelphia
Lewit K 1999 Manipulation in rehabilitation of the motor system, 3rd edn. Butterworth, London
Liebenson C 1996 Rehabilitation of the spine. Williams and Wilkins, Baltimore
Lum L C 1994 Hyperventilation syndromes: physiological considerations in clinical management. In: Timmons B (ed) Behavioural and psychological approaches to breathing disorders. Plenum Press, New York
McPartland J 1996 Cranial iatrogenesis. Journal of Bodywork and Movement Therapies 1(1): 2–5
Murray J F 1986 The normal lung, 2nd edn. WB Saunders, Philadelphia
Myers T 1997 Anatomy Trains. Journal of Bodywork and Movement Therapies 1(2): 91–101
Naifeh 1994 Basic anatomy and physiology of the respiratory system and the autonomic nervous system. In: Timmons BH, Ley R (eds) Behavioral and psychological approaches to breathing disorders. Plenum Press, New York
Norris C M 1999 Functional load abdominal training. Journal of Bodywork and Movement Therapies 3(3): 150–158
Page L 1952 Academy of Applied Osteopathy Yearbook
Platzer W 1992 Color atlas/text of human anatomy. Vol. 1: Locomotor system, 4th edn. Thieme, Stuttgart
Richardson C, Jull G 1995 Muscle control: pain control. Manual Therapy 1(1): 2–10
Richardson C, Jull G, Hodges P, Hides J 1999 Therapeutic exercise for spinal segmental stabilization in low back pain. Churchill Livingstone, Edinburgh
Scanlan C L, Spearman C B, Sheldon R L 1995 Egan's fundamentals of respiratory care, 6th edn. Mosby, St Louis
Seeley R R, Stephens T D, Tate P 1995 Anatomy and physiology, 3rd edn. McGraw-Hill, New York
Simons D, Travell J, Simons L 1998 Myofascial pain and dysfunction: the trigger point manual, 2nd edn. Williams and Wilkins. Baltimore, Vol. 1
Snyder S H 1992 Nitric oxide: first in a new class of neurotransmitters? Science 257: 494
Stone C 1999 The science and art of osteopathy. Stanley Thornes, Cheltenham
Thibodeau G A, Patton K T 1996 Anatomy and physiology, 3rd edn. Mosby, St Louis
Timmons B (ed) 1994 Behavioral and psychological approaches to breathing disorders. Plenum Press, New York
Weibel E R 1963 Morphometry of the human lung. Springer-Verlag, Berlin
West J B 2000 Respiratory physiology: the essentials. Lippincott/Williams and Wilkins, Philadelphia
White A, Panjabi M 1978 Clinical biomechanics of the spine. J B Lippincott, Baltimore

2

Patterns of breathing dysfunction in hyperventilation syndrome and breathing pattern disorders

Dinah Bradley

INTRODUCTION

This chapter covers both normal breathing patterns and what happens to individuals when breathing patterns become dysfunctional. The consequences of disordered breathing patterns are not only distressing to the patient but also expensive to our health care systems if they are not diagnosed and treated (once more serious pathologies have been ruled out).

Too often, patients present to emergency rooms or to general practitioners with frightening symptoms which mimic serious disease (Lum 1987), though blood tests, heart checks such as electrocardiographs (ECGs), and thorough physical examinations reveal nothing out of the ordinary. Breathing pattern abnormalities and their sequelae (see below) are commonly missed by doctors and health care professionals, or else dismissed as 'over anxiousness', and no treatment options are offered.

The incidence of hyperventilation syndrome (HVS) and breathing pattern disorders (BPDs) is as follows:

● Up to 10% of patients in general internal medicine practice are reported to have HVS/ BPD as their primary diagnosis, although equivalent data are not available for emergency department presentations.

- There is a female preponderance in HVS/BPD that ranges from 2:1 to 7:1. The peak age of incidence is 15–55 years, although other ages can be affected. Women may be more at risk because of hormonal influences: progesterone is a respiratory stimulant and in the luteal phase (post ovulation to the onset of menstruation) CO_2 on average drops 25%. Added stress would 'increase ventilation at a time when carbon dioxide levels are already low' (Damas-Mora et al 1980).

- One study reported a series of 45 patients with chest pain who had normal coronary arteries on angiography and who were ultimately diagnosed as HVS. Over a 3.5 year average follow-up, 67% had made subsequent emergency department visits for chest pain and 40% had been readmitted to rule out myocardial infarction. Consequently, not only do HVS/BPDs produce severe and genuine discomfort for patients, they also account for considerable medical expense in excluding more serious pathology (Newton 2000).

- Acute hyperventilation is only about 1% of all cases of hyperventilation, and is well outnumbered by chronic hyperventilation (Lum 1975).

NORMAL BREATHING

Normal resting breathing rates are between 10 and 14 breaths per minute, moving between 3 and 5 liters of air per minute through the airways of the chest. During the active inspiratory phase, air flows in through the nose, where it is warmed, filtered, and humidified before being drawn into the lungs by the downward movement of the diaphragm and the outward movement of the abdominal wall and lower intercostal muscles. The upper chest and accessory breathing muscles remain relaxed. The expiratory phase is effortless as the abdominal wall and lower intercostals relax downward and the diaphragm ascends back to its original domed

position aided by the elastic recoil of the lung. A relaxed pause at the end of exhalation releases the diaphragm briefly from the negative and positive pressures exerted across it during breathing (see Ch. 4, p. 93). Under normal circumstances people are quite unaware of their breathing. Breathing rates and volumes increase or fluctuate in response to physical or emotional demands, but in normal subjects return to relaxed low-chest patterns after the stimuli cease.

DEFINITION OF HVS/BPDs

Hyperventilation is a pattern of overbreathing, where the depth and rate are in excess of the metabolic needs of the body at that time. Breathlessness usually occurs at rest or with only mild exercise. Physical, environmental, or psychological stimuli override the automatic activity of the respiratory centers, which are tuned to maintain arterial carbon dioxide (Pa_{CO_2}) levels within a narrow range. At that particular time, the body's CO_2 production is set at a certain level, and the exaggerated breathing depth and rate eliminates CO_2 at a faster pace resulting in a fall in Pa_{CO_2}, or arterial hypocapnia. This results in the arterial pH (acid/alkaline balance) rising into the alkaline region to induce respiratory alkalosis (Fig. 2.1).

ORGANIC CAUSES OF INCREASED BREATHING

It is important to exclude organic causes, where breathlessness is an appropriate respiratory response to a physical disease causing diminished arterial oxygen saturation (Pa_{O_2}) and elevated arterial carbon dioxide (Pa_{CO_2}) levels. In true breathlessness, tachypnea (rapid breathing) or hyperpnea (increase in respiratory rate proportional to increase in metabolism), the respiratory centers are responding *automatically* to rising CO_2 production due to exercise or organic disease, and deeper and faster breathing response is appropriate.

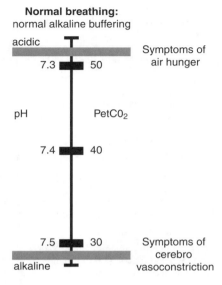

Normal breathing:
normal alkaline buffering

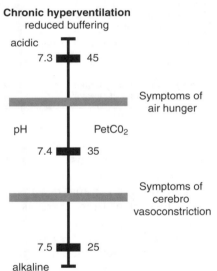

Chronic hyperventilation
reduced buffering

Figure 2.1 When hyperventilation continues for several hours or more, there is a drive to restore normal pH by excreting more alkaline buffer. This compensation permits CO_2 at a level of 35 mmHg to coexist with 7.4 pH. Such an individual becomes subject to reduced capacity to tolerate acidosis from any source, including breath-holding, and is also closer to the symptom line for reduced CO_2. (Reproduced from Gilbert 1999.)

⚠ **CAUTION:** It is dangerous to embark on a course of treatment for hyperventilation where the cause is an organic disease requiring *prompt* investigation and medical therapy. Table 2.1 lists the organic causes which should first be excluded, along with the main appropriate investigation(s) for them.

HISTORICAL BACKGROUND

The first description of hyperventilation in Western medical literature dates back to the USA, during the Civil War, when a surgeon published a paper entitled 'On irritable heart: a clinical study of a form of functional cardiac disorder and its consequences' (Da Costa 1871). The series of 300 soldiers studied suffered breathlessness, dizziness, palpitations, chest pain, headache, and disturbed sleep. The symptoms improved when the soldiers were removed from the front line, but their recovery was slow. Although Da Costa recognized the symptoms as functional in origin, he did not identify hyperventilation as the primary cause.

Physiologists Haldane & Poulton (1908) associated numbness, tingling, and dizziness with overbreathing. A year later. Vernon (1909) added an additional symptom, muscular hypertonicity. These symptoms occurred with respiratory alkalosis when patients were hyperventilating.

Kerr and colleagues (1937) introduced the term 'hyperventilation syndrome' (HVS) and pointed out the diversity and variability of symptoms in many systems of the body. Before these publications, a number of cardiologists following up Da Costa's syndrome had debated whether the heart was involved and coined phrases to fit in with their own views. Thomas Lewis (1940) used the terms 'soldier's heart' and 'effort syndrome' in relation to British soldiers in and after the First World War, whereas US cardiologists were reluctant to label the symptoms as cardiac or related to effort. They preferred the term 'neuro-circulatory asthenia'.

These arguments were largely settled when Soley & Shock (1938) found that all the manifestations of 'soldier's heart' and 'effort syndrome' could be induced by hyperventilation and consequent respiratory alkalosis. Since then, many names have been given to this complex set of symptoms – changing with the fads of the time.

Table 2.1 Organic causes of breathlessness

System	Disease	Investigations
Respiratory	Asthma	Peak expiratory flow (PEF) and other lung functions
	Chronic obstructive respiratory disease	X-ray, PEF, and other lung functions
	Interstitial lung disease	X-ray, biopsy, and lung functions
	Pneumonia	X-ray, sputum, and white blood count
	Pulmonary embolus	X-ray, arterial blood gases, V/Q scan
	Pneumothorax	X-ray
	Pleural effusion	X-ray and aspiration
Cardiovascular	Acute and chronic left heart failure	X-ray, ECG, cardiac enzymes, and echocardiogram
	Right heart failure	
	Tachyarrhythmias	X-ray, ECG, cardiac enzymes, and echocardiogram, plus Holter monitor
	Pulmonary hypertension	X-ray, ECG, cardiac enzymes, and echocardiogram, Holter monitor, plus catheter studies
Hemopoietic	Anemia	Blood count and bone marrow
Renal	Nephrotic syndrome	Urine and serum albumin, chest X-ray
	Acute and chronic renal failure	Arterial blood gases, serum creatinine. Ultrasound of kidneys and urinary tract
Endocrine	Diabetes with ketoacidosis	Blood glucose, arterial blood gases, urine ketones
	Pregnancy	Pregnancy test and ultrasound
	Progesterone therapy	Identify medication
Metabolic	Liver failure	Liver function tests and serum albumin
Drugs	Aspirin	Identify drug and overdose
	Caffeine	Identify drug and daily intake
	Amphetamine	Identify drug and daily intake
	Nicotine	Identify drug and daily intake

With thanks to David Scott MB ChB BMedSc FRCP(Lond) FRACP

'Designer jeans syndrome' (Perera 1988) was popular in the 1970s, and the current so-called Gulf and Balkan War syndromes include many of the same signs and symptoms. Broadly speaking, HVS/BPD was accepted as being of psychiatric origin in the USA and readily diagnosed, whereas in the UK physicians were reluctant to recognize it. A number of factors may have been operating. Most of the reports were in psychological and psychiatric literature, unnoticed by general practitioners and physicians. Influential UK cardiologist Paul Wood (1941) had reviewed Da Costa's syndrome and firmly placed it in the hands of the psychiatrists. Sadly there was little dialogue between the two specialties.

More recently, chest physician Claude Lum (1977), writing from the Addenbrooke and Papworth hospitals in Cambridge, England, with physiotherapists Diana Innocenti (1987) and Rosemary Cluff (1984), who developed assessment and treatment programs, has done much to enlighten the medical practitioners in the UK and reignite scientific interest and research into the condition. Since that time there has been a flowering of literature on the subject as more sophisticated and accessible research equipment has become available. Recommended reviews are listed in Box 2.1.

Despite such progress, there are still considerable numbers of cardiologists, general and specialist physicians, or general practitioners who are reluctant to diagnose or seek treatment for their patients with hyperventilation. Endless, increasingly sophisticated, tests are carried out. Or, alternatively, patients are referred to further specialists for symptoms related to other fields, or they are told 'nothing is wrong' with them. As hyperventilation has no reliable, repeatable, or easily performed diagnostic tests, investigations are protracted, the diagnosis is avoided, and the

Box 2.1 Recommended reviews of hyperventilation disorders
Brashear R E 1983 Hyperventilation syndrome. Lung 161: 257–273 Cowley D S, Roy-Byrne P R 1987 Hyperventilation and panic disorder. American Journal of Medicine 83: 929–937 Gardner W N 1996 The pathophysiology of hyperventilation disorders. Chest 109: 516–534 Grossman P 1983 Respiration, stress, and cardiovascular function. Psychophysiology 20(3): 284–300 Nixon P G F 1993 The grey area of effort syndrome and hyperventilation. Journal of the Royal College of Physicians of London 27(4): 377–383 Timmons B H, Ley R (eds) 1994 Behavioural and psychological approaches to breathing disorders. Plenum, New York

patient's file is often relegated to the 'too hard' basket. This puts patients at great risk of invalidism or of being labeled as malingerers. Medical historians have suggested, for example, that the chronic invalidism of Florence Nightingale and Charles Darwin in the 19th century was more likely chronic hyperventilation, rather than heart disease resulting from infections picked up in the Crimea and the Andes respectively, as was previously believed (Timmons & Ley 1994).

SYMPTOMS AND SIGNS OF HYPERVENTILATION

Table 2.2 lists the diverse symptoms and signs of hyperventilation. None is absolutely diagnostic. Consequently, clinicians rely on a suggestive group of symptoms. Each patient has a characteristic set of symptoms which can be amplified during an acute episode or when hyperventilation is exaggerated. The intermittent nature and variable intensity of the symptoms adds to the difficulty of diagnosis. In addition, many patients fail to mention some of their symptoms, either because they think they are unrelated or because they are ashamed to discuss them. Examples are hallucinations, phobias, sexual problems, fear of impending death or madness, and nightmares. Careful interrogation about the relationship of breathlessness to exercise usually reveals a variation in severity from day to day.

ACUTE HYPERVENTILATION

The diagnosis of an acute episode, either witnessed by the clinician or recalled by the patient, is relatively easy. The patient appears distressed, the pattern of respiration involves deep and rapid breaths using the accessory muscles visible in the neck and the upper chest. Wheezing may be heard as a result of bronchospasm triggered by hypocapnia. Oxygen saturations (measured by pulse oximetry, see p. 178) are within normal ranges (95–98%), and are commonly up to full saturations of 100%. A stressful precipitating event is usually reported.

Neurological signs

Hypocapnia reduces blood flow to the brain (2% decrease in flow per 1 mmHg reduction in arterial CO_2), causing frightening central nervous system symptoms. Poor concentration and memory lapses may result, with tunnel vision and onset in those susceptible of migraine-type headaches or tinnitus. Sympathetic dominance brings on tremors, sweating, clammy hands. Palpitations, and autonomic instability of blood vessels causing labile blood pressures (Magarian 1982). Bilateral perioral and upper extremity paresthesiae and numbness may be reported. Unilateral tingling is most often confined to the left side. Dizziness, weakness, visual disturbances, tremor, and confusion – sometimes fainting or even seizures – are typical symptoms. Spinal reflexes become exaggerated through increased neuronal activity caused by loss of CO_2 ions from the neurons. Tetany and cramping may occur in severe bouts (Fried & Grimaldi 1993).

Metabolic disturbances

Two tests of nerve hyperexcitability produced by hypocapnia-induced hypocalcemia are

Table 2.2 Symptoms and signs of hyperventilation

System	Symptom/sign	Probable cause
Neurology	Headache	Cerebrovascular constriction
	Numbness and tingling	Neuronal excitability from alkalosis
	extremities, more often the left hand and perioral	or hypocalcemia, or flux in ionized calcium
	Positive Trousseau's and Chvostek's signs	Neuronal excitability from alkalosis
		or hypocalcemia or flux in ionized calcium
	Giddiness and dizziness	Vasoconstriction of the vertebral
		arteries and reduced O_2 availability
	Ataxia and tremor	Vasoconstriction of the vertebral
		artery and reduced O_2 availability
	Blurred and tunnel vision	Vasoconstriction of the carotid
	Anxiety and panic	arteries and reduced O_2 availability
	Phobias	
	Irritability	
	Depersonalization	
	Detachment from reality	
	Impaired concentration, thinking, performance, and affect	
	Poor stamina	
	Disturbance of sleep, nightmares	
	Hallucinations	
Cardiovascular	Chest pains and angina	Reduced coronary blood flow
	Palpitations and arrhythmias	Changed excitability of SA and AV
		nodes and cardiac muscle
	Tachycardia	Compensatory for reduced cardiac
		output and reduced blood pressure
	Lightheadedness and syncope	Reduced cardiac output and blood
		pressure from peripheral vasodilatation
	ECG changes with ST depression	Reduced coronary blood flow
	or elevation and prolonged QT	
	interval and sometimes T wave inversion	
	Associated conditions:	Reduced coronary blood flow
	— Mitral valve collapse	
	— Prinzmetal's angina	
Respiratory	Breathlessness and inability to take a deep breath,	
	often nocturnal	
	Sighing and yawning	
	Upper-chest breathing and use of accessory muscles	
	in the neck	
	Chest wall tenderness	Muscle fatigue
	Two hand test, one on upper sternum and the other on upper	
	abdomen – top one moves more	
	Voluntary hyperventilation and end-tidal $P\text{CO}_2$ measurement	
	Dry, non-productive cough and mannerism of clearing	
	the throat	
	Wheezing	Bronchospasm from dry air and activation
		of eicosanoid and muscarinic receptors
Muscular	Aching and stiffness due to hypertonicity	The motor nerve hyper-excitability
	Limb weakness	Muscle fatigue
	Cramps, carpopedal spasm and tetany	Hyper-excitability of motor nerves
Gastrointestinal	Lower chest and epigastric discomfort	
	Esophageal reflux and heartburn	
	Upper abdominal distension	Air swallowing and stomach distension
	Dry mouth	Mouth breathing
	Mannerism of air swallowing and belching	
Skin	Sweating	Cutaneous vasoconstriction

With thanks to David Scott MB ChB BMedSc FRCP(Lond) FRACP

Trousseau's sign and Chvostek's sign. The Trousseau test consists of occluding the brachial artery into the arm by pumping the blood pressure cuff above the systolic pressure for 2.5 minutes. A positive sign is where paresthesia is felt severely within the period and the wrist and fingers arch in carpopedal spasm – termed 'main d'accoucheur' or obstetrician's hand. The Chvostek sign is when tapping the facial nerve at the point where it emerges through the parotid salivary gland elicits a contraction of the facial muscle which twitches the side of the mouth. This is also a test for magnesium deficiency (Werbach 2000).

Acute hypophosphatemia also contributes to weakness and tingling.

Cardiac signs

Chest pain is another alarming symptom challenging the clinician to exclude heart disease. Epinephrine-induced ECG changes can occur in hyperventilation uncomplicated by coronary heart disease. One study suggests that up to 90% of non-cardiac chest pain is thought to be induced by HVS/BPD (De Guire et al 1992).

In older patients, established coronary artery disease can be exacerbated by vasoconstriction arising from hypocapnia, putting these patients at risk of coronary occlusion and myocardial damage. Alternatively, hyperventilation can trigger spasming of normal caliber coronary arteries. This type of variant angina (Prinzmetal's angina) occurs without provocation, usually at rest. This phenomenon is prevented by calcium channel blockers, which reduce calcium ion migration from the cells. To date, no specific studies of breathing retraining and outcome measurements for this type of angina have been done.

Syndrome X refers to those patients with a history of angina and a positive exercise test (chest pain within 6 minutes or less), yet who have normal angiography. Thought to be a functional abnormality of coronary microcirculation, it is much more common in women than in men (Kumar & Clark 1998).

Gastrointestinal signs

Rapid and/or mouth breathing instigates aerophagia from air gulping, causing bloating, burping, and extreme epigastric discomfort. Irritable bowel syndrome (IBS) is listed as a common symptom of chronic overbreathing. Fear and anxiety may induce abdominal cramps and diarrhea (Lum 1987). The median swallowing rate in healthy, non-dyspeptic controls is 3 or 4 per 15 minutes. In the absence of food, up to 5 ml of air accompanies saliva into the gastrointestinal tract with each swallow (Calloway & Fonagy 1985).

Some clinicians think aerophagia may exacerbate hiatus hernia (part of the stomach passes up through a weakened esophageal valve

---

Case study 2.1 Acute hyperventilation

A 39-year-old man with profound deafness from past middle ear infections came into the emergency department with a severe headache, abdominal pain, and an inability to stand and walk. Numbness and pins and needles also affected his legs. He looked and felt distressed. Five doctors assessed him in the course of the 12 hours he spent in the department. The history obtained was fragmentary because a person skilled in sign language was not sought. The medical registrar called in the physician, who ordered a CT scan of the patient's head because of the headache, paresthesiae, and paraparesis. The CT scan was normal. They noted an increased respiratory rate but dismissed this finding, as both chest X-ray and ECG were normal and there were no abnormal cardiac signs. The surgical registrar and surgeon considered the abdominal pain warranted an ultrasound of the patient's abdomen and were relieved that this was normal. As the day wore on the symptoms improved, and the patient and the fifth doctor were reassured by the normal investigations. It was therefore decided to send him to the ward pending an investigation of a spinal cord lesion. Overnight, a sympathetic nurse found out that the man had just lost his 48-year-old partner. Her grown-up children had removed a lot of the patient's furniture from his house, believing it to be their mother's, and one of her sons had written off the patient's (uninsured) car in a crash. This set of misfortunes – bereavement, loss and depression – set up the acute hyperventilation, less apparent on admission, when the consequent symptoms were dominant. Eventually a signer was brought in and the symptoms and hyperventilation explained. The patient responded to this explanation and to counseling.

in the diaphragm into the chest cavity), or may even be the cause in susceptible people. Case study 2.1 describes a patient with abdominal pain following acute hyperventilation.

CHRONIC HYPERVENTILATION

The diagnosis of chronic and intermittent hyperventilation is more difficult, as the patient will often only present when having an acute episode on top of chronic hyperventilation.

Often the patient will dwell on one symptom in a particular system and will be referred to a specialist, for example a cardiologist, gastroenterologist, neurologist, psychiatrist, or respiratory physician. Each will diagnose and investigate within the particular speciality, delaying the diagnosis for months, or even years. Some patients have such a thick folder of notes, including all their previous tests, that this in and of itself is considered diagnostic by some experienced physicians – the 'fat folder syndrome' (Lum 1975).

A careful history and systemic inquiry, checking all other symptoms in the other body systems, usually highlights a suspicious pattern, particularly to the experienced clinician who can think beyond his own special interest. There are often some symptoms which do not fit with the referred complaint and provisional diagnosis.

Careful inquiries as to the precipitating causes of attacks helps both with the diagnosis and with focusing on choice of treatment. There are often attacks where there is no preceding stressful event. It is thought that in those with chronic hyperventilation the respiratory centre is reset to tolerate a lower than normal partial pressure of arterial carbon dioxide ($Pa\text{CO}_2$) in the blood (Nixon 1993). In such patients a single sigh or one deep breath will reduce the $Pa\text{CO}_2$ enough to bring on symptoms.

Examination must exclude organic diseases of the brain and nervous system, diseases of the heart (particularly angina and heart failure), respiratory disease, and gastrointestinal conditions, especially if there are suspicious symptoms in these systems.

SPECIAL AND LABORATORY TESTS

The following tests are usually carried out by the patient's doctor, or in a laborotary setting as requested by the doctor:

- There are preliminary tests to exclude respiratory and cardiac disease: peak expiratory flow (PEF) rate, chest X-ray, and electrocardiogram (ECG). Where chest pain is a presenting symptom an exercise ECG is done, and during the hyperventilation provocation test (HVPT) (in which the patient is asked to voluntarily overbreathe to bring on symptoms) the ECG should be monitored.

- Arterial blood gas determination is an invasive and painful test (arterial puncture) appropriate in the emergency room where the diagnosis of acute hyperventilation is required. With patients in whom chronic hyperventilation is suspected, the end-tidal carbon dioxide ($PET\text{CO}_2$) can be measured. $PET\text{CO}_2$ is equivalent to $Pa\text{CO}_2$ in subjects unstressed and with normal lungs. It can be measured non-invasively from a continuous sampling through nasal prongs, with the mouth occluded, or for those with nasal obstruction the tube can be sited in an oral airway to monitor CO_2 deficits.

The patient can be put through a 4-minute quiet breathing rest period, followed by exercise and recovery, or one may do an HVPT test in the recovery period. Most patients with chronic hyperventilation will have a $PET\text{CO}_2$ at or below 30 mmHg and a markedly delayed recovery from hypocapnia after overbreathing (Chambers et al 1988).

- Some clinicians place a 'think test' (Nixon & Freeman 1988) 3–4 minutes into the recovery period. The patient is asked to recall a painful emotional experience where symptoms developed. If the $PET\text{CO}_2$ drops 10 mmHg, the test supports hyperventilation. In a non-laboratory setting a modified version of this test may also be used to provoke symptoms, as breathing patterns change during disclosure of emotionally charged events. Subjective symptoms are recorded instead of CO_2 levels (see Ch. 8).

Table 2.3 Respiratory function tests and exercise tests (from Kumar & Clark 1998 with permission)

Test	Use	Advantages	Disadvantages
PEFR	Monitoring changes in airflow limitation in asthma	Portable Can be used at the bedside	Effort-dependent Poor measure of airflow limitation
FEV, FVC, FEV$_1$/FVC	Assessment of airflow limitation The best single test	Reproducible Relatively effort-independent	Bulky equipment but smaller portable machines available
Flow–volume curves	Assessment of flow at lower lung volumes Detection of large airway obstruction both intra- and extra-thoracic (e.g. tracheal stenosis, tumor)	Recognition of patterns of flow–volume curves for different diseases	Sophisticated equipment needed
Airways resistance	Assessment of airflow limitation	Sensitive	Technique difficult to perform
Lung volumes	Differentiation between restrictive and obstructive lung disease	Essential adjunct to FEV$_1$	Sophisticated equipment needed
Gas transfer	Assessment and monitoring of extent of interstitial lung disease and emphysema	Non-invasive (compared with lung biopsy or radiation from repeated chest X-rays and CT)	Sophisticated equipment needed
Blood gases	Assessment of respiratory failure	Can detect early lung disease when measured during exercise	Invasive
Pulse oximetry	Postoperative, sleep studies, and respiratory failure	Continuous monitoring Non-invasive	Measures saturation only
Exercise tests (6 min walk)	Practical assessment for disability and effects of therapy	No equipment required	Time consuming Learning effect At least two walks required
Cardiorespiratory assessment	Early detection of lung/heart disease Fitness assessment	Essential in differentiating breathlessness due to lung or heart disease	Expensive and complicated equipment required

In some patients with hyperventilation the $PaCO_2$ and the $PETCO_2$ may be in the normal range. In those who are asymptomatic at the time of testing, this finding could be accepted. However, a normal level while experiencing symptoms negates hypocapnia as the cause of symptoms. It prompts a search for an alternative explanation.

- A peak expiratory flow (PEF) measurement (compared with age, sex, and height tables) provides a simply done, quick exclusion of significant respiratory restriction in the clinic room. Further lung function tests would be scheduled if signs of respiratory obstruction or restriction or cardiac disease was suspected. These might include the tests listed in Table 2.3. Examples of the first common initial tests are described in Figure 2.1.

- Resting ECG and chest X-rays are usually routinely done in patients presenting to emergency medical centers with chest pain.
- The breath-holding time test is done in the clinic and does not require additional measurements or equipment. The time a hyperventilating patient can breath-hold is usually greatly reduced, often not beyond 10–12 seconds – 30 seconds has been used as the approximate dividing line between hyperventilators and normals by some clinicians. It is worth noting that breathless patients *without* hyperventilation may have equal difficulty in breath-holding (Gardner 1996).
- Voluntary overbreathing is a useful test to reproduce symptoms – the hyperventilation provocation test (HVPT) – in a laboratory setting. If there is simultaneous measurement of end-tidal $PETCO_2$ during the test and recovery, the

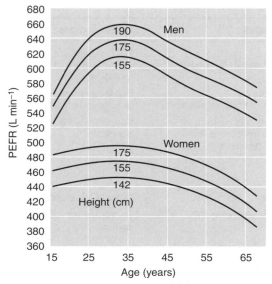

Figure 2.2 Graph of normal readings (from Kumar & Clark 1998 with permission).

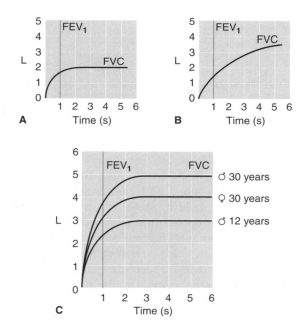

Figure 2.3 Graphs showing **A** restrictive pattern FEV$_1$ and FVC reduced **B** airflow limitation (FEV$_1$ only reduced) and **C** normal patterns for age and sex (from Kumar & Clark 1998 with permission).

slow return of this measurement from hypocapnia can be diagnostic. If chest pain is a presenting symptom, ECG monitoring is desirable.

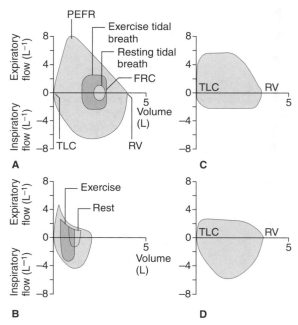

Figure 2.4 **A and B.** Maximal flow volume loops, showing the relationship between maximal flow rates of expiration and inspiration (a) in a normal subject (b) in a patient with severe airflow limitation. **C and D.** Flow volume loops of patients with large airway (tracheal) obstruction showing plateauing of maximal expiratory flow high in the lung volume (from Kumar & Clark 1998 with permission).

⚠ **CAUTION:** As this test can provoke cardiac arrhythmias, with the possibility of a coronary event in those with perhaps undiagnosed coronary artery disease, it is best used *only* where there is medical back-up on site.

The test is best done before explanations of symptoms, to prevent suggestion and bias. Patients need to be warned only of a dry mouth. The patient is asked to concentrate on how they feel during the 1–2 minute period when they are overbreathing at the rate of 30–40 per minute. The rate is set by the examiner's hand movements. The operator must stress the importance of the test and the need to continue for as long as the patient can. An arterial blood gas determination at the end of the test can be of use to establish the depth of hypocapnia. Some clinicians rely on as little as 12 deep breaths which the patient can recover from easily, and subjective symptoms produced are recorded.

Case study 2.2 An example of chronic HVS

A 38-year-old woman was referred for an exercise ECG because of chest pain at rest and on exercise, though its relation to exercise was variable. The test was normal, but a detailed history was suspicious. She was a happily married woman with two children who were doing well. A senior bank officer, she had been promoted to a position for which she had had no past experience, nor was she given any orientation. She was meticulous in her work and it frustrated her that immediate mastery of the new job eluded her. This promotion and the move into a new house had coincided with the onset of the chest pain. The pain was left sub-mammary, coming on mainly during rest, but sometimes with light exercise. It was associated with breathlessness and some tingling of the left arm and around her mouth. She had previously enjoyed walking and keeping fit by going to the gym 2 days a week, but she had to give up these pastimes because of the chest pain and breathlessness. She had an anxious air. Though her respiratory rate was normal, the two-hand test revealed an intercostal breathing pattern. Significant respiratory and cardiac disease was excluded by a normal PEF, chest X-ray, and normal resting and exercise ECGs. An HVPT was positive in producing chest pain and paresthesiae, and the ECG during the pain was normal.

She was relieved by the normal tests and quickly saw the logic of the multiple stressors generating symptoms from hyperventilation. Over 6 weeks her attacks diminished and eventually stopped as she reduced her working hours and had breathing retraining with an experienced respiratory physiotherapist.

- In both the breath holding and voluntary over breathing tests, the skills of the clinician are important for maintaining the trust and cooperation of patients.

DIAGNOSIS

Clinical diagnosis of primary HVS/BPD would be made on the findings of specific or relevant tests done, and after exclusion of organic disease. Case study 2.2 gives an example of a patient with chronic HVS.

When considering the myriad of balanced biochemical reactions which make up normal metabolism, and their dependence on the careful maintenance of an optimal pH, it is not surprising that respiratory alkalosis resulting from hyperventilation causes such widespread distur-

bances and symptoms (Fig. 2.5; see also Ch. 3). Out of the mass of data some major threads emerge – changes in vasomotor tone, mainly reducing cerebral, coronary, and cutaneous blood flow, diminished oxygen availability to tissues, and increased neuronal excitability of the peripheral nervous system:

- Buffering mechanisms protect the pH by renal excretion of bicarbonate (HCO_3). If this compensation is prolonged chronic loss of buffer base reserves further stimulates respiration to avoid metabolic acidosis.
- Oxygen uptake is impaired by a leftshift of the oxyhaemaglobin dissociation curve (Bohr effect) leading to sensations of breathlessness (Fig. 2.6). As $PaCO_2$ is depleted, there is a linear reduction in cerebral blood flow (see above). The respiratory centre becomes reset to a lower CO_2 threshold. A chronic exhausting circle is established (Nixon 1993).
- Proton magnetic resonance spectroscopy reveals increased levels of brain lactate in patients with hyperventilation. These abnormalities would explain all the profound neurological symptoms except tingling, numbness, muscle hypertonicity, and carpopedal spasm.
- Neuronal hyperexcitability is related again to falling CO_2 levels. These result in elevated sensory and motor nerve potentials and bursts of spontaneous discharges, giving rise to paresthesiae of the hands, trunk, and around the mouth as well as hypertonicity, cramps, and carpopedal spasm of the muscles. The mechanism is uncertain. There is a dramatic lowering of serum phosphate which may influence calcium flux; calcium ions stabilize the nerve membrane potential. The same symptoms occur with hypocalcemia, but there is no evidence of reduced serum calcium levels in respiratory alkalosis (Magarian 1982).
- Hyperexcitability of cardiac muscle fibers and electrical conducting systems may cause atrial cardiac arrhythmias.
- As $PaCO_2$ falls there is a reduced coronary blood flow with myocardial hypoxia due to vasoconstriction, and sometimes spasming of coronary arteries. This may be one cause of

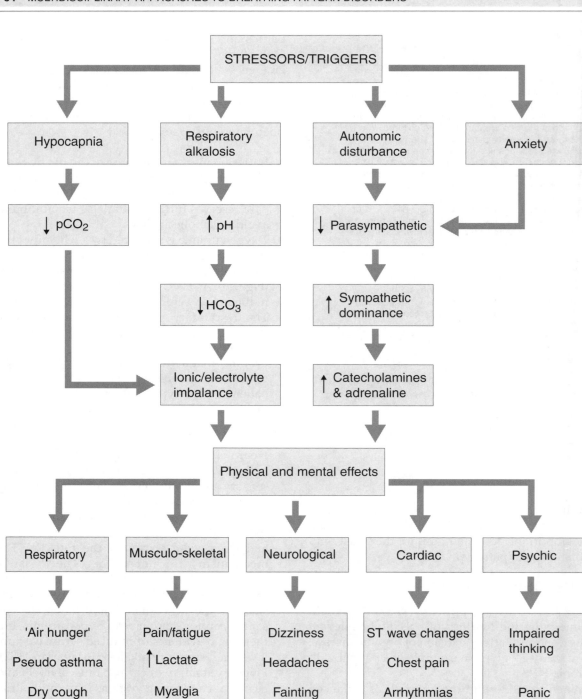

Figure 2.5 Pathophysiological explanations of the symptoms. (Adapted from Bradley 1994.)

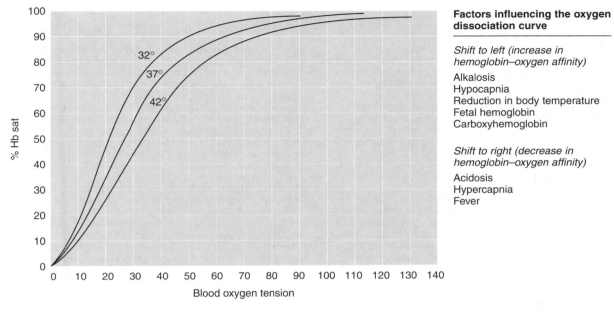

Figure 2.6 Oxygen dissociation curve of blood at a pH of 7.4 showing variations at three temperatures. For a given oxygen tension, the lower the blood temperature the more the hemoglobin holds onto its oxygen, maintaining higher saturation. (Reproduced from Wilkins et al 2000.)

anginal chest pain, which is of particular relevance to those with pre-existing coronary artery disease, with the risk of dislodging plaque and precipitating occlusion/infarction/death.

Chest pain in hyperventilation may also stem from:

- Sharp pains felt on inspiration from *pressure on the diaphragm* from aerophagia ('air gulping' from mouth breathing) (Evans & Lum 1981).
- A typical dull and diffuse pain due to *intercostal muscle fatigue and spasm* (Evans & Lum 1981; see also Ch. 6).
- Heavy retrosternal pain, sometimes radiating to the neck and arms, which mimics angina, lasts longer, and does not abate at rest nor become worse with continued activity as with classic angina; nor does it respond to nitrolingual sprays (anti-anginal medications) (Magarian 1982).

- *Esophageal reflux* is another source of central chest discomfort outside the respiratory system.

Case study 2.3 gives an example of panic breathing.

Hyperventilation may initiate bronchoconstriction in non-asthmatic subjects. As hyperventilators are often mouth breathers, air entering the bronchi is dry and increases the airway fluid osmolarity, rendering it more sticky and tenacious. This stimulates nicotinic and muscarinic receptors, releasing prostanoids and leukotrienes, which cause bronchospasm and mucosal damage.

During hyperventilation there is an additional reduction in peripheral vascular resistance, with a drop in mean arterial blood pressure. This can result in fainting or extreme light-headedness. However, compensatory increases in heart rate and cardiac output supervene with blood pressure (BP) rising above baseline, causing elevated or fluctuating BP levels.

Case study 2.3 Example of panic breathing (adapted from Gilbert (1998)).

A middle-aged woman presented with panic attacks specific to driving, severe enough to limit her to about a 3-mile radius from her home. Her first panic attack had occurred 2 weeks previously as she was driving in light traffic on a city street. Her symptoms had a large component of hyperventilation, with consequent dizziness, anxiety, and chest tightness. She feared that she might lose control of the car if she went too far from her home, and believed that her overbreathing was a consequence of the anxiety rather than contributing to it. Medical examination had not provided any explanations and she had been given a minor tranquilizer, but medication frightened her and so she refused it.

Since the panic had started only 2 weeks before, she was questioned closely about the context of the first attack, in the expectation that her memory would still be fresh. Her general account of how the problem started shifted gradually from 'It came out of nowhere' to 'I was just driving to the hospital to visit my husband. I was a bit frustrated with him that day. I was furious with him, but couldn't admit it. I guess.' This history-gathering over two sessions was alternated with instruction on how to regulate her breathing (mouth closed, abdominal inhale, slow exhale, pause and relax) and suggestions to gradually expand her driving range while practicing this procedure.

The whole story finally emerged. Her husband had been hospitalized for investigation of a mild cardiac incident and was actually enjoying his hospital stay, but did not have the good judgment to keep this to himself. While his wife struggled to carry out the family chores, care for the children, work part-time, and dutifully visit her husband every day, he was telling her how pretty the nurses were and how he could watch all the TV he wanted. She brought him special treats and diversions from home, but apparently felt in competition with the nurses. Her rage grew and swelled against the containment of her prohibition against expressing anger at a sick man. This, it was surmised, had stimulated the ragged, frustrated breathing so typical of anger in conflict with niceness. As she related her feelings about her husband, her breathing style changed to thoracic, open-mouthed, and hyperinflating, and she felt at times some of the familiar dizziness and disorientation.

She finally accepted the probability that, by her own testimony, her first panic attack had definitely not come out of nowhere. The panic had solved her immediate conflict by curtailing her hospital visits until her husband was sent home (the hospital was about a mile beyond the edge of her safe perimeter). But her overbreathing had probably become conditioned to the experience of driving, and she still felt unsafe behind the wheel. During weekly sessions she discussed how symptoms of panic could emerge from suppressed rage affecting her breathing, and spoke more freely about her marriage and about how she managed feelings of anger in general. She continued to practice the breathing control. Within a month the panic attacks subsided and her driving ability returned to normal.

BREATHING PATTERN DISORDERS SECONDARY TO OTHER HEALTH PROBLEMS

Observation of changes to patients during primary hyperventilation and disordered breathing patterns also needs to extend to disorders in which hyperventilation prevails as a coexisting complication. The aim is to provide a broad overview of common conditions and alert clinicians to secondary breathing pattern dysfunctions in patients which may complicate the original disorder and/or add unwarranted stressors.

Obstructive disorders

Starting with the most common obstructive lung disorders (asthma, chronic obstructive airways disease (COAD) and emphysema), airways obstruction may be due to:

- Reversible factors (as in asthma), e.g. inflammation, bronchospasm, or mucus plugging
- Irreversible factors (as in emphysema and chronic bronchitis) e.g. damaged alveoli leading to loss of elastic recoil of adjacent lung tissue, or scarred airway walls (Hough 1996).

Careful viewing of Figure 2.7 shows that there is a great deal of overlapping between these disorders, with mixing and matching of signs and symptoms. Clear definitions are sometimes elusive.

Restrictive disorders

Restrictive lung disorders, with reductions in both lung volumes and lung compliance, include:

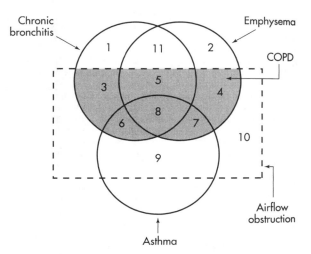

Figure 2.7 Schema of chronic obstructive pulmonary disease (COPD). This nonproportional Venn diagram shows subsets of patients with chronic bronchitis, emphysema, and asthma. The subsets composing COPD are shaded. Subset areas are not proportional to actual relative subset sizes. Asthma is by definition associated with reversible airflow obstruction, although in variant asthma special maneuvers may be necessary to make the obstruction evident. Patients with asthma whose airflow obstruction is completely reversible (*subset 9*) are not considered to have COPD. Because in many cases it is virtually impossible to differentiate patients with asthma whose airflow obstruction does not remit completely from persons with chronic bronchitis and emphysema who have partially reversible airflow obstruction with airway hyperreactivity, patients with unremitting asthma are classified as having COPD (*subsets 6, 7, and 8*). Chronic bronchitis and emphysema with airflow obstruction usually occur together (*subset 5*), and some patients may have asthma associated with these two disorders (*subset 8*). Individuals with asthma who are exposed to chronic irritation, as from cigarette smoke, may develop a chronic, productive cough, a feature of chronic bronchitis (*subset 6*). Such patients are often referred to as having *asthmatic bronchitis* or the *asthmatic form of COPD*. Persons with chronic bronchitis and/or emphysema without airflow obstruction (*subsets 1, 2, and 11*) are not classified as having COPD. Patients with airway obstruction caused by diseases with known etiology or specific pathology, such as cystic fibrosis or obliterative bronchiolitis (*subset 10*), are not included in this definition. (From Scanlan et al 1999.)

- Acute inflammations such as pleurisy or pneumonia
- Chronic disorders, often under the collective term, interstitial lung disease (ILD) which covers over 200 variants. Examples of these are fibrosing alveolitis, sarcoidosis, asbestosis, bird fancier's lung, pneumoconiosis ('coal miners lung')

Breathing patterns

Breathing patterns often provide clues as to the type of condition involved:

- Rapid shallow upper-chest breathing suggests loss of lung volume seen in restrictive diseases, where the work of breathing is increased to maintain ventilation
- Prolonged exhalation time as witnessed in someone having an asthma attack indicates acute intrathoracic obstruction
- Prolonged exhalation (perhaps 'pursed-lip' in severe cases) caused by chronic intrathoracic obstruction in patients with COAD
- Prolonged inspiratory time occurs in acute upper airway obstruction as in croup or globus (throat spasm) (Wilkins et al 2000).

In all the above, accessory muscle use would be clearly visible, and mouth breathing would probably be the chosen route to move air in and out of the lungs. Assisting patients to reduce the work of breathing and diffuse anxiety, with the use of rest positions and relaxation techniques, may be of benefit (see Ch. 8).

Case study 2.4 describes the experience of a patient with a breathing disorder mistakenly diagnosed as chronic hyperventilation.

Patients who are recovering from acute chest infections or asthma attacks require 'debriefing' to ensure correct breathing patterns are restored. This is particularly important in those with asthma, as hyperventilation is a very common secondary problem which may trigger attacks. Lowered CO_2 levels from chronic hyperventilating encourage catecholamine and histamine release into the blood, which in turn stimulates mast cells in the lung parenchyma, promoting bronchoconstriction and hyperinflation. Inhaling cold air via the mouth has also been shown to trigger bronchoconstriction (Gardner 1996).

Those working in pulmonary rehabilitation programmes with COAD patients need to be aware of breathing retraining measures to help maximize respiratory function and encourage relaxed breathing. Mild to moderately affected patients benefit more than those with more severe disease with diaphragm flattening and

---

Case study 2.4 An example of a non-HVS/BPD diagnosis

A 44-year-old woman was referred to physiotherapy by her family doctor for assessment and treatment of chronic hyperventilation following a very stressful period at work, and the decision to leave her marriage. Her main symptoms were chest pain and exertional shortness of breath, and overt upper thoracic breathing. Her doctor had carried out an ECG which was normal, as were the results of a routine blood test.

The woman ran her own successful business, exercised regularly at a gym, and looked extremely fit and well. She had a history of smoking (from the age of 14) but had stopped 6 years ago (aged 38). She had no children, and her periods were regular with no history of low blood iron levels or PMS (premenstrual syndrome). She complained of increasing shortness of breath during exercise and noticed this particularly at work climbing stairs. She was clearly worried by this, and was generally anxious and tearful.

The patient had no history of wheeze or productive cough. Her Nijmegen score (see p. 176) was negative at 20/64, the highest scores across the listed symptoms were breathing related. Her upper thoracic trigger points were exquisitely tender and she was a habitual mouth

breather. Her PEF was slightly lower at 370 liters a minute (l/min) than the normal predicted for her age and height (420 l/min).

The patient's resting O_2 saturations were 93% and she desaturated down to 90% on a preliminary exercise test walking upstairs. She was immediately re-referred on to a respiratory specialist physician for further lung function tests and investigations. Spirometry revealed a moderate loss of lung volume and special blood tests revealed she had an α_1-antitrypsin deficiency (sometimes called *genetic emphysema*. This deficiency prevents the protective effect of the protein α_1-antitrypsin against break-down of lung elastin which supports the alveolar walls of the lung. Her hyperventilation apart from her social stressors signaled a serious underlying obstructive lung disease. During a follow up telephone conversation the woman wondered why her doctor had not sent her straight to a specialist in the first place and considered that it might be sex stereotyping, pigeonholing her as a highly anxious and neurotic woman. The irony of this case was that her soon-to-be-ex husband, who had also been experiencing chest pain, had been sent straight to a cardiologist by his doctor, and was diagnosed as having hyperventilation syndrome.

---

reduced respiratory competence. But breathing assessment and retraining where necessary make a useful adjunct to pharmacological therapies and in some cases help patients safely to reduce anxiety levels and medications.

PRE- AND POST-SURGICAL BREATHING PROBLEMS

Patients waiting to undergo an operation may hyperventilate in response to fear and pain, which may persist after surgery. Those who have been in chronic pain for long periods (waiting for hip replacement, for instance) may be especially vulnerable to HVS/BPDs.

Coronary bypass patients facing open-chest surgery are often briefed beforehand on the importance of deep breathing exercises to expand and clear the lungs of mucus secretions in order to prevent chest infection. Some at-risk patients (perhaps with coexisting COAD from smoking) are given incentive inspirometers – hand-held devices to breathe through which make the work of inhalation harder, encouraging air entry down to the lung bases.

Part of the debriefing before the patient leaves hospital (and as part of any coronary rehabilitation programs) should be the restoration of normal, relaxed nose/abdominal breathing. Closure of coronary bypass grafts may be a consequence of vasoconstrictive or vasospastic influences of chronic hyperventilation (Nixon 1989).

CONCLUSION

HVS/BPDs are common problems affecting the health of 10% of the normal population (Newton 2000). Doctors and other health care professionals need to be aware of the effects of depletion of the body's buffering systems in response to chronic hyperventilation. They can be alerted by clearly visible abnormal changes in breathing patterns and postural changes, and this should prompt a search for symptoms and signs. (The subsequent application of diagnostic tests and the establishment of diagnoses and treatments are discussed in later chapters.) Checking respiratory rates and breathing patterns should be an essential part of all health care investigations, with treatment options offered to those with this omnipresent debilitating disorder.

REFERENCES

Baldry P 1993 Acupuncture, trigger points and muscular pain. Churchill Livingstone, Edinburgh

Bradley D 1994 Discussion paper. Physiotherapy Conference. New Zealand

Calloway S P, Fonagy P 1985 Aerophagia and irritable bowel syndrome. Lancet 14 December, p. 1368 [letter]

Chambers J B, Kiff P J, Gardner W N 1988 The value of measuring end-tidal partial pressure of carbon dioxide as an adjunct to treadmill exercise testing. British Medical Journal 296: 1281–1285

Cluff R A 1984 Chronic hyperventilation and its treatment by physiotherapy: discussion paper. Journal of the Royal Society of Medicine 77: 855–862

Da Costa J M 1871 On irritable heart: a clinical study of a form of functional cardiac disorder and its consequences. American Journal of Medicine 61: 17–51

Damas-Mora J, Davies L, Taylor W, Jenner F A 1980 Menstrual respiratory changes and symptoms. British Journal of Pyschiatry 136: 492–497

De Guire S, Gervitz R, Kawahara Y, Maguire W 1992 Hyperventilation syndrome and the assessment and treatment for functional cardiac symptoms. American Journal of Cardiology 70: 673–677

Evans D W, Lum L C 1981 Hyperventilation as a cause of chest pain mimicking angina. Practical Cardiology 7(7): 131–139

Fried R, Grimaldi J 1993 The psychology and physiology of breathing. Plenum, New York, pp 186–187

Gardner W N 1996 The pathophysiology of hyperventilation disorders. Chest 109: 516–534

Gilbert C 1998 Emotional sources of dysfunctional breathing. Journal of Bodywork and Movement Therapies 2(4): 224–320

Gilbert C 1999 Hyperventilation and the body. Accident and Emergency Nursing 7: 130–140

Haldane J S, Poulton E P 1908 The effects of want of oxygen on respiration. Journal of Physiology 37: 390

Hough A 1996 Physiotherapy in respiratory care. Stanley Thornes, London, pp 53–88

Innocenti D M 1987 Chronic hyperventilation syndrome. Cash's textbook of chest heart and vascular disorders for physiotherapists, 4th edn. Faber and Faber, London, pp 537–549

Kerr W J, Dalton J A, Gliebe P A 1937 Some physical phenomena associated with the anxiety states and their relation to hyperventilation. Annals of Internal Medicine 11: 961

Kumar P, Clark M 1998 Clinical medicine, 4th edn. W B Saunders Edinburgh

Lewis T 1940 The soldier's heart and the effort syndrome. Shaw, London

Lum L C 1975 Hyperventilation: the tip and the iceberg. Journal of Psychosomatic Research 19: 375–383

Lum L C 1977 Breathing exercises in the treatment of hyperventilation and chronic anxiety states. Chest Heart and Stroke Journal 2: 6–11

Lum L C 1987 Hyperventilation syndromes in medicine and psychiatry: a review. Journal of the Royal Society of Medicine: 229–231

Magarian G J 1982 Hyperventilation syndromes: infrequently recognised common expressions of anxiety and stress. Medicine 62: 219–236

Newton E 2000 Hyperventilation from the emergency department. <www.emedicine.com/EMERG/topic 270.htm> (accessed 5/5/01)

Nixon P G F 1989 Hyperventilation and cardiac symptoms. Internal Medicine 10(12): 67–84

Nixon P G F 1993 The grey area of effort syndrome and hyperventilation: from Thomas Lewis to today. Journal of the Royal College of Physicians of London 27(4): 377–383

Nixon P G F, Freeman L J 1988 The 'think test': a further technique to elicit hyperventilation. Journal of the Royal Society of Medicine 81: 277–279

Perera J 1988 The hazards of heavy breathing. New Scientist 3 Dec 1988, pp 46–49

Scanlan C L, Wilkins R L, Stoller J K 1999 Egan's fundamentals of respiratory care, 7th edn. Mosby, St Louis

Soley M H, Shock N W 1938 The aetiology of effort syndrome. American Journal of Medical Science 196: 840

Timmons B H, Ley R (eds) 1994 Behavioral and psychological approaches to breathing disorders. Plenum, New York, p 115

Vernon H M 1909 The production of prolonged apnea in man. Journal of Physiology 38: 18

Werbach M 2000 Adult attention deficit disorder: a nutritional perspective. Journal of Bodywork and Movement Therapies 4(3): 182–183

Wood P 1941 Da Costa's syndrome (or effort syndrome). British Medical Journal [Vol?]: 767

Wilkins, Kreder, Sheldon 2000 Clinical assessment in respiratory care, 4th edn. Mosby, St Louis

3

Biochemical aspects of breathing

Christopher Gilbert (notes on food sensitivities and nutrition: Leon Chaitow)

This chapter will present aspects of the biochemistry of respiration relevant to breathing pattern disorders, including psychological, allergic, and nutritional factors. The focus will be on the processes of the delivery of oxygen (O_2) to the tissues and the removal of carbon dioxide, and the powerful function that carbon dioxide performs on its way out of the body. The utilization of oxygen after it reaches the cells is not so important here. There are a number of texts which provide a comprehensive picture of the biochemistry of breathing, including Comroe 1974, West 1995, Taylor et al 1989, Nunn 1993, and general physiology textbooks.

THE BIOCHEMISTRY OF BREATHING

Breathing itself – the mechanical, muscle-powered part of respiration – is a major focus of this book. With its functioning grossly visible, many variables of breathing can be assessed fairly easily from moment to moment. However, it is important to outline what happens deeper down in the system, in association with the actual gas exchange that takes place, since respiration is ultimately a chemical matter. Here, as so often happens, the most important events are invisible.

Simply put, the body extracts oxygen from the inhaled air and excretes carbon dioxide to be exhaled. That formulation suggests that all we need to remember is that oxygen is good and carbon dioxide is bad. Yet if one considers that life-giving oxygen can also be corrosive and toxic, and that a deficiency of the waste gas carbon dioxide (CO_2) can cause fainting, seizures, or even death, then the good/bad distinction must be restated as good within certain limits and bad within certain limits.

Maintaining these two gases within those limits is a complex task for the body, even more so because the supply of each gas fluctuates with each breath. This tidal oscillation must be smoothed out so that the brain and bodily tissues receive a steady supply of O_2, and also so that CO_2 in the body remains at a stable level. This need for CO_2 stability may be less familiar than the need for stability of O_2, but with respect to both of these gases, we live in a narrow zone of homeostasis bordered on both sides by physiological disaster. Much of what goes wrong with breathing involves attempts to avoid this disaster, and that sometimes misguided regulation is the focus of this chapter.

In understanding the biochemistry underlying breathing, one must keep several factors in mind simultaneously because they all interact. A newcomer first experiencing a basketball or soccer game would have the advantage of viewing the whole game at once, and would be able to pick out certain factors at will for special observation, thereby building up an understanding of how the game works. In studying the process of respiration, however, achieving such a simultaneous view requires imagination. For one thing, the scales of the various factors are vastly different, ranging from the atomic, to the molecular, to the cellular, to the circulatory, to microscopic membrane action, to the large muscle movements of the chest and abdomen. Moreover, these factors do not all change simultaneously; some are slower to react than others. There are layers of security operating, safeguards to ensure a steady supply of O_2 to the brain and the heart.

In considering aberrations in the breathing pattern, it is helpful to keep the following rough classification in mind:

1. Adequate and inadequate compensations for pathology elsewhere (e.g. acidosis from diabetes or kidney problems)
2. Responses to extrinsic factors (such as allergy or drugs)
3. Responses to intrinsic factors (such as progesterone)
4. Truly pathological disorders of the breathing system itself
5. Psychogenic or functional breathing problems.

All of these must be compared to the idealized normal picture of breathing, which is presented below. The following are the main factors involved in the biochemical regulation:

- Saturation of blood with oxygen – how much it is carrying; and the chemical status of hemoglobin – how much oxygen it is able to carry
- Saturation of the blood with carbon dioxide, mostly dissolved as carbonic acid
- The amount of the alkaline buffer bicarbonate in the blood
- The pH of the blood, the cerebrospinal fluid, and the body in general
- The retention or disposal of acid and alkaline components by the kidneys
- The breathing 'drive' – with multiple competing inputs
- The amount of actual and expected metabolic demand, especially physical exertion
- The mechanical actions of breathing – rate per minute, depth, nose vs. mouth breathing.

pH

The story might best begin with pH, as this factor influences every organ of the body. To review briefly:

- The pH scale runs from 1 to 14, with 1 being acidic and 14 alkaline. The neutral midpoint is at 7. The more acidic a solution, the higher its proportion of hydrogen ions, which are positively charged and ready to combine with other molecules ('pH' designates partial pressure of hydrogen). It may be easier to think of the pH scale as an alkalinity scale, since higher numbers indicate higher alkaline content.

- The variable of relative acidity facilitates many metabolic exchanges and it must be kept in careful balance. Since pH describes the proportion of hydrogen ions available for combination, and the pH is on a log scale, a small change in pH, for example from 7.4 to 7.2, means doubling the number of hydrogen ions present. The binding of hydrogen to negative sites helps to regulate enzymatic action, endocrine secretion, integrity of protein molecules, and cellular metabolism, including oxygen absorption and release. A pH of 7.2 would seriously compromise many physiological functions.

- The physiological normal pH in the arterial blood is around 7.4, with an acceptable range from 7.35 to 7.45. Outside these limits lie ill effects of many kinds. The body will sacrifice many other things in order to maintain proper pH. A rise to 7.5 means more alkalinity, a drop to 7.3 more acidity. The term 'acidosis' means an excess of acid in the blood and tissues.

Carbon dioxide

The acidity of the blood is determined mainly by carbon dioxide, and so now we get to breathing. Carbon dioxide (CO_2) is the end product of aerobic metabolism, and comes primarily from the mitochondria (site of energy production within the cytoplasm) inside cells. It is the biological equivalent of smoke and ash. It is odorless, heavier than air, and puts out fires, including ours – if breathed in its pure form, it will quickly cause suffocation. It is present in the atmosphere at a concentration of around $\frac{2}{100}$ of 1% – low enough to be innocuous to us, but still at a level which sustains plant life.

Of all our excretions, CO_2 is the most lethal. For transport of this dangerous substance from the tissues into the blood and then into the lungs for exhalation, the body converts CO_2 to carbonic acid (H_2CO_3), of which we have a perpetual surplus. Breathing saves us from poisoning: the human lungs exhale around 12 000 mEq carbonic acid per day, compared to less than 100 mEq of fixed acids from the kidneys. An increase in bodily activity produces even more CO_2, which means the blood becomes more acidic unless more CO_2 is excreted.

Therefore, changes in breathing volume relative to CO_2 production regulate the moment-to-moment concentration of pH in the bloodstream (longer-term regulation of pH is shared with the kidneys). There is a tight interaction between the breathing volume, the amount of CO_2 production, the partial pressure of CO_2 in the arterial blood (indicated as Pa_{CO_2}), and blood pH. Note that the concentration of CO_2 in the blood, not the amount of oxygen, is the major regulator of breathing drive. Higher CO_2 level *immediately* stimulates more breathing, apparently on the assumption that abundance of CO_2 means that one is breathing oxygen-poor air, or that breathing has stopped, or that something else is happening which is an antecedent to suffocation.

During exercise, more CO_2 is produced, but more oxygen is needed also, so the need to keep pH constant is nicely linked with a greater drive to breathe:

High CO_2 = high acidity = low pH = higher breathing drive

Conversely, reduced exertion reduces oxygen need, and also lowers CO_2 production, which lessens the drive to breathe:

Low CO_2 = low acidity = high pH = lower breathing drive

The effects of different pH values, from acidosis to alkalosis, are shown in Table 3.1. Under normal circumstances, Pa_{CO_2} and pH are linked as shown in the table. Changes in breathing rate and volume adjust pH of the blood up or down. This relationship can be altered by metabolic acidosis or alkalosis and by renal compensation, offsetting one scale relative to the other.

Breath-holding does not produce more CO_2, but its blood level will rise anyway because it is not being exhaled; meanwhile more is being dumped into the bloodstream every second. To feel the urgency of this drive to resume breathing we need only hold the breath to breaking point. It is not really oxygen deficiency that we are feeling but rather the accumulation of CO_2; we are exquisitely sensitive to its build-up in the bloodstream. In underwater swimming, hyperventilating before the plunge will permit a longer

Table 3.1 Relationship between arterial pH and $Paco_2$, with effects

	pH	$Paco_2$	Effects
Acidosis			
	7.1	90–100+	Coma
	7.2	70	Hypercapnia symptoms (drowsiness, confusion)
	7.3	50	Breathing reflex stimulated
	7.4	**40**	**Normal**
	7.5	30	Mild hypocapnia symptoms (light-headedness, weakness), breathing reflex suppressed
	7.6	20	Moderate hypocapnia symptoms (paresthesias, confusion, twitches)
	7.7	10	Coma
	7.8+	0	Death
Alkalosis			

stay beneath the surface before the urge to breathe becomes unbearable. The reason is that the alarm substance has been depleted. The danger here is of brain hypoxia and underwater blackout, because the lack of an urge to breathe is mistakenly taken as a sign that there is still sufficient oxygen in the bloodstream.

Why do we have this complicated system which gives a waste gas on its way out of the body such a prime role in regulating breathing drive? Sensitivity to oxygen itself would appear to be a more direct way to regulate the breathing. However, the body's safeguards to preserve oxygen supply dictate against this. For one thing, there is a large reserve of oxygen in the bloodstream, such that under normal conditions about 75% of the oxygen inhaled is carried through the system and then exhaled without being utilized. Even with maximal exercise perhaps 25% of the inhaled oxygen is exhaled again. This enormous reserve, plus other factors which labor to maximize blood saturation, make direct indexing of oxygen a poor candidate for regulation of breathing drive. The pool of available oxygen is 'slushy' in the sense that it does not change quickly. The Pao_2 (partial pressure of oxygen in the arterial blood) must drop from 100 torr (mmHg) to about 50 before the brain's hypoxia detectors are moved to demand an increase in breathing. Low oxygen level does prime the CO_2 receptors to increase sensitivity if there is a drop in CO_2 however, so the systems are in communication.

The fact that carbon dioxide is the major regulator of the acid-base balance is linked to its role in regulating breathing, since breathing is the regulator of CO_2. The body can apparently afford fluctuations in CO_2 better than it can afford oxygen fluctuations. Fine adjustments of breathing rate and depth can change CO_2 rapidly, and this serves to maintain both adequate oxygen and proper pH (Figs 3.1 and 3.2).

Metabolic alkalosis and acidosis

When alkalosis or acidosis are caused primarily by aberrations in breathing, they are described as respiratory alkalosis/acidosis. But many physiological conditions associated with illness or dysregulation affect pH as well, and can cause an

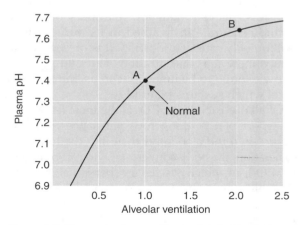

Figure 3.1 Change in plasma pH associated with relative alveolar ventilation. Normal alveolar ventilation = 1. Point A is normal pH and point B represents the change in pH associated with a two-fold increase in alveolar ventilation.

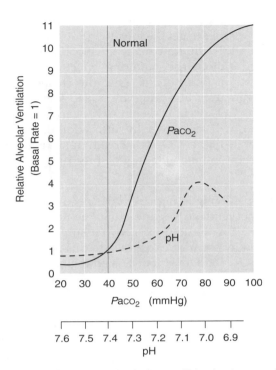

Figure 3.2 Stimulation of alveolar ventilation by decreased arterial pH or increased Pa_{CO_2}. (From Guyton 1971.)

alkaline or acidic condition for which the body tries to compensate by adjusting rate and depth of breathing. Distinguishing metabolic alkalosis/acidosis from respiratory is best done by blood analysis and careful consideration of medical factors. For example:

• In the case of ketoacidosis (excess metabolism of fats combined with insufficient carbohydrates, as in some drastic weight-loss diets or poorly controlled diabetes), the acidic state of the blood will promote deeper, faster breathing because the breathing centers are responding to the higher CO_2 content. This is hyperventilation, but not of the anxiety-based type. It represents instead the body's attempt to compensate for the blood imbalance by overbreathing in order to excrete CO_2 and bring the blood pH closer to normal.

• Diarrhea results in loss of plasma bicarbonate ion, which is alkaline, and if the diarrhea goes on too long acidosis is the result. This stimulates corrective overbreathing in order to remove CO_2

(as carbonic acid) and normalize the pH. (See Ch. 2 for fuller coverage of metabolic acidosis as a source of hyperventilation.)

• Excessive vomiting, on the other hand, causes loss of hydrochloric acid, shifting the body's overall balance toward alkalosis and depressing breathing enough to allow CO_2 to build up and restore pH. Hypoventilation is the result.

• Use of steroids and diuretics can also bring on alkalosis.

Normal values are listed in Box 3.1.

Bicarbonate buffer

The bicarbonate ion (HCO_3^-) is derived from CO_2 during its ride in the bloodstream; CO_2 dissociates into hydrogen ions (H^+) and HCO_3^-. This bicarbonate reserve is adjustable as needed, up to a point, and constitutes a major alkaline buffer system which opposes rises in acidity. The kidneys regulate the regulators by adjusting amount of bicarbonate returned to the bloodstream. If the kidneys detect excess acidity (a surplus of positively-charged hydrogen ions) they will try to retain more bicarbonate to balance the acid, but it is not fast; adjusting their filtration characteristics takes hours to days.

In the short run, meanwhile, if bicarbonate buffering of excess acid is not sufficient or if the bicarbonate is depleted, a faster back-up buffering system is available – hyperventilation. Excessive breathing exhales more CO_2 (acid), thereby raising pH closer to normal. In this case, one system's goals are subordinated to those of another system: the value of keeping Pa_{CO_2} near 40 is sacrificed so that pH can be kept around 7.4. This happens with acidosis, as in the above examples, and with alkalosis in the reverse.

Box 3.1 Normal values for breathing

• Pa_{CO_2} at 35–40 torr (mmHg)
• Bicarbonate around 24 mEq/liter
• pH at 7.4
• Pa_{O_2} close to 100 mmHg
• Breathing rate at 10–14 cycles per minute through the nose, with primarily diaphragmatic movement

Breathing more to compensate for metabolic acidosis has side-effects which are the consequence of both low CO_2 and high pH. In the short term these might include widespread vasoconstriction, interference with nerve function, cognitive and sensory disturbances, muscle weakness, and fatigue (see Ch. 2). Part of this effect will subside once the renal compensation sets in and the pH normalizes, but the low CO_2 may remain depressed in order to maintain the proper pH, and so the consequences of low CO_2 cannot be avoided.

Conditions which disrupt bodily pH are not rare, and the body has systems to compensate for them so that pH stays as stable as possible. Since these conditions vary in duration and chronicity, the body must be able to adapt both quickly and in the long term. An analogy with the suspension system of an automobile conveys some of the complexity of this system-of-systems: on a rough road, the rubber tires flex but are buffered by the contained air pressure. The shock absorbers further absorb and dispel the bumps; the leaf and coil springs continue the task, the upholstery of the car further cushions what comes through, until finally the individual passenger experiences a minimum of road bumps and shocks – in a serene state of homeostasis.

Hyperventilation clearly has many possible causes, which may be as varied as kidney failure and anxiety. Blood analysis of pH, bicarbonate, O_2 and CO_2 saturation all together will help distinguish the reason for any abnormalities. Medical determination of acid-base disorders is beyond the scope of this chapter, but if dire pathophysiology is ruled out, the distinction between compensated and non-compensated at least is important for a practitioner to know when working with hyperventilation:

- If the Pa_{CO_2} is low, the pH is high (alkaline) and the bicarbonate level is normal, it is uncompensated, and the hyperventilation could be transitory, perhaps easily remedied.
- If the Pa_{CO_2} is low but the pH is normal and the bicarbonate is low, this means that the kidneys have excreted more bicarbonate than usual to bring the pH down to normal. The person is then stuck in a more chronic compen-

sated or adapted state of hyperventilation, and it will be harder to get the breathing back to normal because this will now make the blood a little too acidic, without the buffering effect of normal amounts of bicarbonate. Since the chemoreceptors regulating breathing are sensitive to pH as well as CO_2 itself, a rise in CO_2 even if toward normal, will feel closer to suffocation. Learning to tolerate higher CO_2 (less breathing) is therefore important in rehabilitating the breathing pattern (Fig. 3.3).

People living at high altitudes need constantly to hyperventilate to some extent in order to compensate for the low oxygen pressure, and they eventually seem able to adjust to this necessarily low CO_2 blood level, but this adaptation is variable among individuals and not always successful. According to West (1995): 'Those born at high altitude have a diminished ventilatory response to hypoxia that is only slowly corrected by subsequent residence at sea level. Conversely, those born at sea level who move to high altitudes retain their hypoxic response intact for a long time. Apparently therefore ventilatory response is determined very early in life' (p. 138).

OXYGEN TRANSPORT AND DELIVERY

The blood carries oxygen mainly in molecules of hemoglobin which are contained in red blood cells. The value of oxygen saturation refers to how close to maximal the hemoglobin is loaded with oxygen; near sea level, this is generally 97–8%, and above 95% considered normal.

Within the red blood cell there occurs an exquisite regulation of oxygen transport. The readiness of hemoglobin to combine with oxygen (to form the compound oxyhemoglobin) varies according to local pH as well as Pa_{O_2}. The changes are designed to ensure adequate oxygen supply. This readiness to combine ('affinity') is important not only for absorbing oxygen in the lungs through the delicate walls of the alveoli, but also for releasing oxygen through the capillary walls, where oxygen diffuses into the tissues. These two properties seem destined to oppose one other, but the system adjusts to local conditions so that when

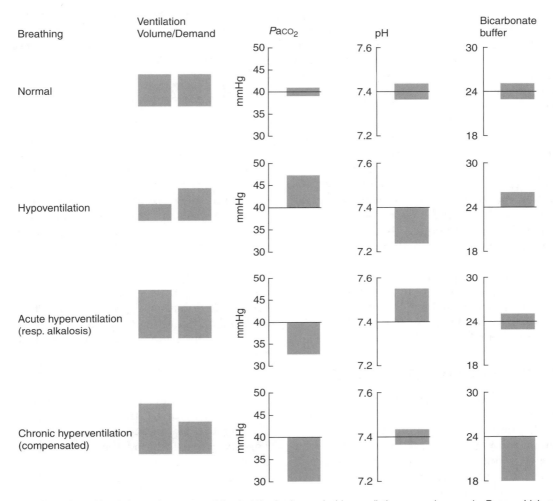

Figure 3.3 When breathing volume does not match what the body needs (demand) there are changes in Pa_{CO_2} which affect pH. The bars are meant to show directional shifts rather than exact values.

pH is low and the blood more acidic, hemoglobin in that area is stimulated to release more oxygen. This is true of metabolically active tissues in general, but especially of muscles. An exercising muscle needs all the oxygen it can get, and this is facilitated by its chemical nature: 'an exercising muscle is acid, hypercarbic, and hot, and it benefits from increased unloading of O_2 from its capillaries' (West 1995, p. 75). Heat acts like acidity in reducing hemoglobin's affinity for oxygen.

In the lungs the need is to bind oxygen to hemoglobin, not to release it. Since the lungs are a more alkaline environment, the chemistry favors affinity between hemoglobin and O_2, and so oxygen is easily absorbed through the pulmonary capillary walls and is combined with hemoglobin. This general effect of pH on oxyhemoglobin dissociation is called the Bohr effect.

Regulating oxygen delivery through changes in pH may seem like a complicated mechanism, but it works well, and it is fast: a red blood cell coming from the heart is exposed to oxygen in the lung for about $\frac{3}{4}$ second. There are about 280 million molecules of hemoglobin in a single red blood cell, and each hemoglobin molecule can carry four molecules of oxygen. The saturation of the available hemoglobin with oxygen normally stays at around 97–8%. Conditions such as high altitude (lower barometric pressure), or inadequate ventilation from any cause, will lower the saturation figure.

A shift of the blood toward acidity promotes dissociation and release of oxygen from the hemoglobin, while alkalinity encourages retention of oxygen. This is particularly relevant to the matter of hyperventilation: the resulting alkalinity causes the hemoglobin molecule to retain more oxygen than usual, making the metabolically active tissues resemble the lungs, where conditions encourage the blood to absorb oxygen rather than release it. Under conditions of uncompensated hyperventilation, SaO_2, the measure of oxygen saturation, may reach 100%. This sounds good to a patient, but it really means less oxygen available to the tissues. Increased breathing only makes the situation worse.

PSYCHOGENIC HYPERVENTILATION

Hyperventilation is a natural compensatory activity when the blood is too acidic, and illustrates the importance of both CO_2 level and breathing for regulating the body's pH on a minute-to-minute basis. But hyperventilation need not be a compensatory activity; it may be initiated and maintained by strictly mental stimuli, so that whatever factors drive anxiety also drive the breathing. Thus strong emotions such as chronic anxiety, apprehension, time urgency, resentment, and anger manifest somatically in some people as excess breathing, as if preparing for exertion. One of the biochemical aspects of strong emotion is a rise in adrenaline and noradrenaline, and under these conditions Heistad et al (1972) established that the body's sensitivity to CO_2, shown as increased ventilation, rises about 30%. In the absence of muscle exertion, respiratory alkalosis is the likely result. If this becomes a chronic state, the same renal compensation occurs as with metabolic alkalosis – dumping of bicarbonate into the urine. As will be explained later, this adjustment constitutes a

new equilibrium based on the assumption that the overbreathing will continue. This adaptation most likely adds to the difficulty in restoring normal breathing habits.

Cerebral blood flow

The effect of hyperventilation in the cortex of the brain is to reduce blood flow. This is partly through the vasoconstrictive effect of low CO_2 on smooth muscle, and partly through the effect of elevated pH. Lactic acid rises in the brain under conditions of respiratory alkalosis; this local change may act as a brake on the effects of rise in pH, but it also stimulates respiratory centers in the medulla to increase breathing, which may contribute to maintaining a hyperventilatory breathing pattern.

Cerebral blood flow has been found to be linearly related to arterial $PaCO_2$ (Hauge et al 1980), showing a 2% decline for each 1 mmHg drop in $PaCO_2$. A typical transient drop in CO_2 in a person prone to hyperventilation who is experiencing an anxious moment might be from 40 to 30 torr. This translates to a 20% drop in cerebral circulation. The precise effects of such a change have not been studied, apart from findings such as a slowing in EEG frequency (Gotoh et al 1965). This reduction in blood flow is in the opposite direction from what is most efficient for alertness and effective thinking (Fig. 3.4).

The biochemistry of anxiety and activity

Anxiety is not merely a mental phenomenon. Perception of threat is supported by bodily changes designed to enhance readiness for action. Increased breathing is often one of those changes, and it is reasonable in the short term because it creates a mild state of alkalosis. This would help offset a possible surge of acid in the blood (not only carbonic acid but also lactic acid if muscle exertion is drastic enough, since lactic acid is given off by anaerobic metabolism). Long-distance runners, sprinters, and horse trainers have experimented successfully with doses of sodium bicarbonate, which supplements the

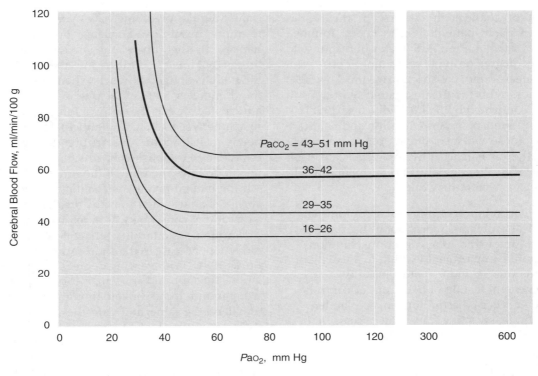

Figure 3.4 Changes in cerebral blood flow as a function of Pa_{CO_2} at different Pa_{CO_2}s. The heavy line represents the normal Pa_{CO_2} range. Note that both hypercapnia (higher Pa_{CO_2}) and hypoxemia (lower Pa_{O_2}) increase blood flow, and that hypocapnia causes a sharp decrease.

natural bicarbonate buffer and opposes the lactic acid load created by exercising muscles (Schott & Hinchcliff 1998, McNaughton et al 1999).

But if action does not occur within a minute or two, homeostasis is disrupted. No action means no surge in CO_2 production, even though the breathing is expecting it. If the perception of threat continues, the physiological alarm condition continues also, often boosted more by perception of the bodily changes which are the shadow of the anxious thinking. The chemical cascade (and eventual imbalance) then becomes an additional disturbance to the person seeking safety by worrying and hypervigilance – the human body is not really equipped to deal with chronic anxiety.

A likely sequence of events in the person prone to panic with hyperventilation, showing changes in the chemical, behavioral, and cognitive realms, is shown below:

- Initial threat perception (anxiety)
- Increased breathing, mirroring the mind
- Respiratory alkalosis and cerebral hypoxia
- Appearance of symptoms in several body systems
- Impairment of thought processes, disrupted mental stability
- Hyperemotionality, sustained anxiety, restricted reality orientation, and limited awareness of available options for coping with the anxiety trigger.

Some people are more susceptible than others to this sequence, and this variability may reflect constitutional factors which predispose some people to greater vasoconstriction for a given degree of hypocapnia. Using Doppler ultrasound to monitor changes in the size of the basilar artery in panic patients, Gibbs (1992) found a wide variance in arterial diameter in response to the same degree of hyperventilation. Those with the strongest artery constriction (as much as 50%) were those with the greatest panic symptoms (a finding confirmed by Ball & Shekhar in 1997).

Few sufferers of hyperventilation and panic are aware of the 'vicious circle' phenomenon in which the off-balance physiological state itself stimulates further anxiety. Several mental mechanisms can sustain this cycle:

1. Misinterpretation of physical symptoms as medical problems (worry about heart attack, brain tumor, and lung cancer are common)
2. Cognitive impairment leading to a feeling of 'losing one's mind' – fear of insanity
3. The general feeling of being out of control – such effects as disequilibrium, accelerated heart rate, sweating, muscle weakness, and paresthesias are alarming when they have no obvious source.

Unstable breathing

L. C. Lum (1976, 1981) proposed that the most drastic neurological consequences of hyperventilation result not from a low level of CO_2 but from sudden drops or fluctuations. Irregular breathing has been shown to accompany anxiety states (Han et al 1997). The increased variability from breath to breath may appear in rate, volume, or CO_2 level; the exact effects of this on the stability of cortical functions has not been studied systematically, but given the close relationship between the mechanical and the chemical variables of breathing, one could postulate what such study would reveal: namely, a loose, ragged coupling in which pH, hemoglobin oxygen-retention characteristics, respiratory drive, and $Paco_2$ struggle to adjust to each other because of the entry of anticipatory anxiety into the system.

Patel (1989, 1991) describes a common pattern during stress and anxiety of hyperventilation alternating with brief apnea. Attention to sensory input or to sudden memory intrusion or indeci-

sion is likely to suspend the breath. The restoration of regular breathing may overshoot, leading to more instability. Focusing on what might happen in the future, the anxious individual brings that imagined future into the present, and the body is obliged to react. When the conscious mind invokes a 'manual override' because of anticipated threat, the body is forced into a mismatch between actual and anticipated metabolic needs. Distraction interrupts the state; a reminder re-establishes it. Physiology for many people follows the play of thoughts and feelings – if the mental process is chaotic and jerky with abrupt changes, then so is the breathing, causing a cascade of consequences in many systems.

Neuronal excitability increases with CO_2 reduction, at least in the short term (Macefield & Burke 1991). With varying degrees of hyperventilation, sensory and muscular evoked potentials were found to rise even though the stimulus remained the same, and paresthesias and muscle twitches occurred if CO_2 dropped far enough. Yet those who live at high altitudes do not generally complain of paresthesias, dizziness, weakness, and rapid heartbeat, even though their CO_2 levels may be suboptimal. Their systems seem able to adjust, given time, as long as there is stability.

Neural regulation of breathing

Acute shifts in CO_2, however, seem to challenge homeostasis. The regulation of breathing is effected by two types of chemoreceptors: those in the medulla (central) and those in the carotid and aortic bodies (peripheral). Both are sensitive to CO_2 concentration, but the central receptors are slower. It seems that the medulla handles the minute-to-minute adjustments while the peripheral receptors handle the second-to-second adjustments. Animal experimentation has shown that breathing drive can even be altered in midbreath by exposing the peripheral receptors to rapid changes in CO_2 content.

Having two separate sources of control may provide safeguards, but it also opens the way for discoordination, in the same way that two musicians playing together create the chance for discord that would not occur with one alone. The irregularity of breathing and of CO_2 level in anxious individuals, particularly those with panic disorder, may reflect difficulty in coordination between these two neural control centers. The sub-threshold (sub-symptom) effects in response to sudden shifts in breathing may contribute to the pervasive uneasiness and restlessness common in chronic hyperventilators, and could feed back into the mental state to compound the anxiety. Add to this the restricted cortical circulation, and critical thinking and discrimination are further compromised.

Persistence of hyperventilation

Hyperventilation tends to persist in many people, and once a pattern of overbreathing is established it can be maintained by only a 10% increase in minute volume, which could be achieved by a combination of 10% deeper breaths, 10% faster breathing, or an occasional sigh (Saltzman et al 1963). Such subtle differences are difficult to detect without instrumentation. A clear marker of chronic hyperventilation is a delayed return to baseline after hyperventilation provocation (Hardonk & Beumer 1979). This test is covered more fully in Chapter 8.

Persistence of emotion may explain the persistence of hyperventilation, or there may be a physiological factor. In one study, 90 patients diagnosed with hyperventilation syndrome were asked to hyperventilate for a few minutes, focus on a negative emotional memory, and then resume normal breathing and indicate when they thought their breathing was actually back to normal. More than half of them signalled 'normal' when their CO_2 was less than 80% of their baseline, or resting level, while only 4% of the control subjects did so (King 1990).

This study, by including the 'think test' (induced negative emotion) confounded the effect of emotional persistence with the effect of hyperventilation itself, but it still offers valuable observations about a possible trait in hyperventilators (see Ch. 8 for more on the 'think test'). It may be that enough experience with this hypocapnic state creates a habituation to this compromised chemical condition and changes

the threshold for normality. Gardner (1996) found chronic hyperventilation to be a very persistent, stubborn pattern, subsiding only during the later stages of sleep. If such individuals routinely perceive their breathing as normal when it is not, this 'lowering of standards' would work against improvement. It is the same in principle as acceptance of poor posture or chronic muscle tension, reaching a stage of not even noticing the problem, yet being constrained by it in some way. Breathing rehabilitation therefore should include help in recognizing optimal breathing, as well as learning to create and sustain it without constant attention.

Panic attacks during relaxation

Panic attacks which happen suddenly, without apparent reason, are a frequent experience for those with panic disorder. Sitting quietly watching television or driving long distances are often associated with a sudden onset of breathlessness. Nocturnal panic attacks which awaken the individual from deep sleep may seem to challenge any psychological explanation, unless one postulates possible dream content, but such speculation is hard to confirm objectively.

Ley (1988a, 1988b) has offered a plausible explanation for this phenomenon based on the body's adaptation to chronic hyperventilation. The long-term reduction in bicarbonate buffer concentration is an attempt to offset the lowered $PaCO_2$, which increases alkalinity. This returns pH to normal, but the equilibrium is an uneasy one, dependent on the continuation of hyperventilation. This situation makes the individual more susceptible than ever to a rise in CO_2 (more acidity) because the alkaline buffer has been reduced. As a consequence, a change in breathing toward normal, away from hyperventilation, may feel closer to suffocation than it would if the person possessed normal bicarbonate buffering capacity.

Ley's proposal is that during certain deep sleep stages (not paradoxical sleep) and during sedentary states, the breathing is most likely to slow, and since the system has been set to expect a certain amount of hyperventilation, it is caught by surprise by the more normal breathing. Core temperature drops between 1.5 and 2°F. Lowered metabolism reduces the production of CO_2, adding to the already low level created by hyperventilation. Timing is important; if the breathing volume does not keep pace exactly with shifting metabolic requirements, there will be a period of mismatch. In Ley's words:

The chronic hyperventilator … is vulnerable to the effects of *decreases* in metabolism because a decrease in CO_2 may lower an already abnormally low resting level of $PaCO_2$ beyond the threshold of severe respiratory alkalosis and thereby produce those sensations of hypocapnia (e.g. dyspnea) that mark the panic attack. Thus, the chronic hyperventilator teeters on the brink of calamity. If the metabolic production of CO_2 drops suddenly, as when one sits down or lies down to relax, *while minute volume remains constant*, the sensations of hypocapnia will increase in intensity and thereby lead to the familiar symptoms which mark the panic attack. (Ley 1988b, p. 255)

General summary

High body priorities are to maintain pH around 7.4 and ensure adequate oxygen supply and delivery. Excess breathing excretes more CO_2 than is being produced, so pH moves higher, toward the alkalinity end (low $PaCO_2$ promotes alkalosis). Insufficient breathing retains more CO_2 than is being produced, so pH drops toward the acidic end. The pH in the short term is adjusted by increases or decreases in breathing volume.

Bicarbonate is an alkaline buffer which cushions abrupt rises in acidity. With the continued respiratory alkalosis created by chronic hyperventilation, the kidneys attempt to return pH to normal, excreting bicarbonate. This creates a new false equilibrium which works against resuming normal ventilation, which now creates sensations of breathlessness as $PaCO_2$ rises, less buffered by bicarbonate.

Muscle contraction, or any increase in metabolism, produces more CO_2, but normally the breathing increases also, resulting in more exhalation of CO_2. When respiration is matched to metabolic need, the level of $PaCO_2$ and pH stays stable. However, anticipated metabolic production (set off by apprehension, anxiety, preparation for exertion, discomfort, or chronic pain) will raise breathing volume. If the exertion does not occur, $PaCO_2$ will drop because the anticipatory increased breathing is not followed by increased muscle activity.

With higher $PaCO_2$ (lower pH), hemoglobin is stimulated to release more oxygen to the tissues. But a deficit of CO_2 promotes oxygen retention by the hemoglobin molecule. Thus, at a time when vasoconstriction is being promoted by alkalosis and high pH, release of oxygen is further inhibited by the Bohr effect. The system does not seem to have a mechanism for handling anticipatory anxiety unaccompanied by exertion, and this may constitute a functional, chemical loophole suffered by sentient beings able to project into the future.

ALLERGIC, DIETARY, AND NUTRITIONAL FACTORS

Food allergy is an immunological event, involving immunoglobulin E (IgE), whereas food intolerance involves adverse physiological reactions of unknown origin, without immune mediation. Food intolerance may involve food toxicity or idiosyncratic reactions to foods, sometimes related to enzyme deficiency or pharmacological responses (Anderson 1997).

It would certainly be helpful to be able to make a clear distinction between frank food allergy (hypersensitivity) reactions and food intolerance responses; however, these terms are a source of much confusion and little certainty. Mitchell (1988) states that in the UK the Royal College of Physicians and the British Nutrition Foundation have directly addressed the problem of terminology. They recommend that the general term 'food intolerance' be used, and that other terms such as food allergy and hypersensitivity be reserved for those situations where a pathogenetic mechanism is known or presumed. By definition (Royal College of Physicians 1984), food intolerance is a reproducible, unpleasant (i.e. adverse) reaction to a specific food or food ingredient which is not psychologically based.

MECHANISMS

Foodstuff in the gut is usually reduced enzymatically to molecular size (short chain fatty acids, peptides, and disaccharides) for absorption or elimination; however, it has been noted for some years that food antigens and immune complexes also find their way across the mucosal barrier to enter the bloodstream. The rate of entry seems to relate directly to the load of antigenic material in the gut lumen (Walker 1981, Mitchell 1988). Mitchell states: 'The presence of specialised membranous epithelial cells ... appears to allow active transport of antigen across the mucosa even when concentrations of antigen are low.' Box 3.2 lists the factors which can damage the gut wall. Permeability is retarded by defensive mechanisms, including enzyme and acid degradation, mucus secretion, and gut movement and barriers, which reduce absorption and adherence.

Gut wall irritation resulting from bacterial or yeast overgrowth (Gumowski 1987), or from higher levels of toxic load (dysbiosis), can increase the rate of transportation of undesirable molecules into the bloodstream – the so-called 'leaky-gut syndrome.' A variety of immunological defensive strategies occur to counter the entry of toxins and antigens into the system; however, a degree of adaptive tolerance seems to be a common outcome. Mitchell states that animal studies suggest strongly that the liver, along with

the age of first exposure, the degree of the antigenic load, and the form in which the antigen is presented, all play roles in regulation of the antigen specific tolerance (hyporesponsiveness) which emerges from this process (Mitchell 1988, Roland 1993). Early feeding patterns seem to be a critical factor in determining subsequent antibody responses to foods, with eggs, milk, fish, and nuts rating as among the greatest culprits (Mitchell 1988, Brostoff 1992). Apparently most people show the presence of serum antibody responses to food antigens, involving all classes of immunoglobulins. It is assumed that antibodies assist in elimination of food antigens via the formation of immune complexes which are subsequently phagocytosed. Failure to remove these complexes may result in tissue deposition and subsequent inflammation (Brostoff 1992). Sometimes the immune response to food antigens involves IgE, and sometimes not. The true food allergy exists, as do other responses which fall short of the criteria which would attract this label, and these are the food intolerances. An approach to the food intolerant patient is shown in Figure 3.5.

Mast cells

Mast cells in the lung, intestines, and elsewhere are critical to the allergic response, occurring as mucosal and connective tissue variants. Mast cells have surface receptors with a high affinity to IgE, but, critically, also to non-immunological stimuli including food antigens. How violent an allergic reaction is, involving the interaction of mast cells with IgE or other stimuli, depends on the presence of a variety of mediators such as histamine and arachidonic acid (and its derivatives such as leukotrienes) which augment inflammatory processes (Wardlaw 1986, Holgate 1983).

Histamine is secreted by mast cells during exposure to allergens, and the level of circulating histamine rises during prolonged hyperventilation (Kontos et al 1972). Histamine causes local inflammation and edema as well as bronchiole constriction. This last effect is especially relevant to asthmatics, but can affect anyone to some degree, adding to breathing difficulty.

Box 3.2 What damages the gut wall? (Deitch 1990, Iocono 1995, Jenkins 1991, O'Dwyer 1988, Isolauri 1989, Hollander 1985, Bjarnason 1984)

- Drugs (antibiotics, steroids, alcohol, NSAIDs)
- Age
- Allergies (specific genetically acquired intolerances)
- Infections of the intestine – bacterial, yeast, protozoal, etc.
- Chemicals ingested with food (pesticides, additives, etc.)
- Maldigestion, constipation (leading to gut fermentation, dysbiosis, etc.)
- Emotional stress which alters the gut pH, negatively influencing normal flora
- Major trauma such as burns (possibly due to loss of blood supply to traumatized area)
- Toxins which are not excreted or deactivated may end up in the body's fat stores

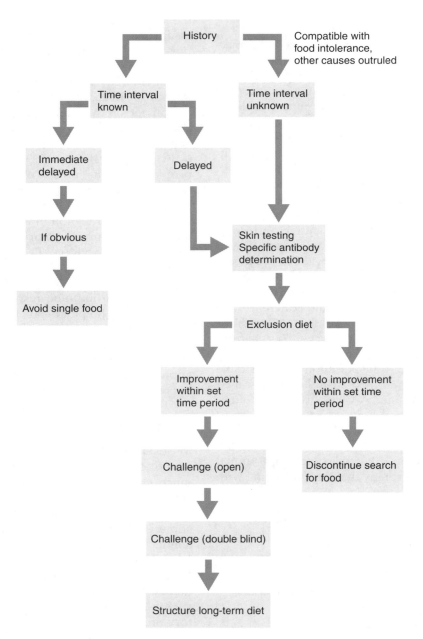

Figure 3.5 Approach to food intolerant patient.

At times a rapid response is noted to ingested and absorbed antigens; however, hours or days may elapse before a reaction manifests (Mitchell 1988). In the context of this text the relation between food intolerance and respiratory symptoms is of particular relevance. Both allergic rhinitis and bronchial asthma may result from a reaction to food (Box 3.3). Wilson and colleagues demonstrated (1982) that even in the absence of an immediate episode of bronchospasm, a reac-

---

Box 3.3 Food sensitivity and its relation to bronchial conditions

A summary of the evidence relating food sensitivity to asthma and other bronchial conditions is given below:

- Avoidance by lactating mothers of milk, eggs, fish, and nuts – and avoidance by the infant (up to 12 months) of the same foods plus soy, wheat, and oranges – reduced allergic disease (including asthma) in 58 cases compared with 62 controls (Spector 1991)
- In adults who have asthma the prevalence of food allergy in one double-blind, placebo controlled study was 2%, and in children 6.8%. Where asthma is poorly controlled, food allergy should be suspected. The main culprits identified are egg, milk, peanuts, soy, fish, shellfish, and wheat (Onorato 1986, James 1997).
- Another study showed that up to 10% of asthma may involve food allergy. This is more likely if the patient has a history of atopic dermatitis (egg, peanuts, and milk were identified as the main foods to cause a reaction). If asthma is refractory to standard medication, food allergy should always be considered (Plaut 1997)
- Food intolerance is identified in various studies to be a trigger in up to 50% of asthma patients (Anthony 1994, Warner 1995, Sheldon 1991, Metcalf 1989, Wilson 1988, Bahna 1991)
- Double blind food challenge provoked asthmatic response in two of four patients aged between 6 and 17 (Watson 1992)

---

tion to foods (cola drinks were being tested) can modify the function of the bronchial wall, although the mediating pathways are unclear.

Testing for intolerances and even frank allergies is not straightforward. Various factors may cause confusion, including the following (Roberson 1997):

- Demonstration of IgE antibodies in serum may be confounded because of the presence of other antibody classes
- Cytotoxic blood tests commonly produce false positive results
- Skin testing is an effective means of demonstrating the presence of inhaled allergens; however, this is not the case for food allergens (Rowntree et al 1985)
- Early in life the skin test response to food may be lost even though IgE antibodies are present in serum.

- Skin testing is inefficient in assessing delayed sensitivities and fails to accurately evaluate metabolic intolerances to foods (Hamilton 1997)

It is suggested that, following positive skin tests and/or radio-allergo-sorbant (RAST) tests, an *elimination diet* should be introduced to assess for food intolerances (James 1997) (see also Fig. 3.5).

An elimination diet involves a food or food family being excluded for a period – commonly 3 weeks – during which time symptoms are assessed. If there is an improvement, a challenge is initiated as the food is reintroduced. If there is benefit when the food is excluded, and symptoms emerge when it is reintroduced, the food is then excluded for not less than 6 months. This process offers the simplest, safest, and most accurate method of assessing a food intolerance, but only when it is applied strictly.

Strategies

Oligoallergenic diets, elimination diets, challenge studies, and rotation diets are variations which attempt to identify and then minimize the exposure of an individual to foods which provoke symptoms. Some recommended strategies are described in Chapter 10. Evidence of the value of such approaches is listed in Box 3.4.

Summary

Breathing disorders as severe as asthma, and as mild but irritating as chronic rhinitis, may be aggravated, or at times triggered, by food intolerances which are not frank allergies. Reduction or avoidance of factors in the diet which load the defensive mechanisms of the body is a choice patients may make if the evidence is presented to them in a coherent way, and strategies are offered which allow them to possibly enhance their quality of life. Clinical experience suggests that after a period of exclusion (6 months at least), cautious reintroduction of previously poorly tolerated foods may no longer provoke symptoms, especially if the foods are rotated (i.e. not eaten on a daily basis). Other strategies include desensitization, using homeopathic injection or orally

---

Box 3.4 Dietary strategies and asthma

- 74% of 50 patients with asthma experienced significant improvement without medication following an elimination diet. 62% were shown to have attacks provoked by food alone and 32% by a combination of food and skin contact (Borok 1990)
- When 113 individuals with irritable bowel syndrome were treated by an elimination diet, marked symptomatic improvement was noted. 79% of the patients who also displayed atopic symptoms, including hay fever, sinusitis, asthma, eczema and urticaria, showed significant improvements in these symptoms as well (Borok 1994)
- A moderate to high intake of oily fish has been shown to be associated with reduced risk of asthma, presumably due to high levels of eicosapentaenoic acid (EPA) which inhibits inflammatory processes (Hodge 1996, Thien 1996)
- A vegan diet which eliminated all dairy products, eggs, meat, and fish as well as coffee, tea, sugar, and grains (apart from buckwheat, millet, and lentils) was applied to 35 asthmatics, of whom 24 completed the 1-year study. There was a 71% improvement in symptoms within 4 months and 92% after 1 year (Lindahl 1985)

---

administered dilutions of the food(s) in question (Reilly 1994, Kahn 1995).

DIETARY LINKS TO ANXIETY, PANIC ATTACKS, AND PHOBIC BEHAVIOR

Ley (Timmons & Ley 1994) states that emotional arousal gives rise to conditionable changes in ventilation, and it appears that the connection between the emotions and breathing is a reciprocative relationship, in which changes in one lead to corresponding changes in the other (p. 82; see Ch. 5 for further coverage of conditioning). This suggests that feelings of anxiety may predispose to hyperventilation, which behavior then reinforces the feelings of anxiety, forming a potentially destructive cycle. Ley's statement, of course, also suggests that hyperventilation predisposes towards feelings of apprehension and anxiety. Opinions differ as to the relative hierarchy of importance between these two factors, i.e. which comes first, anxiety or hyperventilation, making this a very practical chicken and egg conundrum. And although Gardner (in Timmons & Ley 1994, p. 102) expresses the view

that there is ample evidence that 'chronic hyperventilation can occur in the absence of manifest anxiety' – which suggests the possibility of eggs without chickens, or vice versa – the fact remains that anxiety is established as a common instigator of hyperventilation.

Anxiety as an emotional state usually attracts psychosocial therapeutic attention. If, however, it could be shown that there exist common dietary factors which encourage anxiety, these triggers could be seen to be precursors to the breathing pattern changes which follow. This would offer the opportunity, in such individuals, for relatively simple dietary interventions (exclusions) which could potentially reduce or eliminate the anxiety state which may represent the main precursor to hyperventilation. A variety of such dietary triggers have been identified (Werbach 1991) and some of the key features of this phenomenon are summarized below:

- Buist (1985) has demonstrated a direct connection between clinical anxiety and elevated blood lactate levels, as well as an *increased lactate: pyruvate ratio*. This ratio is increased by alcohol, caffeine, and sugar. Experimentally infused lactate is likely to provoke panic attacks, including hyperventilation, in people prone to panic, but not in those who are not prone to panic. The lactate leads to peripheral alkalosis by being converted to bicarbonate. This lactate effect is paralleled by that of breathing 5% CO_2 for a short time: panickers are more likely to panic, but not those who are not panickers. The hypothesis proposed by some researchers is that sensitivity to lactate and CO_2 comes from the fact that both are precursors of suffocation; panickers are more sensitive to build-up of these chemicals for reasons that may be either chemical or psychological (Gorman et al 1984).

- *Glucose* loading has been shown to elevate blood lactate : pyruvate ratio in anxiety-prone individuals (Wendel & Beebe 1984). In a study involving 15 psychoneurotics (seven with anxiety), 28 schizophrenics (eight with anxiety), and six healthy controls the subjects consumed a cola drink containing 100 g of glucose. Blood lactate levels were markedly elevated during the

3rd, 4th, and 5th hours post-glucose only in the anxiety-prone psychoneurotic and schizophrenic patients (p<0.001). Blood pyruvate was shown to be significantly depressed by the 2nd hour post-glucose in all the psychoneurotic and schizophrenic patients, with the ratio of lactate to pyruvate increasing to a maximum of + 29.1 in the anxiety-prone group. The ratio did not exceed +4.0 for the non-anxiety group. The implication is that in dealing with anxiety prone people, sugar intake should be moderated, if at all possible.

• *Alcohol* inhibits gluconeogenesis from blood lactate, which directly raises the lactate : pyruvate ratio (Alberti & Natrass 1977). In an experimental placebo-controlled study involving 90 healthy male volunteers, an increase was shown in state anxiety following administration of ethanol as compared with placebo (Monteiro 1990). In this study separate infusions were made of either ethanol or diazepam. The Spielberger State Anxiety Inventory was applied, demonstrating significant increases in state anxiety following ethanol infusion, as compared to significant reductions in feelings of tension which were reported after the placebo administration. The implication is that in dealing with anxiety-prone people, alcohol intake should be moderated or eliminated, if at all possible.

• *Caffeine* was shown to have anxiogenic effects on patients with anxiety, particularly those suffering panic disorders. In an experimental controlled study (Charney 1985) 21 agoraphobic patients with panic attacks or panic disorder and 17 controls ingested caffeine 10 mg/kg of body weight. Caffeine was found to produce significantly greater increases in subject-rated anxiety, nervousness, fear, nausea, palpitations, restlessness, and tremors in the patients compared with the controls. 71% of the patients reported that the behavioral effects were similar to those experienced during panic attacks. The implication is that in dealing with anxiety-prone people, caffeine intake should be moderated or eliminated, if at all possible.

In a separate experimental double-blind study (Uhde 1984) it was shown that following a caffeine challenge, plasma cortisol levels, but not plasma MHPG levels, increased significantly, as did anxiety levels, in both panic disorder patients and controls. Two normal control patients experienced panic attacks accompanied by a 5-fold increase in plasma cortisol after a challenge dose of 720 mg of caffeine. MHPG is a metabolite of noradrenaline, and is often found lowered during depression.

Deficiency in various minerals, vitamins, and amino acids has been associated with anxiety disorders:

• In an experimental study (Hoes 1981), 13 patients who had suffered at least two hyperventilation attacks a week for between 6 months and 3 years were supplemented with *pyridoxine* (vitamin B_6) (125 mg three times daily) and *L-tryptophan* (2 g daily) for 4 weeks. After 3 weeks, nine patients (70%) were free of attacks. The researchers noted that baseline xanthurenic acid excretion (an index of peripheral tryptophan metabolism) had initially been either elevated or depressed in eight of the nine patients who improved, while the baseline in the non-responding four and in one of the responders was normal. Following the loading with pyridoxine and tryptophan, xanthurenic acid excretion normalized in all patients after 4 weeks. The responders remained symptom free at 3-month follow-up with no further supplementation.

⚠ **CAUTION:** Tryptophan is an amino acid which has been widely used to treat stress symptoms and insomnia. The Food and Drug Administration (FDA) removed tryptophan from over-the-counter sale in the early 1990s when Japanese manufacturers used a genetically engineered bacterial process to produce tryptophan, leading to eosinophilia-myalgia syndrome (Belongia 1990).

5-HTP: a safe form of tryptophan

A plant source of *5-hydroxy-L-tryptophan* (5-HTP), the immediate precursor to serotonin (5-hydroxitryptamine) is found abundantly in an African bean (*Griffonia simplicifolia*). Research has confirmed that this form of tryptophan safely converts into serotonin when it reaches the brain, and is at least as effective as L-tryptophan in encouraging sleep and reducing anxiety levels (Zmilacher 1988). 5-HTP is available from health food stores and pharmacists.

In an experimental double-blind study, 50 patients with primary fibromyalgia syndrome, with anxiety as one of their presenting symptoms, randomly received either 5-hydroxy-L-tryptophan 100 mg three times daily or placebo. After 30 days there were significant declines in the number of tender points and in the intensity of subjective pain, and significant improvements in morning stiffness, sleep patterns, anxiety and fatigue, in the patients receiving 5-HTP compared with the placebo group. Only mild and transient gastrointestinal side-effects were reported by some individuals (Caruso et al 1990, Puttini & Caruso 1992).

⚠ **CAUTION:** Vitamin B_6 (pyridoxine) in doses in excess of 200 mg daily, taken for extended periods, has been shown to be capable of producing sensory neuropathy (Waterston & Gilligan 1987). This risk can be avoided by using the active coenzyme form of pyridoxal phosphate, or by ensuring a short duration of supplementation (a month or less) at moderate dosages (under 200 mg).

Magnesium deficiency has been shown to increase the lactate to pyruvate ratio and is commonly associated with anxiety (Buist 1985). Supplementation (250–750 mg daily) is claimed to be useful for anxiety, especially if taken with calcium (Werbach 1991).

The glucose–hyperventilation connection

Diet has another effect on breathing disorders, namely that the level of glucose in the blood moderates the effect of low CO_2. These two factors are independent: that is, an individual may be in a hypoglycemic state and may or may not be hypocapnic also. The combination amplifies the negative effects of each on the brain by diminishing cerebral circulation and therefore interfering with neural metabolism. The brain requires both glucose and oxygen to function,

and the cortex is more sensitive to fuel interruptions than any other area. The brain uses approximately 20% of the glucose available in the blood at any one time.

Engel and colleagues (1947) studied this relationship most thoroughly, and used dominant EEG frequency as an index of cortical functioning. Their subjects hyperventilated for 3 minutes with their blood glucose at different levels, manipulated by fasting or glucose infusion. There were drastic differences in the EEG effects of hyperventilation depending on the glucose concentration, with a level of 72 mg (100 is considered normal, 80 is borderline) dropping the dominant EEG frequency to less than half of normal, into the delta-wave range normally associated with coma or sleep. This would translate into very poor cortical functioning.

The interesting point to note is that even a small reduction in blood glucose is sufficient to potentiate significantly the effects of hyperventilation. Many people will drop often into the mildly hypoglycemic range of 80–90 mg without much effect other than hunger. But add to that an episode of overbreathing and the effect may be drastic reduction of cognitive skills, reaction time, concentration, memory, and general orientation.

Wyke (1963) summarized: 'Engel and co-workers found that the disturbances of consciousness associated with hyperventilation correlate with the degree of slowing in the electroencephalogram, and that both sets of phenomena are enhanced by coincident hypoxia and hypoglycaemia and minimized by a high arterial PaO_2 and a high blood glucose concentration' (p. 63). The effect of low glucose on dominant EEG frequency is to slow it, causing rapid interference with attention, orientation, and cognition. Serum glucose in adequate concentration compensates for the vasoconstrictive, oxygen-robbing effect of hypocapnia to some extent; higher CO_2 maintains cerebral vasodilation and compensates for low glucose. When these two deficits occur together, both sources of brain fuel are threatened.

This means two things primarily to the clinician: first, if episodes of hyperventilation are reported to occur in late morning or late afternoon, or any time relatively far removed from a previous meal, the coincidence of hypoglycemia and hyperventilation should be considered. A partial remedy would consist of prescribing a hypoglycemic diet (high protein, frequent meals).

Second, an individual's response to a hyperventilation challenge test will vary according to the blood sugar level. To maximize the chance of obtaining a positive test (duplicating the conditions under which the symptoms are more likely to appear), request fasting for at least 4 hours before the challenge is carried out. Depending on the efficiency of a person's insulin regulation, fasting may make little difference for the effects of hyperventilation, or it may make a very large difference.

The progesterone–hyperventilation connection

During the latter half of the menstrual cycle, progesterone begins to rise and peaks around the 22nd day, or a week after ovulation. Apart from promoting thickening of the uterine wall, progesterone also stimulates respiration. Some research suggests that it first stimulates acidosis, which in turn increases breathing to compensate. Other research supports progesterone's direct stimulation of breathing. Either way, hyperventilation is the result. Apart from increasing minute volume, progesterone also increases the sensitivity of CO_2 receptors in the respiratory centers of the brain (increased sensitivity implies that an urge to breathe would develop sooner).

Pa_{CO_2} level is systematically related to the menstrual cycle, reaching its highest point before ovulation and its lowest point when progesterone has peaked. The average drop during the luteal phase is around 20–25%. Pa_{CO_2} remains depressed for many days, with all the potentially symptom-generating effects on vasoconstriction, nerve conduction, muscle tension, anxiety, etc. Hyperventilation may contribute to severity of other premenstrual symptoms; there is much

individual variability (Damas-Mora et al 1980). When a woman's breathing pattern is essentially normal, the premenstrual drop may not be enough to cause disruption because it is still in the low-normal range. But if a woman already has a tendency toward hyperventilation, a safety reserve is absent and the Pa_{CO_2} may drop into the zone which can cause symptoms (Fried 1993).

Progesterone helps to maintain pregnancy and so also remains high throughout pregnancy, continuing to stimulate breathing. Some degree of hyperventilation is common, if not universal, during pregnancy, and this chronically depressed CO_2 may, if added to an already existing pattern, aggravate anxiety and other symptoms. Altered levels of progesterone during menopause may disrupt stability further by its effect on breathing.

Women are at higher risk for anxiety disorders, and there may be a contribution to this liability by their periodic hormonal shift which disrupts their breathing pattern and thus their biochemistry. The progesterone effect is independent of other factors; in one study in which men were given either progesterone or a control substance, only the progesterone produced a higher basal temperature and decreased Pa_{CO_2}.

Exercise

Another peril of chronic hyperventilation is poor tolerance of exercise. The increased activity creates more carbonic acid (with aerobic exercise) and lactic acid once the anaerobic threshold is reached. But hyperventilators have a smaller buffer zone as a result of loss of bicarbonate, so blood acidity of any sort is relatively unopposed. This increases the chance of premature fatigue, feelings of breathlessness, dyspnea, and muscle pain. In addition, the large exercise-induced swings in metabolism create lag times and increase the chance of mismatches between metabolic demand and breathing volume.

REFERENCES

Alberti K, Natrass M 1977 Lactic acidosis. Lancet 2: 25–29

Anderson J 1997 Allergic diseases: diagnosis and treatment. Henry Ford Health System, Allergy Division, Detroit

Bahna S 1991 Asthma in the food sensitive patient. Journal of Allergy and Clinical Immunology 87(1), part 11: 174, abstract 144

Ball S, Shekhar A 1997 Basilar artery response to hyperventilation in panic disorder. American Journal of Psychiatry 154(11): 1603–1604

Belongia E 1990 An investigation of the cause of the eosinophilia-myalgia syndrome associated with tryptophan use. New England Journal of Medicine 323(6): 357–365

Bjarnason I 1984 The leaky gut of alcoholism – possible route for entry of toxic compounds. Lancet i: 79–182

Borok G 1990 Childhood asthma – foods that trigger? South African Medical Journal 77: 269

Borok G 1994 IBS and diet. Gastroenterology Forum (April): 29

Brostoff J 1992 Complete guide to food allergy. Bloomsbury, London

Buist R 1985 Anxiety neurosis: the lactate connection. International Clinical Nutrition Review 5(1): 1–4

Caruso I, Sarzi Puttini P, Cazzola M, Azzolini V 1990 Double-blind study of 5-hydroxytryptophan versus placebo in the treatment of primary fibromyalgia syndrome. Journal Internal Medical Research 18(3): 201–209

Charney D 1985 Increased anxiogenic effects of caffeine in panic disorders. Archives of General Psychiatry 42: 233–243

Comroe J H 1974 Physiology of respiration, 2nd edn. Year Book Medical Publishers, Chicago

Damas-Mora J, Davies L, Taylor W, Jenner F A 1980 Menstrual respiratory changes and symptoms. British Journal of Psychiatry 136: 492–497

Deitch E 1990 Intestinal permeability increased in burn patients shortly after injury. Surgery 107: 411–416

Engel G L, Ferris E B, Logan M 1947 Hyperventilation: analysis of clinical symptomatology. Annals of Internal Medicine 27: 683–704

Fried R 1993 The psychology and physiology of breathing. Plenum, New York, pp 174–176

Gardner W N 1996 The pathophysiology of hyperventilation disorders. Chest 109: 516–534

Gibbs D M 1992 Hyperventilation-induced cerebral ischemia in panic disorder and effects of nimodipine. American Journal of Psychiatry 149: 1589–1591

Gorman J M, Askanazi J, Liebowitz M R, Fyer A J, Stein J, Kinney J M, Klein D F 1984 Response to hyperventilation in a group of patients with panic disorder. American Journal of Psychiatry 141(7) (July): 857–861

Gotoh F, Meyer J S, Takagi Y 1965 Cerebral effects of hyperventilation in man. Archives of Neurology 12: 410–423

Gumowski P 1987 Chronic asthma and rhinitis due to *Candida albicans*, epidermophyton and trichophyton. Annals of Allergy 59: 48–51

Guyton A C 1971 Textbook of medical physiology, 4th edn. W B Saunders, Philadelphia

Hamilton K 1997 Allergy/hypersensitivity/intolerance. In: Roberson K (ed) Asthma: clinical pearls in nutrition and complementary medicine. I T Services, Sacramento, California

Han J N, Stegen K, Simkens K, Cauberghs M, Schepers R, Van den Bergh O, Clement J, Van de Woestijne K P 1997 Unsteadiness of breathing in patients with hyperventilation syndrome and anxiety disorders. European Respiratory Journal 10: 167–176

Hardonk J, Beumer H 1979 Hyperventilation syndrome. In Vinken P., Bruyn G. (eds) Handbook of clinical neurology. Amsterdam: North Holland, 309–360

Hauge A, Thoresen M, Walloe L 1980 Changes in cerebral blood flow during hyperventilation, and CO_2 rebreathing in humans by a bidirectional, pulsed, ultrasound Doppler blood velocity meter. Acta Physiologia Scandinavia 110: 167–173.

Heistad D, Wheeler R, Mark A, Schmid R, Abboud F 1972 Effects of adrenergic stimulation in man. Journal of Clinical Investigation 51: 1469–1475

Hoes M 1981 Hyperventilation syndrome treatment with L-tryptophan and pyridoxine: predictive values of xanthurenic acid excretion. Journal of Orthomolecular Psychiatry 10(1): 7–15

Hodge L 1996 Consumption of oily fish and childhood allergy risk. Medical Journal of Australia 164: 136–140

Holgate S 1983 Mast cells and their mediators. In: Holborrow E, Reeves W (eds) Immunology in Medicine, 2nd edn. Academic Press, London

Hollander D 1985 Aging-associated increase in intestinal absorption of macro-molecules. Gerontology 31: 133–137

Iocono G 1995 Chronic constipation as a symptom of cow's milk allergy. Journal of Pediatrics 126: 34–39

Isolauri E 1989 Intestinal permeability changes in acute gastroenteritis. Journal of Pediatric Gastroenterology and Nutrition 8: 466–473

James J 1997 Food allergy – what link to respiratory symptoms? Journal of Respiratory Diseases 18(4): 379–390

Jenkins A 1991 Do NSAIDs increase colonic permeability? Gut 32: 66–69

Kahn J 1995 Homeopathic remedy relieves allergic asthma. Medical Tribune, 5 Jan, p 11

Kao F 1972 An introduction to respiratory physiology. Excerpta Medica, Amsterdam

King J 1990 Failure of perception of hypocapnia: physiological and clinical implications. Journal of the Royal Society of Medicine 83 (Dec): 765–767

Kontos H, Richardson D, Raper A 1972 Mechanism of action of hypocapnic alkalosis on limb blood vessels in man and dog. American Journal of Physiology 223: 1296–1307

Ley R 1988a Panic attacks during relaxation and relaxation-induced anxiety: a hyperventilation interpretation. Journal of Behavior Therapy and Experimental Psychiatry 19: 253–259

Ley R 1988b Panic attacks during sleep: a hyperventilation-probability model. Journal of Behavior Therapy and Experimental Psychiatry 19: 181–192

Lindahl O 1985 Vegan regimen with reduced medication in treatment of bronchial asthma. Journal of Asthma 22(1): 44–55

Lum L C 1976 The syndrome of chronic habitual hyperventilation. In: Hill O W (ed) Modern trends in psychosomatic medicine. Butterworth, London

Lum L C 1981 Hyperventilation and anxiety state. Journal of the Royal Society of Medicine 74: 1–4

Macefield G, Burke D 1991 Paraesthesiae and tetany induced by voluntary hyperventilation: increased excitability of human cutaneous and motor axons. Brain 114: 527–540

McNaughton L, Dalton B, Palmer G 1999 Sodium bicarbonate can be used as an ergogenic aid in high-intensity, competitive cycle ergometry of 1 h duration. European Journal of Applied Physiology 80(1): 64–69

Metcalf D 1989 Diseases of food hypersensitivity. New England Journal of Medicine 321(4): 255–257

Mitchell E B 1988 Food intolerance. In: Dickerson W, Lee H (eds) Nutrition in the clinical management of disease. Edward Arnold, London

Monteiro M 1990 Subjective feelings of anxiety in young men after ethanol and diazepam infusions. Journal of Clinical Psychiatry 51(1): 12–16

Nunn J F 1993 Applied respiratory physiology. Butterworth-Heinemann Medical, Oxford

O'Dwyer S 1988 A single dose of endotoxin increases intestinal permeability in healthy humans. Archives of Surgery 123: 1459–1464

Onorato J 1986 Placebo-controlled double-blind food challenge in asthma. Journal of Allergy and Clinical Immunology 878: 1139–1146

Patel C 1989 The complete guide to stress management London: MacDonald Optima; New York: Plenum Press, 1991

Plaut M 1997 New directions in food allergy research. Journal of Allergy and Clinical Immunology April 1997: 7–10

Puttini P S, Caruso I 1992 Primary fibromyalgia syndrome and 5-hydroxy-L-tryptophan: a 90-day open study. Journal of International Medical Research 20(2): 182–189

Reilly D 1994 Is evidence for homeopathy reproducible? Lancet 344: 1601–1606

Roberson K (ed) 1997 Asthma: Clinical pearls in nutrition and complementary medicine. I T Services, Sacramento, California

Roland N 1993 Interactions between the intestinal flora and xenobiotic metabolizing enzymes and their health consequences. World Review of Nutrition and Diet 74: 123–148

Rowntree S, Cogswell J, Platts-Mills T, Mitchell E 1985 Development of IgE and IgG antibodies to food and inhalant allergens in children. Archives of Diseases in Children 60: 727–735

Royal College of Physicians 1984 Food intolerance and food aversion. Journal of the Royal College of Physicians London 18(2)

Saltzman H A, Heyman A, Sieker H O 1963 Correlation of clinical and physiologic manifestations of sustained hyperventilation. New England Journal of Medicine 268: 1431–1436

Schott H C, Hinchcliff K W 1998 Treatments affecting fluid and electrolyte status during exercise. Veterinary Clinics of North America Equine Practice 14(1): 175–204

Spector S 1991 Common triggers of asthma. Postgraduate Medicine 90(3): 50–58

Taylor A, Rehder K, Hyatt R, Parker J 1989 Clinical respiratory physiology. W B Saunders, Philadelphia

Thien F 1996 Oily fish and asthma. Medical Journal of Australia 164: 135–136

Timmons B H, Ley R 1994 Behavioral and psychological approaches to breathing disorders. Plenum Press, New York

Uhde T 1984 Caffeine and behaviour relationship to human anxiety, plasma MPHG and cortisol. Psychopharmacology Bulletin 20(3): 426–430

Walker W 1981 Antigen uptake in the gut. Immunology Today 2: 30–34

Wardlaw A 1986 Morphological and secretory properties of bronchoalveolar mast cells in respiratory diseases. Clinical Allergy 16: 163–173

Warner J 1995 Food intolerance and asthma. Clinical and Experimental Allergy 25 (suppl. 1): 29–30

Waterston J, Gilligan B 1987 Pyridoxine neuropathy. Medical Journal of Australia 146: 640–642

Wendel O, Beebe W 1984 Glycolytic activity in schizophrenia. In: Hawkins D, Pauling L (eds) Orthomolecular psychiatry. W H Freeman, San Francisco

Werbach M 1991 Nutritional influences on mental illness. Third Line Press, Tarzana CA

West J 1995 Respiratory physiology: the essentials. Lippincott, Williams and Wilkins, Philadelphia

Wilson N 1988 Bronchial hyperreactivity in food and drink intolerance. Annals of Allergy 61: 75–79

Wilson N, Vickers H, Taylor G, Silverman M 1982 Objective test for food sensitivity in asthmatic children: increased bronchial reactivity after cola drinks. British Medical Journal 284: 1226–1228

Wyke B 1963 Brain function and metabolic disorders: the neurological effects of hydrogen-ion concentration. Butterworth, London

Zmilacher K 1988 L-5-hydroxytryptophan alone and in combination with a peripheral decarboxylase inhibitor in treatment of depression. Neuropsychobiology 20(1): 28–35

4

Biomechanical influences on breathing

Leon Chaitow

THE STRUCTURE–FUNCTION CONTINUUM

If there is evidence of breathing dysfunction in a patient there will axiomatically be evidence of structural modification related to the functional disturbance. The challenge is to be able to locate, observe, monitor, and, if appropriate, therapeutically modify structural dysfunction in order to initiate functional improvements.

Function and structure are so intimately bound to each other as to ensure that changes in one inevitably lead to, or derive from, the other. When breathing function is being assessed, a complex set of functions, all of which have structural linkages, is being observed. If a pattern of breathing has been disturbed for any length of time, clinical experience suggests that normalization of the musculature and joints associated with the breathing process will require primary attention before normal patterns of use can be restored.

In a different context, involving postural reeducation, structural rehabilitation has been shown to be necessary prior to the reestablishment of more appropriate use patterns.

As Dommerholt (2000) points out:

In general, assessment and treatment of individual muscles must precede restoration of normal posture and normal patterns of movement. Claims that muscle imbalances would dissolve, following lessons in [for example] the Alexander technique are not substantiated in the scientific literature (Rosenthal 1987). Instead muscle imbalances must be corrected through very specific strengthening and flexibility exercises, since generic exercise programs tend to perpetuate the compensatory muscle patterns. Myofascial trigger points must be inactivated using either invasive or non-invasive treatment techniques. Associated joint dysfunction, especially of the cervical and thoracic spine must be corrected with joint mobilizations. Once the musculoskeletal conditions for 'good posture' have been met, postural retraining [using] Alexander or other methods, can proceed.

From an osteopathic perspective (Dommerholt is a physiotherapist), these observations seem appropriate and accurate. Normalization of the structures which support and move those parts involved in a particular function has to precede or accompany rehabilitation and reeducation toward more physiologically functional use patterns.

Whatever efforts are directed towards removal of the causes of any functional imbalance (dysfunction), whether this involves medication, surgery, manual rehabilitation strategies, or behavior modification and reeducation, there is likely to be a more desirable outcome if any identifiable biomechanical structural constraints can first be modified towards normal.

Local and global perspectives

While specific restrictions – shortened muscles, restricted ribs, etc. – may be identified and treated, a wider perspective may also usefully be employed, in order to determine the presence of global restriction patterns.

There are few local biomechanical problems which are not influenced by distant features. For example, a fallen arch may impact, via a sequence of interacting influences, on a stiff neck. Janda (1986) discusses the chain of events which might follow on from the presence of a short leg: this chain might well include such widespread effects as an altered pelvic position, scoliosis, altered head position, changes at the cervicocranial junction, compensatory activity of the small cervico-occipital muscles, increased muscle tone, muscle spasm, probable joint dysfunction, particularly at the cervicocranial junction, and a sequence of compensation and adaptation responses in many muscles, followed by the evolution of a variety of possible syndromes involv-

ing head/neck, temporomandibular joint (TMJ), shoulder/arm, thoracic or other structures.

Conversely, adaptations can reflect inferiorly. Murphy (2000) reports that TMJ dysfunction and cranial distortion, including nasal obstruction, are commonly associated with 'forward head carriage, abnormal cervical lordosis, rounded shoulders, a flattened chest wall and a slouching posture.' We might well ask where such a chain begins – with the facial and jaw imbalance, or in the overall postural distortion pattern which affects the face and jaw? Visual imbalances can likewise create postural disturbances bodywide which remain 'uncorrectable' until the vision factors are addressed (Gagey & Gentaz 1996).

These linkages are no less likely to be evident in respiratory dysfunction (Figs 4.1A and 4.1B).

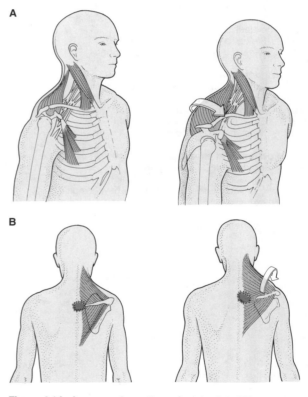

Figure 4.1A A progressive pattern of postural and biomechanical dysfunction develops resulting in, and aggravated by, inappropriate breathing function. **B** The local changes in the muscles of an area being stressed in this way will include the evolution of fibrotic changes and myofascial trigger points. (Reproduced with kind permission from Chaitow 1996b).

Loose–tight

The so-called 'loose–tight' concept is one way of visualizing the three-dimensionality of the body, or part of it, as it is palpated and assessed (Ward 1997). This might involve seeking evidence for large or small areas in which interactive asymmetry exists, involving structures which are inappropriately 'tight' and/or 'loose' relative to each other.

For example:

- A tight sacroiliac (SI) hip is commonly noted on one side, while the contralateral side is loose
- A tight sternocleidomastoid (SCM) and loose scalenes are frequently noted ipsilaterally
- One shoulder may present as tight and the other as loose.

Areas of dysfunction commonly involve vertical, horizontal, and 'encircling' (also described as crossover, or spiral, or 'wrap-around') patterns of involvement. Ward (1997) describes a typical wrap-around pattern associated with a tight left low-back area (which ends up involving the entire trunk and cervical area) as tight areas evolve to compensate for loose, inhibited, areas (or vice versa):

- Tightness in the posterior left hip, SI joint, lumbar erector spinae, and lower rib cage associated with:
- Looseness on the right low back
- Tightness of the lateral and anterior rib cage on the right
- Tight left thoracic inlet, posteriorly
- Tight left craniocervical attachments (involving jaw mechanics).

In relation to breathing function, it is clear that some degree of inhibition of normal excursion of the thoracic cage would coexist with such a pattern.

As tight areas are freed or loosened, even if only to a degree, at any given treatment session, so would inhibiting influences on loose, weak areas diminish, allowing facilitation of a restoration of more normal tone. At such a time rehabilitation, possibly involving proprioceptive educational patterns of use, might beneficially be introduced, and worked with by the patient, so that what subjectively 'feels wrong' in terms of posture and use patterns, become comfortable and starts to feel 'right'.

Pain and the tight–loose concept

- Paradoxically, pain is often noted in the loose rather than the tight areas of the body, which may involve hypermobility and ligamentous laxity at the loose joint or site
- Lax, loose areas are vulnerable to injury and prone to recurrent dysfunctional episodes (SI joint, TMJ dysfunction, etc.)
- More commonly, pain is associated with tight, restricted and bound/tethered structures
- Such changes may be due to local overuse/ misuse/abuse factors, scar tissue, or to reflexively-induced influences, or to centrally mediated neural control
- Myofascial trigger points may exist in either tight or loose structures, but the likelihood is that they will appear more frequently, and be more active, in those tissues which are tethered, restricted, tight and therefore relatively ischemic
- It is established that unless active myofascial trigger points are deactivated they will help to sustain the dysfunctional postural patterns with which they are associated (Simons et al 1998)
- Such deactivation may involve removing the biomechanical and other stress patterns which create and maintain trigger points, or by direct manual or other intervention
- Myofascial trigger points will continue to evolve if the etiological factors which created and maintain them are not corrected.

Barrier terminology

In osteopathic positional release methodology (Strain/counterstrain, Functional technique, etc., discussed in Ch. 6) the terms 'ease' and 'bind' are often used to describe what is noted as unduly tight or loose (Jones 1981). In manual medicine, when joint and soft tissue 'end-feel' is being evaluated, a similar concept is involved in the area being evaluated and it is common practice to make sense of such findings by comparing sides (Kaltenborn 1985).

The characterization of features described as having a 'soft' or 'hard' end-feel, or as being tight or loose, or as demonstrating feelings of 'ease' or 'bind' may be a deciding factor in the choice of therapeutic approach or approaches and the sequence in which they are introduced. The findings loose, tight, etc. have an intimate relationship with the concept of barriers, which need to be identified in preparation for direct – where action is directed towards the restriction barrier, toward bind, tightness – and indirect – where action involves movement away from barriers of restriction, toward ease, looseness – techniques. 'Tightness suggests tethering, while looseness suggests joint and/or soft tissue laxity, with or without neural inhibition' according to Ward (1997). However, it is worth recalling that it is also possible for the tight side to be the normal side, and that tight restriction barriers may sometimes best be left unchallenged in case they are offering some protective benefit.

As an example, van Wingerden and colleagues (1997) report that both intrinsic and extrinsic support for the sacroiliac joint derive in part from hamstring (biceps femoris) status. Intrinsically the influence is via the close anatomical and physiological relationship between biceps femoris and the sacrotuberous ligament (they frequently attach via a strong tendinous link). They state: 'Force from the biceps femoris muscle can lead to increased tension of the sacrotuberous ligament in various ways. Since increased tension of the sacrotuberous ligament diminishes the range of sacroiliac joint motion, the biceps femoris can play a role in stabilisation of the SIJ' (Vleeming et al 1997). They further note that in low back-pain patients, forward flexion is often painful as the load on the spine increases. This happens whether flexion occurs in the spine or via the hip joints (tilting of the pelvis). If the hamstrings are tight and short they effectively prevent pelvic tilting: 'In this respect, an increase in hamstring tension might well be part of a defensive arthrokinematic reflex mechanism of the body to diminish spinal load.'

If such a state of affairs is of long standing, the hamstrings (biceps femoris) will shorten, possibly influencing sacroiliac and lumbar spine dysfunction. The decision to treat tight (tethered) hamstrings should therefore take account of why the hamstring is tight, and consider that in some circumstances it is offering beneficial support to the SIJ, or that it is reducing low-back stress. This example is emphasized because it is so clear and also somewhat surprising. Similar paradoxes exist in relation to the biomechanics of breathing.

Richardson and colleagues (1999) have shown that there may be times when the diaphragm has apparently contradictory roles to play, and where its relative tightness may relate to activities unrelated to respiration. In a study which measured activity of both the costal diaphragm and the crural portion of the diaphragm, as well as transversus abdominis, it was found that contraction occurred in all these areas when spinal stabilization was required (in this instance during shoulder flexion): 'The results provide evidence that the diaphragm does contribute to spinal control and may do so by assisting with pressurization and control of displacement of the abdominal contents, allowing transversus abdominis to increase tension in the thoracolumbar fascia or to generate intra-abdominal pressure.' The involvement of the diaphragm in postural stabilization suggests that situations might occur where conflicting demands become evident – for example where postural stabilizing control is required at the same time that respiratory functions create demands for movement. Richardson and colleagues (1999) state: 'This is an area of ongoing research, but must involve eccentric/concentric phases of activation of the diaphragm.'

Chain reactions and 'tight–loose' changes

Kuchera (1997a) connects gravitational strain with changes of muscle function and structure which lead predictably to observable postural modifications and functional limitations: 'Postural muscles, structurally adapted to resist prolonged gravitational stress, generally resist fatigue. When overly stressed, however, these same postural muscles become irritable, tight, shortened' (Janda 1986). The antagonists to these postural muscles demonstrate inhibitory characteristics described as 'pseudoparesis' (a functional, non-organic, weakness) or 'myofascial trigger points with weakness' when they are stressed.

Observable changes such as those illustrated below in Figures 4.8 and 4.9 (upper and lower crossed syndromes, see later this chapter) emerge through overuse, misuse, and abuse of the postural system, leading to changes in which some muscles shorten and tighten while others are inhibited and weaken and/or lengthen. Common dysfunctional postural patterns emerge with inevitable modification of optimal function, including breathing function.

Current literature does not always agree with Janda's classification of muscles as 'postural' and 'phasic', sometimes confusingly employing different characterizations. Aspects of the muscle debate are summarized in Box 4.1.

MUSCULOSKELETAL– BIOMECHANICAL–STRESSORS

(Janda 1983, Travell & Simons 1992, Basmajian 1974, Dvorak & Dvorak 1984, Lewit 1999, Korr 1978)

The many forms of stress affecting the body in the sequential manner discussed below can be categorized as falling into general classifications of physiological, emotional, behavioral and/or structural. They might include the following types of stress (Barlow 1959):

- Congenital factors such as short or long leg, small hemipelvis, fascial influences such as cranial distortions involving the reciprocal tension membranes (e.g. falx cerebri, tentorium cerebelli) due to birthing difficulties (e.g. forceps delivery)
- Overuse, misuse, and abuse factors such as injury or inappropriate or repetitive patterns of use during work, sport, or other daily activities (Fig. 4.2)

- Immobilization – disuse can lead to irreversible changes after as little as 8 weeks (Lederman 1997)
- Postural stress patterns
- Inappropriate breathing patterns. Lewit (1980) has given due attention to structure and function as it relates to respiration, and states: 'The most important disturbance of breathing is overstrain of the upper auxiliary [accessory breathing] muscles by lifting of the thorax during quiet respiration'
- Chronic negative emotional states such as depression, anxiety, etc. Such emotional states initiate postural changes and muscle bracing, for instance depression is associated with a head-forward posture, hostility with increased shoulder tension and chest breathing; and fear with head 'pulled in'. 'Attitudes' are both physical postures and emotional/cognitive tendencies (personal communication, Gilbert 2001)
- Reflexive influences (including trigger points, facilitated spinal regions).

A BIOMECHANICAL STRESS SEQUENCE (Janda 1983, Travell & Simons 1992, Basmajian 1974, Dvorak & Dvorak 1984, Lewit 1999, Korr 1978)

When the musculoskeletal system is stressed, a sequence of events takes place which can be summarized as follows:

- 'Something' (see the list of possible biomechanical stressors above) occurs, leading to increased muscular tone.
- If this is anything but short term, retention of metabolic wastes commences.
- Increased tone simultaneously causes a degree of localized oxygen deficit, resulting in relative ischemia.
- Ischemia does not produce pain, but an ischemic muscle which contracts rapidly does produce pain (Lewis 1942, Liebenson 1996).
- Increased tone may lead to a degree of edema.
- Retention of wastes/ischemia/edema all contribute to discomfort or pain, which in turn reinforces hypertonicity.

Box 4.1 Muscle designations (Fig. 1.17A, B)

The use of terms such as *postural muscle* and *phasic muscle* requires some elaboration. Physiotherapist Chris Norris (2000) explains his perspective on the classification of muscles as postural, phasic, stabilizer, mobilizer, etc. as follows:

The terms postural and phasic used by Jull and Janda (1987) can be misleading in their categorization, the hamstring muscles are placed in the postural grouping while the gluteals are placed in the phasic grouping. The reaction described for these muscles is that the postural group (represented by the hamstrings in this case) tend to tighten, are biarticular, have a lower irritability threshold and a tendency to develop trigger points. This type of action would suggest a phasic (as opposed to tonic) response, and is typical of a muscle used to develop power and speed in sport for example, a task carried out by the hamstrings. The so called 'phasic group' is said to lengthen, weaken and be uniarticular, a description perhaps better suited to the characteristics of a muscle used for postural holding. The description of the muscle responses described by Jull and Janda (1987) is accurate, but the term postural and phasic do not seem to adequately describe the groupings. Although fibre type has been used as one factor to categorize muscles, its use clinically is limited as an invasive technique is required. It is therefore the functional characteristics of the muscle which is of more use to the clinician. Stabilizing muscles show a tendency to laxity and an inability to maintain a contraction (endurance) at full inner range. Mobilizing muscles show a tendency to tightness through increased resting tone. The increased resting tone of the muscle leads to, or co-exists with, an inclination for preferential recruitment where the tight muscle tends to dominate a movement. The stabilizing muscle in parallel shows a tendency to reduced recruitment or inhibition as a result of pain or joint distention.

Norris continues:

A further categorization of muscles has been used by Bergmark (1989) and expanded by Richardson et al (1999). They have used the nomenclature of local (central) and global (guy rope) muscles, the latter being compared to the ropes holding the mast of a ship. The central muscles are those which are deep or have deep portions attaching to the lumbar spine. These muscles are seen as capable of controlling the stiffness (resistance to bending) of the spine and of influencing intervertebral alignment. The global category includes larger more superficial muscles. Global muscles include the anterior portion of the internal oblique, the external oblique, the rectus abdominis, the lateral fibers of the quadratus lumborum and the more lateral portions of the erector spinae (Bogduk & Twomey 1991). The local categorization includes the multifidus, intertrasversarii, interspinales, transversus abdominis, the posterior portion of the internal oblique, the medial fibers of quadratus lumborum and the more central portion of the erector spinae.

Confusion of nomenclature is currently a feature of muscle categorization. The basic fact is that some muscles behave differently from others, some tending to shortness with others tending to weakness and possibly lengthening. What labels are attached is a matter of convenience and debate. In this chapter the widely used Jull & Janda (1987) terminology will be employed (i.e. postural and phasic).

Among the more important postural muscles which become hypertonic in response to dysfunction are many which have breathing function influences:

- Trapezius (upper), sternocleidomastoid, levator scapulae and upper aspects of pectoralis major in the upper trunk, and the flexors of the arms
- Quadratus lumborum, erector spinae, oblique abdominals and iliopsoas in the lower trunk
- Tensor fasciae latae, rectus femoris, biceps femoris, adductors (longus, brevis, and magnus), piriformis, hamstrings, and semitendinosus in the pelvic and lower extremity region.

Phasic muscles, which weaken in response to dysfunction (i.e. are inhibited), also include some muscles which are involved in breathing function:

- The paravertebral muscles (not erector spinae), scaleni (see notes on scalenes below) and deep neck flexors, deltoid, the abdominal (or lower) aspects of pectoralis major, middle and inferior aspects of trapezius, the rhomboids, serratus anterior, rectus abdominis, gluteals, the peroneal muscles, vasti, and the extensors of the arms.

Muscle groups such as the scaleni are equivocal. Although commonly listed as phasic muscles, they seem to be both postural and phasic (Lin 1994), their status being modified by the type(s) of stress to which they are exposed (for example, people suffering from asthma).

From an osteopathic perspective, thoracic dysfunction will usually be accompanied by evidence of areas of undue tightness and looseness in the soft tissues and joints relating to respiration. Rehabilitation of respiratory function would therefore take account of these imbalances and attempts would be made to restore relative symmetrical tone and freedom of movement. Strategies will be outlined in Chapter 6 for the assessment and treatment of shortness in postural muscles.

- Inflammation, or at least chronic irritation, may evolve.
- Neurological reporting stations in the distressed tissues bombard the central nervous system (CNS) with information regarding their status, resulting in neural sensitization and the evolution of facilitation – a tendency to hyperreactivity.

- Macrophages are activated, as is increased vascularity and fibroblastic activity.
- Connective tissue production increases with cross linkage leading to shortened fascia.
- Chronic muscular stress (a combination of the load involved and the number of repetitions, or the degree of sustained influence) results in the gradual development of hysteresis (the

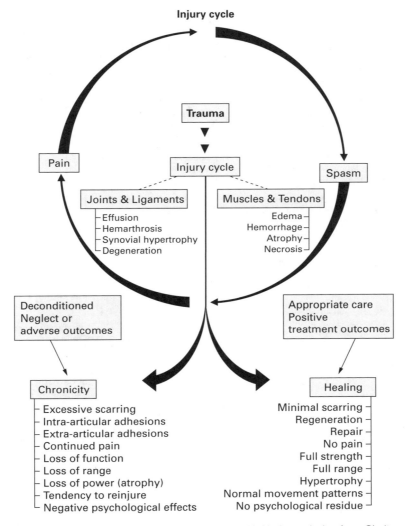

Injury cycle

Figure 4.2 Schematic representation of the injury cycle. (Reproduced with kind permission from Chaitow and DeLany 2000.)

process of energy loss due to friction when tissues are loaded and unloaded) and viscoplastic deformation, in which collagen fibers and proteoglycans are rearranged to produce an altered structural pattern.

- This results in tissues which are more easily fatigued than normal and more prone to damage if strained.
- Since all fascia/connective tissue is continuous throughout the body, any distortions or contractions developing in one region can create fascial deformations elsewhere, negatively influencing structures supported by, or attached to, the fascia (e.g. nerves, muscles, lymph structures, blood vessels).
- Hypertonicity in a muscle leads to reciprocal inhibition of its antagonist(s) and aberrant behaviour in its synergist(s) (Janda 1983).
- Chain reactions evolve in which some muscles (postural) shorten while others (phasic) weaken.
- Because of sustained increased muscle tension, ischemia occurs in tendinous structures, leading to the development of periosteal

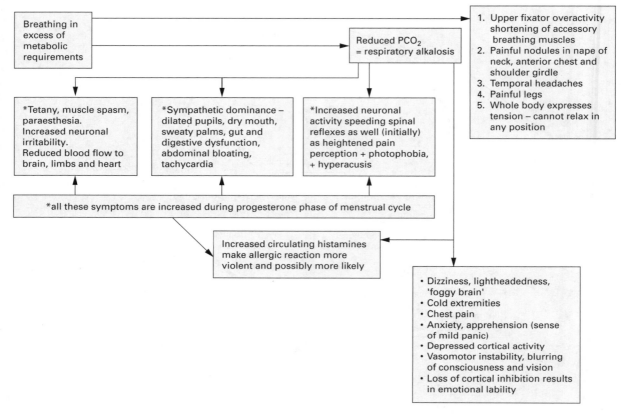

Figure 4.3 Negative health influences of a dysfunctional breathing pattern such as hyperventilation. (Reproduced with kind permission from Chaitow & DeLany 2000.)

pain, and also in localized areas of muscles, leading to myofascial trigger point evolution.

- Compensatory adaptations evolve leading to habitual, 'built-in' patterns of use emerging as the CNS learns to compensate for modifications in muscle strength, length, and functional behavior.
- Abnormal biomechanics result, involving malcoordination of movement (for example erector spinae tighten while rectus abdominis is inhibited).
- The normal firing sequence of muscles involved in particular movements alters, resulting in additional strain.
- Joint biomechanics are directly influenced by the accumulated influences of such soft tissue

changes, and can themselves become significant sources of referred and local pain, reinforcing soft tissue dysfunctional patterns (Schiable 1993).
- Deconditioning of the soft tissues becomes progressive as a result of the combination of simultaneous events involved in soft tissue pain, 'spasm' (guarding), joint stiffness, antagonist weakness, overactive synergists, etc.
- Progressive evolution occurs of localized areas of neural hyperreactivity (facilitated areas) paraspinally, or within muscles (myofascial trigger points).
- Within these trigger points increased neurological activity occurs (for which there is EMG evidence) which is capable of influencing

distant tissues adversely (Simons 1993, Hubbard 1993).

- Energy wastage due to unnecessarily sustained hypertonicity and excessively active musculature leads to generalized fatigue.
- More widespread functional changes develop – for example affecting respiratory function and body posture – with repercussions on the total body economy.
- In the presence of a constant neurological feedback of impulses to the CNS/brain from neural reporting stations indicating heightened arousal (a hypertonic muscle may represent the alarm response of the flight/fight alarm reaction) there will be increased levels of psychological arousal, and a reduction in the ability to relax, with consequent reinforcement of hypertonicity and excessive breathing.
- Functional patterns of use of a biologically unsustainable nature emerge.

At this stage restoration of normal function requires therapeutic input which addresses both the multiple changes which have occurred and reeducation of the individual in how to use the body less stressfully, how to breathe, carry, and use themselves in more sustainable ways. The chronic adaptive changes which develop lead to the increased likelihood of future acute exacerbations as the increasingly chronic, less supple and resilient biomechanical structures attempt to cope with additional stress factors resulting from the normal demands of modern living.

BIOMECHANICAL CHANGES IN RESPONSE TO UPPER-CHEST BREATHING

The general sequence of progressive dysfunction which evolves over time, as described above, can be translated into a sequence directly linked to respiratory dysfunction. Osteopath William Garland (1994) has described the somatic changes which follow from, or which are commonly associated with, a pattern of hyperventilation or chronic upper-chest breathing:

- A degree of visceral stasis and pelvic floor weakness will develop, as will an imbalance between increasingly weak abdominal muscles and increasingly tight erector spinae muscles. (See 'Lower crossed syndrome' discussion later in this chapter.)
- Fascial restriction will be noted from the central tendon via the pericardial fascia, all the way up to the basiocciput.
- The upper ribs will be elevated and there will be sensitive costal cartilage tension on palpation. (See discussion of assessment and treatment of elevated and depressed ribs in Ch. 6.)
- The thoracic spine will be disturbed by virtue of the lack of normal motion of the articulation with the ribs, and sympathetic outflow from this area may be affected (see Fig. 4.4 and notes on assessment and treatment of thoracic spine restrictions in Ch. 6)
- Accessory muscle hypertonia, notably affecting the scalenes, upper trapezius, and levator scapulae, will be palpable and observable.
- Travell & Simons (1992) discuss paradoxical breathing in their *Trigger Point Manual*: 'In paradoxical respiration the chest and abdominal functions oppose each other; the patient exhales with the diaphragm, while inhaling via the thoracic muscles. Consequently a normal effort produces inadequate tidal volume, and the accessory respiratory muscles of the upper chest, including the scalenes, overwork, to exchange sufficient air. The muscular overload results from the failure to coordinate the different parts of the respiratory apparatus.' In order to normalize the resulting dysfunction, a combination of rehabilitation exercise and bodywork is needed. (See notes on trigger points, later in this chapter, notes on assessment and treatment of shortened accessory breathing muscles in Ch. 6 and 'Upper crossed syndrome' discussion later in this chapter.)
- Fibrosis will develop in these muscles, as will myofascial trigger points. Travell & Simons (1992) confirmed that among the many factors which help to maintain and enhance trigger point activity is the low oxygenation of tissues; this is aggravated by muscular tension, stress, inactivity, and poor respiration. (See notes on myofascial trigger points later in this chapter with treatment discussion in Ch. 6.)

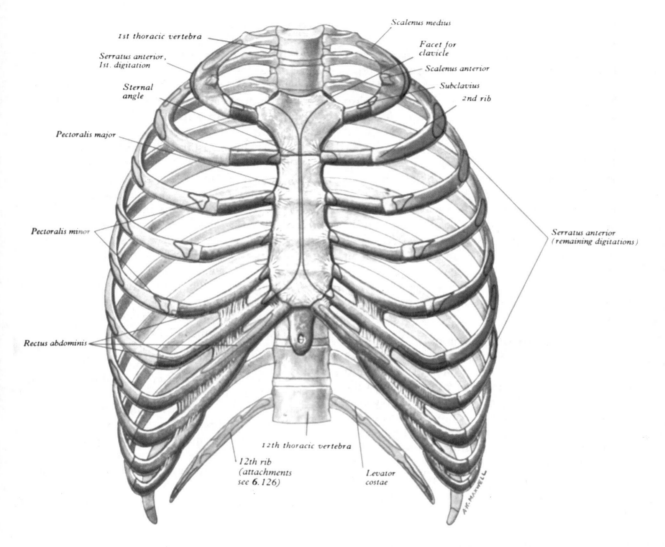

Figure 4.4 The skeleton of the thorax: anterior aspect. (Reproduced with kind permission from Gray 1995).

● The cervical spine will become progressively rigid with a fixed lordosis being a common feature in the lower cervical spine. (See notes on osteopathic treatment methods for restrictions in cervical area in Ch. 6.)

● A reduction in the mobility of the 2nd cervical segment and disturbance of vagal outflow from this region is likely. *Why?*

Although not noted in Garland's list of dysfunction (in which he says, 'psychology overwhelms physiology') we should bear in mind the other likely changes which Janda (1983) has listed in his upper crossed syndrome (see below). They include the potentially devastating effects on shoulder function of the altered position of the scapulae and glenoid fossae as this pattern evolves.

Also worth noting in relation to breathing function and dysfunction are important muscles not included in Garland's list, quadratus lumborum and iliopsoas, and transversus, all of which merge fibers with the diaphragm. Quadratus and psoas are postural muscles, with a propensity to shortening when stressed: the impact of such shortening, uni- or bilaterally, can be seen to have major implications for respiratory function, whether the primary feature of such a dysfunction lies in diaphragmatic or muscular distress. (Assessment and treatment methods for these muscles will be found in Ch. 6.)

Among possible stress factors which will result in shortening of postural muscles is disuse, and a situation in which upper chest breathing has replaced diaphragmatic breathing, would lead to reduced diaphragmatic excursion and consequent reduction in activity for those aspects of quadratus lumborum and psoas which are integral with it, and shortening (of any of these) would result.

Garland concludes his listing of somatic changes associated with hyperventilation as follows: 'Physically and physiologically [all of] this runs against a biologically sustainable pattern, and in a vicious cycle, abnormal function (use) alters normal structure, which disallows return to normal functions'. He also points to the likelihood of counseling (for associated anxiety or depression perhaps) and breathing retraining, being far more likely to be successfully initiated if the structural component(s) – as listed – are dealt with in such a way as to minimize the effects of the somatic changes described (Garland 1994).

Additional biomechanical features

Key areas of biomechanical dysfunction commonly occur at transition junctions, where stable and unstable structures meet, such as the thoracolumbar junction and the cervicothoracic junction. Barring direct trauma, dysfunctional patterns at these junctions are almost always compensatory, adapting to changes which have occurred above or below the region, whether pelvic or cervical/cranial (see Zink's work relating to compensation/decompensation, discussed later in this chapter).

It is important to reinforce the suggestion, based on many years of clinical experience in osteopathic medicine, that thoracic structure and function cannot usefully be considered without account being taken of cervical and lumbar status. The soft tissue links between the thoracic region and the cervical spine include extremely important structures such as levator scapula, upper trapezius, scalenes, and sternocleidomastoid, all of which have a propensity to shorten when stressed (Janda 1983), and all of which are major sites for myofascial trigger point evolution (Simons et al 1998).

Lymphatic considerations

- Drainage occurs via the left and right thoracic lymphatic ducts and the cisterna chyli in the abdomen.
- The integrity of the thoracic inlet is essential to this drainage, as is the efficiency of respiratory function since positive and negative pressure gradients between the thoracic and abdominal cavities is vital to normal movement of lymph (Kuchera 1997b).
- The role of the diaphragm is vital in maintaining the efficient alternation of pressures between the abdominal and thoracic cavities.
- A variety of osteopathic lymphatic pump techniques exist for enhancement of lymph flow and drainage (see Ch. 6).
- Travell & Simons (1992) have identified trigger points which impede lymphatic drainage and flow, particularly in muscles intimately involved in respiration (Travell & Simons 1992; Kuchera 1997b).
- The scalenes (in particular scalenus anterior or anticus) can entrap lymphatic (and other circulatory and neural) structures passing through the thoracic inlet.
- This entrapment can be aggravated by the 1st rib (and clavicular) restrictions, which can be caused by trigger points in the anterior and middle scalenes (Simons et al 1998).

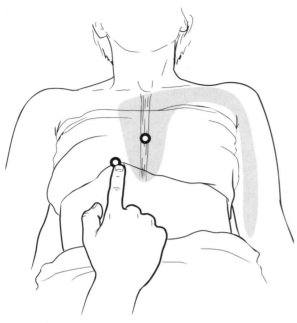

Figure 4.5 The sternalis has a frightening 'cardiac-type' pain pattern independent of movement while the cardiac arrhythmia trigger point (see finger tip) contributes to disturbances in normal heart rhythm without pain referral. (Reproduced with kind permission from Chaitow & DeLany 2000.)

- Scalene trigger points have been shown to reflexively suppress lymphatic duct peristaltic contractions in the affected extremity.
- Trigger points in the posterior axillary folds (involving subscapularis, teres major, latissimus dorsi) influence lymphatic drainage affecting the upper extremities and breasts.
- Trigger points in the intercostal space between 5th and 6th ribs anteriorly, and on the sternum itself can produce alterations in normal cardiac rhythm (Fig. 4.5) when active or compressed, with resultant extreme anxiety symptoms (Simons et al 1998).
- Trigger points in serratus anterior can create a sense of shortness of breath (Simons et al 1998) (Fig. 4.6).
- Similarly, trigger points in the anterior axillary fold (involving pectoralis minor) can be implicated in lymphatic dysfunction affecting the breasts (Fig. 4.7). (Trigger point dysfunction is discussed later in this chapter.)

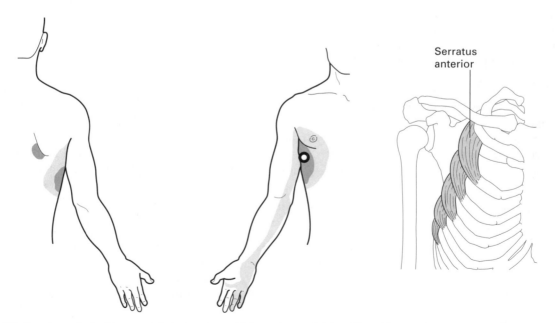

Serratus anterior

Figure 4.6 Serratus anterior trigger points include one which produces a 'short of breath' condition as well as an often familiar interscapular pain. (Reproduced with kind permission from Chaitow & DeLany 2000.)

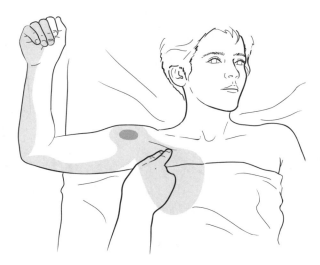

Figure 4.7 Trigger point target zones for pectoralis minor. (Reproduced with kind permission from Chaitow & DeLany 2000.)

POSTURAL PATTERNS WHICH IMPACT ON RESPIRATION

As a result of the stress patterns summarized earlier, in response to multiple biomechanical

(and other) stressors, patterns of dysfunction emerge, two of which are outlined below:

Janda's crossed syndromes
(Janda 1982, 1983)

Upper crossed syndrome (Fig. 4.8)

The upper crossed syndrome involves the following basic imbalance:

Pectoralis major and minor
Upper trapezius
Levator scapulae
Sternomastoid
} All tighten and shorten

while

Lower and middle trapezius
Serratus anterior and rhomboids
} All weaken

As these changes take place they alter the relative positions of the head, neck, and shoulders, as follows:

- The occiput and C1/2 hyperextend, with the head translating anteriorly. Weakness of the deep neck flexors develops along with increased tone in the suboccipital musculature

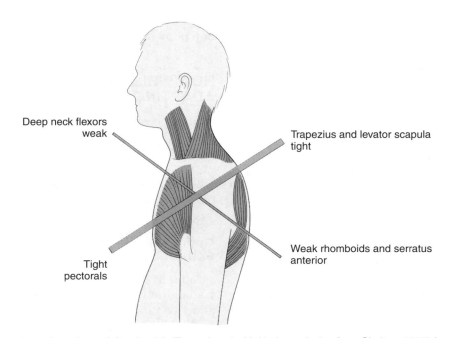

Deep neck flexors weak

Trapezius and levator scapula tight

Weak rhomboids and serratus anterior

Tight pectorals

Figure 4.8 Upper crossed syndrome (after Janda). (Reproduced with kind permission from Chaitow 1996b.)

- The lower cervicals down to the 4th thoracic vertebra will be stressed as a result
- Rotation and abduction of the scapulae occur as the increased tone in the upper fixators of the shoulder (upper trapezius, levator scapula, for example) results in shortening, inhibiting the lower fixators such as serratus anterior and the lower trapezii
- An altered direction of the axis of the glenoid fossa develops resulting in stabilization of the humerus by additional levator scapula and upper trapezius (plus supraspinatus) activity
- Breathing function is negatively influenced because of the crowded and slumped upper body positioning.

The result of these changes is greater cervical segment strain, the evolution of trigger points in the stressed structures, referred pain to the chest, shoulders, and arms. Pain mimicking angina may be noted, as well as a decline in respiratory efficiency.

The solution, according to Janda, is to identify the shortened structures and to release (stretch and relax) these, followed by reeducation towards more appropriate function.

Lower crossed syndrome (Fig. 4.9)

A similar pattern can be observed in the lower trunk, the lower crossed syndrome, in which:

Hip flexors	
Iliopsoas, rectus femoris	All tighten
TFL, short adductors	and shorten
Erector spinae group of the trunk	
while	
Abdominal and gluteal muscles	All weaken

Additional stress commonly appears in the sagittal plane in which:

Quadratus lumborum	Tightens
while	
Gluteus maximus and medius	Weaken

As a result, adaptive demands will focus on the lumbodorsal junction, the diaphragm, and the thorax.

When this 'lateral corset' becomes unstable the pelvis is held in increased elevation, accentuated

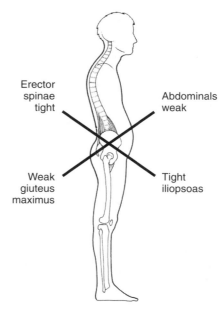

Figure 4.9 Lower crossed syndrome (after Janda). (Reproduced with kind permission from Chaitow 1996b.)

when walking, resulting in L5–S1 stress in the sagittal plane. One result is low back pain. The combined stresses described produce instability at the lumbodorsal junction, an unstable transition point at best.

HOW WELL IS THE PATIENT ADAPTING?

Before focusing on localized dysfunctional patterns which have the potential to add to the patient's stress burden and to have a direct impact on breathing function, a brief diversion will be made to consider questions of assessment of the patient's adaptation status.

Has adaptation reached the point of exhaustion?

As adaptive processes such as those described by Garland and others, above, progress, compensation becomes increasingly difficult, until ultimately, as described in Selye's stress syndrome model (1980), exhaustion is reached and structures break down.

Since (as discussed in Ch. 1) all interventions, including therapeutic interventions, add another layer of adaptive demands, clinical thinking might include questions such as:

- How can we best evaluate this patient's potential for further compensation/ decompensation, adaptation?
- How much more 'elasticity' remains in this patient's adaptive capacity?
- Just how compromised is the patient's adaptive capacity?
- What potential for recovery remains?

Biological rhythms as a guide

A chronically sick person can be described as being in a state of decompensation, where adaptive processes are exhausted and compensation patterns have become pathological. As the adaptive capacities of the body are strained ever further, evidence of a breakdown of compensatory functions manifests as ill health and symptoms.

There are a number of ways in which it is possible to gain a 'snapshot' indication as to how well or how badly an individual is coping with the current load of stressors – whether these are biochemical, biomechanical, or psychosocial, or a combination of these.

The more widely basic biological rhythms fluctuate throughout the day (whether this represents blood pressure, heart rate, blood sugar levels, or anything else which is periodically measurable), the less well homeostatic functions are operating. This is an obvious method for eliciting evidence of homeostatic efficiency (Ringsdorf & Cheraskin 1980).

Additional methods for assessing progress in treatment or for estimating the potential for a positive response – especially in bodywork terms – can be loosely divided into 'narrow' and 'broad' indicators:

Narrow evidence of functional change with treatment

Patients can be said to be capable of improvement if they are seen to improve by virtue of positive objective and subjective changes, over time,

in response to therapeutic intervention and/or rehabilitation protocols. If:

- Painful structures become less so
- Tight structures become looser
- Short structures lengthen
- Weak structures strengthen
- Posture and balance improve or normalize
- Muscle firing patterns approach normal
- Breathing function improves or normalizes
- Functional changes are reported – 'I can now walk 100 yards without too much difficulty' for example, or 'I can now get dressed on my own without help'.

These features are the ones which are commonly measured, sometimes numerically ('give a score out of 10') and sometimes purely verbally. Some are objective and some subjective. If changes of this sort are not realized as a therapeutic program progresses, a review of the strategies involved is called for.

Patient categorization

Therapeutic objectives need to be realistic. It may be possible broadly to categorize patients into those who will recover either with or without intervention (keeping in mind the natural tendency toward normality reflected in recognition of homeostatic function, as discussed in Ch. 1). These individuals may be classified under the heading *fixable*.

Many patients are capable of improvement, although perhaps not to a point of complete symptom-free state. These individuals may be classified as *maintainable*.

The previous group is commonly distinguishable from patients whose condition is such that the best hope is a degree of *containment* – a holding together of an individual in decline, offering some respite from the symptoms, perhaps, and an easing of the downward spiral.

Use of *fix, maintain, and contain* categorizations allows for realistic plans of action to evolve. It should go without saying that there is, in such a model, a need for an inbuilt willingness to modify the assessment, and therefore to alter strategies, should new evidence emerge.

How is one to know, however, at which point in the spectrum of dysfunction and adaptation the patient is currently situated, at the outset or during a course of treatment?

Wider evidence of functional change

The 'breathing wave' (Fig. 4.10)

Lewit (1999) describes the following useful protocol for evaluating the efficiency with which the spine responds to respiratory function:

The patient is prone with head in a face-hole. The practitioner is at waist level, observing from the side, eyes at the same level as the spine.

A full inhalation is performed and the spine is observed to see whether movement commences at the sacrum and finishes at the base of the neck (an ideal, if rare, observation). More often, restricted spinal segments 'rise' simultaneously, as a block, and movement of the spine occurs in two directions, caudally and cephalad, from the 'blocked' movement. Often very little movement occurs above the T7/8 area.

Observation of the wave is not diagnostic, but offers evidence of the current spinal response to breathing.

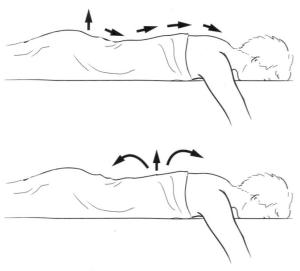

Figure 4.10 Functional (top) and dysfunctional breathing wave movement patterns. (Reproduced with kind permission from Chaitow & DeLany 2000.)

This 'wave' is monitored from treatment session to treatment session, to see whether it slowly normalizes – becoming longer and starting lower both suggest improvement in breathing function and greater mobility of the thoracic cage and spine.

If the breathing wave is other than a movement from the sacrum to the T1 area, a degree of spinal restriction exists, as evidenced by 'flat' segments which may be observed during seated or standing flexion.

Progress is indicated by approximation towards this ideal degree of spinal movement during the programme of treatment and/or rehabilitation.

The wave provides a 'snapshot' of increased, or decreased, or static, functional efficiency of the spinal and thoracic structures in response to a normal function, i.e. breathing.

Zink's postural (fascial) patterns
(Zink & Lawson 1979) (Fig. 4.11)

Relative looseness and tightness, as demonstrated by tissue 'preferences' in different areas, identities adaptation patterns in clinically useful ways:

- *Ideal*: there is minimal adaptive load being transferred to other regions.
- *Well compensated patterns*: there is evidence that compensation patterns alternate in direction from area to area (e.g. atlanto-occipital-cervico-thoracic-thoracolumbar-lumbosacral).
- *Poorly* or uncompensated patterns: there is evidence that compensation patterns do not alternate. This is commonly the result of trauma or of exhustion of biomechanical adaptive capacity. Therapeutic objectives which encourage better compensation are required.

Zink was able to correlate these dysfunctional adaptation patterns with general states of morbidity by evaluating the biomechanical status of over 1000 hospitalized patients. Zink's protocol is described more fully in Chapter 6 (see Box 6.3).

These methods can provide the clinician with means whereby complex situations can be evaluated from the perspective of how well (or how

Well compensated   Poorly compensated
✔   ✘

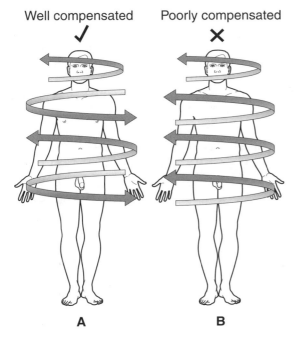

A   **B**

Figure 4.11 Zink's postural (fascial) patterns. Tissue 'preferences' in different areas identify adaptation patterns in clinically useful ways: *ideal* = minimal adaptive load transferred to other regions; *compensated* **A** = patterns alternate in direction from area to area; atlanto-occipital, cervicothoracic, thoracolumbar, lumbosacral; *uncompensated* **B** = patterns which do not alternate. Therapeutic objectives which encourage better compensation are optimal. (Adapted from Zink & Lawson 1979).

poorly) a person is coping (or how well or how poorly a person's spine is coping), and how much/how little the individual or the region being evaluated can handle in terms of additional stress in the form of treatment.

As stated previously, all therapeutic intervention can be seen as yet another form of stress, demanding further adaptive response. There is, therefore, a significant advantage in having tools which can predict possible responses to therapeutic interventions.

TRIGGER POINTS AND RESPIRATION

A trigger point is a localized area of neural sensitization/hyperreactivity which is capable of producing widespread symptoms, mainly of a painful nature, in 'target' tissues some distance from its location. Trigger points have been identified as factors in dysfunctional breathing patterns (Simons et al 1998).

Doctors Simons and Travell (Simons et al 1998) confirm that among the many factors which help to maintain and enhance trigger point activity is the low oxygenation of tissues, aggravated by muscular tension, stress, inactivity, and poor respiration. They also discuss the subject of paradoxical breathing, as outlined earlier in this chapter (Travell & Simons 1983, vol. 1, pp. 364–365):

In paradoxical respiration the chest and abdominal functions oppose each other: the patient exhales with the diaphragm while inhaling via the thoracic muscles, and vice versa [i.e. on inhalation the thorax expands as the abdomen contracts, and on exhalation the abdomen expands]. Consequently a normal effort produces inadequate tidal volume, and the accessory respiratory muscles of the upper chest, including the scalenes, overwork, to exchange sufficient air. The muscular overload results from the failure to coordinate the different parts of the respiratory apparatus.

In order to normalize breathing a combination of retraining exercises and manual therapy is needed.

Trigger points: the Travell and Simons model

Simons, Travell, and Simons (1998) present evidence which suggests that, what they term 'central' trigger points (those forming in the belly of the muscle) develop almost directly in the centre of the muscle's fibers, where the motor endplate innervates it, at the neuromuscular junction. They suggest the following:

- Dysfunctional endplate activity occurs, commonly associated with a strain, causing acetylcholine (ACh) to be excessively released at the synapse, along with stored calcium.
- The presence of high calcium levels apparently keeps the calcium-charged gates open, and ACh continues to be released.
- The resulting ischemia in the area creates an oxygen/nutrient deficit which in turn leads to a local energy crisis.
- Without available adenosine triphosphate (ATP), the local tissue is unable to remove the

calcium ions which are 'keeping the gates open' for ACh to keep escaping.

- Removing the superfluous calcium requires more energy than sustaining a contracture, so the contracture remains.
- The resulting muscle fiber contracture (involuntary, without motor potentials) needs to be distinguished from a contraction (voluntary with motor potentials) and spasm (involuntary with motor potentials).
- The contracture is sustained by the chemistry at the innervation site, not by action potentials from the cord.
- As the endplate keeps producing ACh flow, the actin/myosin filaments attenuate to a fully shortened position (a weakened state) in the immediate area around the motor endplate (at the centre of the fiber).
- As the sarcomeres shorten they begin to bunch and a contracture knot forms. This knot is the 'nodule' which is the palpable characteristic of a trigger point.
- As this process occurs the remainder of the sarcomeres (those not bunching) of that fiber are stretched, creating the taut band which is usually palpable.

This model currently represents the most widely held understanding as to the etiology of trigger points.

Ischemia and muscle pain (Lewis 1931, Lewis 1942, Rodbard 1975)

When the blood supply to a muscle is inhibited, pain is not usually noted unless or until that muscle is asked to contract. In such a case pain is likely to be noted within 60 seconds (as in intermittent claudication). The precise mechanisms are open to debate, but are thought to involve one or more of a number of processes including lactate accumulation and potassium ion build-up.

Pain receptors are sensitized when under ischemic conditions, it is thought due to bradykinin influence. This is confirmed by the use of drugs which inhibit bradykinin release, allowing an active ischemic muscle to remain relatively painless for longer periods (Digiesi 1975). Trigger point activity itself may induce relative ischemia in target tissues and this suggests that any appropriate manual treatment, rehabilitation, or exercise program which encourages normal circulatory function and enhanced oxygenation is likely to modulate these negative effects and reduce trigger point activity.

Facilitation: segmental and local (trigger points) (Korr 1976, Patterson 1976, Ward 1997)

Facilitation is the osteopathic term for the process involved when neural sensitization occurs. There are at least two forms of facilitation, spinal (or segmental) and local (e.g. trigger point). Visceral dysfunction results in sensitization and ultimately facilitation of the paraspinal neural structures at the level of the nerve supply to that organ. Box 4.2 explains this further.

In cardiac disease, for example, the muscles alongside the spine at the upper thoracic level, from which the heart derives its innervation, become hypertonic. The segment becomes facilitated, with the nerves of the area, including those

---

Box 4.2 Facilitation definition

When a pool of neurons (e.g. premotor neurons, motoneurons or preganglionic sympathetic neurons, in one or more segments of the spinal cord) is in a state of partial or subthreshold excitation, less afferent stimulation a required to trigger the discharge of impulses. It is thought that facilitation may result from a sustained increase in afferent input, aberrant patterns of afferent input, or to changes within the affected neurons or their chemical environment. Normal central nervous system activity seems capable of sustaining an area of facilitation once it is established (Ward 1997).

Patterson (1976) explains segmental (spinal) facilitation as follows:

The concept of the facilitated segment states that because of abnormal afferent or sensory inputs to a particular area of the spinal cord, that area is kept in a state of constant increased excitation. This facilitation allows normally ineffectual or subliminal stimuli to become effective in producing efferent output from the facilitated segment, causing both skeletal and visceral organs innervated by the affected segment to be maintained in a state of overactivity. It is probable that the 'osteopathic lesion', or somatic dysfunction with which a facilitated segment is associated, is the direct result of the abnormal segmental activity, as well as being partially responsible for the facilitation.

supplying the heart, becoming hyperirritable. EMG readings of the upper thoracic paraspinal muscles show greater activity in them than in surrounding tissues, and in addition they become hypertonic and more painful to pressure.

Once facilitation occurs, all additional stress impacting the individual, of any sort – whether emotional, physical, chemical, climatic, mechanical – leads to an increase in neural activity in the facilitated segments and not in the rest of the (unfacilitated) spinal structures. Korr has called such an area a 'neurological lens', since it concentrates neural activity in the facilitated area, so creating more activity and also a local increase in muscle tone at that level of the spine. Similar segmental (spinal) facilitation occurs in response to any visceral disease affecting the segments of the spine from which the neural supply to that particular organ derive.

Other causes of segmental (spinal) facilitation include biomechanical stress to that region of the spine, injury, overactivity, repetitive patterns of use, poor posture or structural imbalance (short leg for example).

Korr (1978) tells us that when patients who had had facilitated segments identified 'were exposed to physical, environmental and psychological stimuli similar to those encountered in daily life the sympathetic responses in those segments was exaggerated and prolonged. The disturbed segments behaved as though they were continually in or bordering on a state of "physiologic alarm".'

How to recognize a facilitated area

A number of observable and palpable signs indicate an area of segmental (spinal) facilitation (see also notes on viscerosomatic reflexes in Ch. 6).

Beal (1983) tells us that such an area will usually involve two or more segments, unless traumatically induced, in which case single segments are possible. The paraspinal tissues will palpate as rigid or 'board-like'. With the patient supine and the palpating hands under the patient's paraspinal area to be tested (standing at the head of the table, for example, and reaching under the shoulders for the upper thoracic area),

any ceilingward 'springing' attempt on these tissues will result in a distinct lack of elasticity, unlike more normal tissues above or below the facilitated area (Beal 1983).

Palpable or observable features

Grieve, Gunn and Milbrandt, and Korr have all helped to define the palpable and visual signs which accompany facilitated dysfunction (Baldry 1993, Grieve 1986, Gunn & Milbrandt 1978, Korr 1948):

- A 'goose flesh' appearance is observable in facilitated areas when the skin is exposed to cool air – as a result of a facilitated pilomotor response
- A palpable sense of 'drag' is noticeable as a light touch contact is made across such areas, due to increased sweat production due to the sudomotor reflexes (see description of 'drag' palpation method in Ch. 6 and Box 6.3)
- There is likely to be cutaneous hyperesthesia in the related dermatome, as the sensitivity is increased – for example to a pin prick – due to facilitation
- An 'orange peel' appearance is noticeable in the subcutaneous tissues when the skin is rolled over the affected segment, due to subcutaneous trophedema
- There is commonly localized spasm of the muscles in a facilitated area, which is palpable segmentally as well as peripherally in the related myotome. This is likely to be accompanied by an enhanced myotatic reflex due to the process of facilitation.

Local (trigger point) facilitation in muscles

A process of local facilitation occurs when particularly vulnerable sites of muscle (origins and insertions for example) are overused, abused, misused, disused. Localized areas of hypertonicity develop, sometimes accompanied by edema, sometimes with a stringy feel, but always with a sensitivity to pressure. Many of these palpably painful, tender, sensitive, localized, facilitated points are myofascial trigger points, which are not only painful themselves when pressed, but when active will also transmit or activate pain (and other) sensations some distance away from themselves, in 'target' tissues. Melzack & Wall (1988) have stated that there are few if any chronic pain problems which do not have trigger point activity as a major part of the picture, perhaps not always as a prime cause but almost always as a maintaining feature.

In the same manner as the facilitated areas alongside the spine, trigger points will become more active when stress, *of whatever type*, makes adaptive demands on the body as a whole, not just on the area in which they are found.

When not actively directing *recognizable* pain to a distant area, trigger points (locally tender or painful to applied pressure) are said to be 'latent'. The same signs as described for spinal, segmental, facilitation can be observed and palpated in these localized areas.

Selective motor unit involvement

The effect of psychogenic influences on muscles may be more complex than a simplistic 'whole' muscle or region involvement. Researchers at the National Institute of Occupational Health in Oslo, Norway, have demonstrated that a small number of motor units in particular muscles may display almost constant, or repeated, activity when influenced psychogenically (a normal individual performing a reaction time task) (Waersted et al 1993). Using the trapezius muscle as the focus of attention the researchers were able to demonstrate low amplitude levels of activity (using surface EMG) when individuals were inactive. They explain this phenomenon as follows:

In spite of low total activity level of the muscle, a small pool of low-threshold motor units may be under considerable load for prolonged periods of time. Such a recruitment pattern would be in agreement with the 'size principle' first proposed by Henneman (1957), saying that motor units are recruited according to their size. Motor units with Type I [postural] fibers are predominant among the small, low threshold, units. If tension provoking factors are frequently present and the subject, as a result, repeatedly recruits the same motor units, the hypothesized overload may follow, possibly resulting in a metabolic crisis and the appearance of Type I fibers with abnormally large diameters, or 'ragged-red' fibers, which are interpreted as a sign

of mitochondrial overload. (Edwards 1988, Larsson et al 1990)

The researchers report that similar observations were noted in a pilot study (Waersted et al 1992).

The implications of this information are profound, since they suggest that emotional stress can selectively involve postural fibers of muscles, which shorten over time when stressed (Janda 1983). The possible 'metabolic crisis' suggested by this research has strong parallels with the evolution of myofascial trigger points as described by Wolfe & Simons (1992).

Notes on trigger points

Primary activating factors for trigger points include:

- Persistent muscular contraction (emotional or physical cause)
- Trauma (local inflammatory reaction)
- Adverse environmental conditions (cold, heat, damp, draughts, etc.)
- Prolonged immobility
- Febrile illness
- Systemic biochemical imbalance (e.g. hormonal, nutritional)
- Factors such as age and general health status (including genetically acquired characteristics) will influence the degree of trigger point activity.

Secondary activating factors include (Baldry 1993):

- Compensating synergist and antagonist muscles to those housing primary triggers may develop triggers
- Satellite triggers evolve in referral zone (from primary triggers or visceral disease referral, e.g. myocardial infarct).

Underlying stressors

Travell & Simons state that the following stressors help to maintain and enhance trigger point activity (Travell & Simons 1983):

- Nutritional deficiency (especially vitamins C, B-complex, and iron)

- Hormonal imbalances (thyroid in particular)
- Infections
- Allergies and intolerances (wheat and dairy products in particular) (Ogle et al 1980, Gerrard 1966, Nsouli et al 1994, Hurst 1996)
- Low oxygenation of tissues (aggravated by tension, stress, inactivity, poor circulation and respiration).

Active and latent trigger point features

- Trigger points may be either active or latent
- Active trigger points refer a pattern that is recognizable to the person, whether pain, tingling, numbness, itching or other sensation
- Latent trigger points are locally painful and only refer on pressure, or they refer a pattern which is not familiar, or perhaps one the patient reports he used to have in the past, but has not experienced recently
- Latent trigger points may become active trigger points if sufficiently stressed
- Activation may occur when the tissue is overused, strained by overload, chilled, stretched (particularly abruptly), shortened, traumatized (as in a motor vehicle accident or a fall or blow), or when other perpetuating factors (such as poor nutrition or shallow breathing) provide less than optimal conditions for tissue health
- Active trigger points may become latent trigger points with their referral patterns subsiding for brief or prolonged periods of time
- They may then become reactivated with their referral patterns returning for no apparent reason, a condition which confuses the practitioner as well as the patient (see notes on facilitation).

Autonomic effects as result of trigger point activity (Travell & Simons 1982/1993)

- Vasoconstriction (blanching)
- Coldness
- Sweating
- Pilomotor response
- Ptosis
- Hypersecretion.

Clinical symptoms other than pain as result of trigger point activity (Kuchera 1997b)

- Diarrhea, dysmenorrhea
- Diminished gastric motility
- Vasoconstriction and headache
- Dermatographia
- Proprioceptive disturbance, dizziness
- Excessive maxillary sinus secretion
- Localized sweating
- Cardiac arrhythmias (especially pectoralis major triggers)
- 'Goose flesh'
- Ptosis, excessive lacrimation, conjunctival reddening.

Trigger point deactivation

- Acupuncture, manual methods, and removal of the stressor factors maintaining them are all options for trigger point deactivation
- If hypertonia is a major etiological feature in the evolution of trigger points, then those muscles which have the greatest propensity towards hypertonia, the postural, Type I muscles, should receive closest attention (Liebenson 1996, Jacob & Falls 1997)
- Trigger points may be used as monitors of improved oxygenation (including via breathing retraining), rather than being directly treated to deactivate them:
  - as oxygenation improves trigger points become less reactive and painful
  - normalized or enhanced breathing function represents a reduction in overall stress, reinforcing the concepts associated with neural facilitation (see above), that as stress of whatever kind reduces, trigger points react less acutely
  - direct deactivation tactics are therefore not the only way to treat trigger points; the removal of stress factors maintaining them offers an alternative approach
  - trigger points can be perceived to be acting as alarm signals, virtually quantifying the current levels of adaptive demand being imposed on the individual (Bradley 1999).

Trigger point deactivation variations are discussed in detail in Chapter 6.

POSTURAL AND EMOTIONAL INFLUENCES ON MUSCULOSKELETAL DYSFUNCTION
(Fig. 4.6)

An insightful Charlie Brown cartoon has him standing in a pronounced stooping posture, while he philosophizes to Lucy that it is only possible to get the most out of being depressed if you stand in this way. Standing up straight, he asserts, removes all sense of being depressed.

Australian (Sydney) based British osteopath Philip Latey has found a useful metaphor to describe observable and palpable patterns of distortion which coincide with particular clinical problems (Latey 1996). He uses the analogy of clenched fists because, he says, the unclenching of a fist correlates with physiological relaxation, while the clenched fist indicates fixity, rigidity, over-contracted muscles, emotional turmoil, withdrawal from communication, and so on: 'The "lower fist" is centred entirely on pelvic function. When I describe the "upper fist" I will include the head, neck, shoulders and arms with the upper chest throat and jaw. The "middle fist" will be focused mainly on the lower chest and upper abdomen.'

A restrained expression of emotion itself results in suppression of activity and, ultimately, chronic contraction of the muscles which would be used were these emotions to be expressed, including rage, fear, anger, joy, frustration, sorrow.

Latey's descriptions of the emotional background to physical 'guarding' offers a meaningful vehicle with which to accompany more mechanistic interpretations as to what may be happening in any given dysfunctional biomechanical pattern.

Emotional patterns: postural interpretations

One of Latey's concepts involves a mechanism which leads to muscular contraction as a means of disguising a sensory barrage resulting from an emotional state. He describes:

- A sensation which might arise from the pit of the stomach being hidden by contraction of the muscles attached to the lower ribs, upper abdomen, and the junction between the chest and lower spine
- Genital and anal sensations which might be drowned out by contraction of hip, leg, and low back musculature
- Throat sensations which might be concealed with contraction of the shoulder girdle, neck, arms, and hands.

Latey's 'middle fist' (Latey 1996)

When considering the 'middle fist' Latey concentrates his attention on respiratory and diaphragm function and the many emotional inputs which affect this region. He challenges the conception that breathing is produced by contraction of the diaphragm and the muscles which raise the rib cage, with exhalation being but a relaxation of these muscles. He states: 'The even flow of easy breathing should be produced by dynamic interaction of two sets of muscles.' The active exhalation phase of breathing is the result, he suggests, of transversus thoracis, which lies inside the front of the chest, attaching to the back of the sternum and fanning out inside the rib cage, and then continuing to the lower ribs where they separate. This is the inverted 'V' below the chest (it is known as transversus abdominis in this region). This, he says, has direct intrinsic abilities to generate all manner of uniquely powerful sensations, with even light contact sometimes producing reflex contractions of the whole body, or of the abdomen or chest, feelings of nausea and choking, all types of anxiety, fear, anger, laughter, sadness, weeping, and so on. He discounts the idea that its sensitivity its related to the 'solar plexus,' maintaining that its closeness to the internal thoracic artery is probably more significant, since when it is contracted it can exert direct pressure on it. Latey believes that physiological breathing has as its central event a rhythmical relaxation and contraction of this muscle. Rigidity is often seen in the patient with 'middle fist' problems, where 'control' dampens the emotions which relate to it.

The other main exhalation muscle is serratus posterior inferior which runs from the upper lumbar spine, fanning upwards and outwards over the lower ribs which it grasps from behind, pulling them down and inward on exhalation. These two muscles mirror each other, working together. Latey states that it is common to find a static overcontracture of this muscle, with the underlying back muscles in a state of fibrous shortening and degeneration, reflecting the fixity of the transversus, and the extent of the emotional blockage. There is a typical associated posture, with the shoulder girdle raised and expanded, as if any letting go would precipitate a crisis. Compensatory changes usually include very taut deep neck and shoulder muscles (see earlier discussion of Janda's upper crossed syndrome description: Janda 1983).

In treating such a problem, Latey starts by encouraging function of the 'middle fist' itself, then after extending into the neck and shoulder muscles, encouraging them to relax and drop, he goes back to this 'middle fist'. Dramatic expressions of alarm, unease, and panic may be seen. Patients might report sensations of being smothered, drowned, choked, engulfed, crushed.

Latey's 'upper fist'

The 'upper fist' involves muscles which extend from the thorax to the back of the head, where the skull and spine join, extending sideways to include the muscles of the shoulder girdle. These muscles therefore set the relative positions of the head, neck, jaw, shoulders, and upper chest, and to a large extent the rest of the body follows this lead. It was F. M. Alexander, another Australian, who showed that the head–neck relationship is the primary postural control mechanism (Alexander 1984). This region, says Latey, is 'the centre, *par excellence*, of anxieties, tensions and other amorphous expressions of unease.'

In chronic states of disturbed 'upper fist' function, Latey asserts, the main physical impression is one of restrained, over-controlled, damped-down expression. The feeling of the muscles is that they are controlling an 'explosion of affect.' Those experiences which are not allowed free play on the face are expressed in the muscles of the skull and the base of the skull. This is, he believes, of central importance in problems of headache, especially migraine. Says Latey: 'I have never seen a migraine sufferer who has not lost complete ranges of facial expression, at least temporarily.'

Effects of 'upper fist' patterns

Latey states:

The medical significance of 'upper fist' contracture is mainly circulatory. Just as 'lower fist' contraction contributes to circulatory stasis in the legs, pelvis, perineum and lower abdomen; so may 'upper fist' contracture have an even more profound effect. The blood supply to the head, face, special sense, the mucosa of the nose, mouth, upper respiratory tract, the heart itself and the main blood vessels are controlled by the sympathetic nervous system and its main 'junction boxes' (ganglia) lie just to the front of the vertebrae at the base of the neck.

Thus headaches, eye pain, ear problems, nose and throat, as well as many cardiovascular troubles may contain strong mechanical elements relating to 'upper fist' muscle contractions. Latey reminds us that it is not uncommon for cardiovascular problems to manifest at the same time as chronic muscular shoulder pain (avascular necrosis of the rotator cuff tendons) and that the longus colli muscles are often centrally involved in such states.

A biomechanical–biochemical–psychological example

Consider someone who habitually breathes in an upper-chest mode (for postural, habitual, emotional, or other reasons), the stress of which will place adaptive demands on the accessory breathing muscles, with consequent hypertonicity, shortness, reciprocal inhibition, malcoordination, stiffness and pain, probably involving trigger point activity as well as joint dysfunction.

The biomechanical changes which evolve from this functional chaos will modify the structure of the breathing apparatus to the extent that

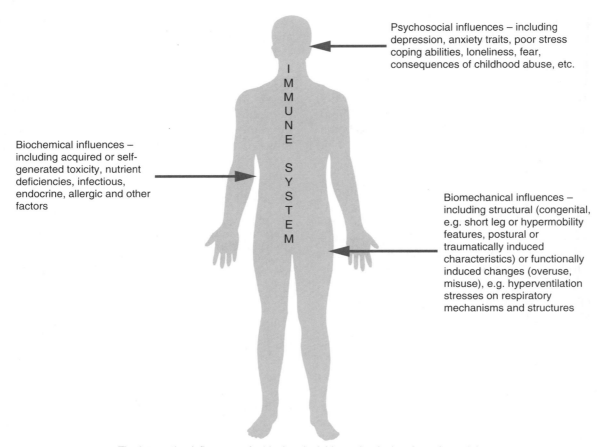

Psychosocial influences – including depression, anxiety traits, poor stress coping abilities, loneliness, fear, consequences of childhood abuse, etc.

Biochemical influences – including acquired or self-generated toxicity, nutrient deficiencies, infectious, endocrine, allergic and other factors

I M M U N E   S Y S T E M

Biomechanical influences – including structural (congenital, e.g. short leg or hypermobility features, postural or traumatically induced characteristics) or functionally induced changes (overuse, misuse), e.g. hyperventilation stresses on respiratory mechanisms and structures

The interacting influences of a biochemical, biomechanical and psychosocial nature do not produce single changes. For example:
- a negative emotional state (e.g. depression) produces specific biochemical changes, impairs immune function and leads to altered muscle tone.
- hyperventilation modifies blood acidity, alters neural reporting (initially hyper and then hypo), creates feelings of anxiety/apprehension and directly impacts on the structural components of the thoracic and cervical region – muscles and joints.
- altered chemistry affects mood; altered mood changes blood chemistry; altered structure (posture for example) modifies function and therefore impacts on chemistry (e.g. liver function) and potentially on mood.

Within these categories – biochemical, biomechanical and psychosocial – are to be found most major influences on health.

Figure 4.12 Biochemical, biomechanical, and psychosocial influences on health. (Reproduced with kind permission from Chaitow & DeLany 2000.)

normal breathing function becomes difficult or impossible.

In addition, the individual will probably display evidence of anxiety as a direct result of respiratory alkalosis, deriving from CO_2 imbalance (see Ch. 3) caused by the breathing pattern. Or the breathing pattern may have been created because of a predisposing anxiety (Timmons 1994). This pattern of breathing, and the anxiety it encourages, feed back into a cycle of aggravated upper-chest breathing, reinforcing the pattern, so that what may have started as an emotional state evolves into a chronic biochemical imbalance and a state of relative biomechanical rigidity.

It is easy to see how interventions which focus on the anxiety would be helpful, as would focus on the biomechanical/structural imbalances:

- Interventions which reduce anxiety will help all associated symptoms. Such interventions might also involve biochemical modification (medication, etc.), stress coping approaches, or psychotherapy.
- Interventions which improve breathing function, probably involving easing of soft tissue distress (including deactivation of trigger points) and/or joint restrictions should also help to reduce the symptoms by allowing, with retraining, a more normal breathing pattern to be practiced.

The most appropriate approach will be the one which most closely deals with causes rather than effects, and which allows for long-term changes which will reduce the likelihood of recurrence. Biochemistry, biomechanics, and the mind are seen, in this example, to be inextricably bonded with each other.

CAUTIONS AND QUESTIONS

⚠ **CAUTION:** There is, justifiably, intense debate regarding the question of the induction by bodywork therapists of emotional release. The following aspects need to be considered:

- If the most appropriate response an individual can make to the turmoil of his life is to 'lock away' emotions in his musculoskeletal system, we should ask ourselves whether it is advisable to unlock the emotions the tensions and contractions hold.
- If there exists no current ability mentally to process the pain that these somatic areas hold, are they not best left where they are until counseling or psychotherapy or self-awareness lead to the individual's ability to reflect, handle, deal with, and eventually work through the issues and memories?
- What is the advantage of triggering a release of emotions, manifested by crying, laughing, vomiting, or whatever – as described by Latey and others – if neither the individual nor the practitioner can then take the process further?

It is suggested that each patient and each therapist/practitioner should reflect on the issues listed above before removing (however gently and however temporarily) the defensive armouring that life may have obliged vulnerable individuals (i.e. most of us) to erect and maintain. At the very least we should all learn skills which allow the safe handling of emotional releases, which may occur with or without deliberate effort on our part to induce them. If the handling of emotional features is outside the scope of practice of the practitioner/therapist, appropriate referral is a better option.

REFERENCES

Alexander F 1984 The use of the self. Centerline Press, Dourney, California [first published 1932]

Baldry P 1993 Acupuncture, trigger points and musculoskeletal pain. Churchill Livingstone, Edinburgh

Barlow W 1959 Anxiety and muscle tension pain. British Journal of Clinical Practice 13(5): 339

Basmajian J 1974 Muscles alive. Williams and Wilkins, Baltimore

Beal M 1983 Palpatory testing of somatic dysfunction in patients with cardiovascular disease. Journal of the American Osteopathic Association (July)

Bergmark A 1989 Stability of the lumbar spine. Acta Orthopaedica Scandinavica 230(Suppl): 20–24

Bogduk N, Twomey L 1991 Clinical anatomy of the lumbar spine, 2nd edn. Churchill Livingstone, Edinburgh

Bradley D 1991 In: Gilbert C (ed) Breathing retraining advice from three therapists. Journal of Bodywork & Movement Therapies 3: 159–167

Chaitow L 1996a Modern neuromuscular techniques. Churchill Livingstone, Edinburgh

Chaitow L 1996b Muscle energy techniques. Churchill Livingstone, Edinburgh

Chaitow L, DeLany J 2000 Clinical application of neuromuscular techniques. Vol 1: the upper body. Churchill Livingstone, Edinburgh

Digiesi V 1975 Effect of proteinase inhibitor on intermittent claudication. Pain 1: 385–389

Dommerholt J 2000 Posture. In: Tubiana R, Camadio P (eds) Medical problems of the instrumentalist musician. Martin Dunitz, London

Dvorak J, Dvorak V 1984 Manual medicine: diagnostics. Georg Thiem Verlag, Thieme-Stratton, Stuttgart

Edwards R 1988 Hypotheses of peripheral and central mechanisms underlying occupational muscle pain and injury. European Journal of Applied Physiology 57: 275–281

Gagey P-M, Gentaz R 1996 Postural disorders of the body. In: Liebenson C (ed) Rehabilitation of the spine. Williams and Wilkins, Baltimore

Garland W 1994 'Somatic changes in hyperventilating subject'. Presentation to the International Society for Advancement of Respiratory Psychophysiology Congress, France, 1994

Gerrard J W 1966 Familial recurrent rhinorrhea and bronchitis due to cow's milk. Journal of the American Medical Association 198: 605–607

Gray's Anatomy 1995 37th edn, ed. P. Williams. Churchill Livingstone, Edinburgh

Grieve G (ed) 1986 Modern manual therapy of the vertebral column. Churchill Livingstone, Edinburgh

Gunn C, Milbrandt W 1978 Early and subtle signs in low back sprain. Spine 3: 267–281

Henneman E 1957 Relation between size of neurons and their susceptibility to discharge. Science 126: 1345–1347

Hubbard D 1993 Myofascial trigger points show spontaneous EMG activity. Spine 18: 1803

Hurst D S 1996 Association of otitis media with effusion and allergy as demonstrated by intradermal skin testing and eosinophil protein levels in both middle ear effusions and mucosal biopsies. Laryngoscope 106: 1128–1137

Jacob A, Falls W 1997 Anatomy. In: Ward R (ed) Foundations for osteopathic medicine. Williams and Wilkins, Baltimore

Janda V 1982 Introduction to functional pathology of the motor system. Proceedings of the Seventh Commonwealth and International Conference on Sport. Physiotherapy in Sport 3: 39

Janda V 1983 Muscle function testing. Butterworths, London

Janda V 1986 Extracranial causes of facial pain. Journal of Prosthetic Dentistry 56(4): 484–487

Janda V 1988 Muscle weakness and inhibition (pseudoparesis in back pain syndromes). In: Grieve G (ed) Modern manual therapy of the vertebral column. Churchill Livingstone, Edinburgh

Jones L 1981 Strain and counterstrain. Academy of Applied Oesteopathy. Colorado Springs

Jull G, Janda V 1987 Muscles and motor control in low back pain. In: Twomey L, Taylor J (eds) Physical therapy for the low back. Clinics in physical therapy. Churchill Livingstone, New York

Kaltenborn F 1985 Mobilization of the extremity joints. Olaf Norlis Bokhandel, Universitetgaten 24, N-0162 Oslo 1, Norway

Korr I 1948 The emerging concept of the osteopathic lesion. Journal of the American Osteopathic Association 48: 127–138

Korr I 1976 Spinal cord as organiser of disease process. Academy of Applied Osteopathy. Yearbook, Newark, Ohio

Korr I 1978 Neurologic mechanisms in manipulative therapy. Plenum Press, New York

Kuchera M 1997a Treatment of gravitational strain pathophysiology. In: Vleeming A et al (eds) Movement, stability and low back pain. Churchill Livingstone, Edinburgh

Kuchera M 1997b Travell and Simons myofascial trigger points. In: Ward R (ed) Foundations for osteopathic medicine. Williams and Wilkins, Baltimore

Larsson S-E et al 1998 Chronic trapezius myalgia: morphology and blood flow studied in 17 patients. Acta Orthopedica Scandinavica 61: 394–398

Latey P 1996 Feelings, muscles and movement. Journal of Bodywork and Movement Therapies 1(1): 44–52

Lederman E 1997 Fundamentals of manual therapy: physiology, neurology and psychology. Churchill Livingstone, Edinburgh

Lewis T 1931 Observations upon muscular pain in intermittent claudication. Heart 15: 359–383

Lewis T 1942 Pain. Macmillan, London

Lewit K 1980 Relation of faulty respiration to posture. Journal of the American Osteopathic Association 79(8): 525–529

Lewit K 1999 Manipulative therapy in rehabilitation on the locomotor system, 3nd edn. Butterworths, London

Liebenson C 1996 Rehabilitation of the spine. Williams and Wilkins, Baltimore

Lin J-P 1994 Physiological maturation of muscles in chilhood. Lancet (June 4): 1386–1389

Melzack R, Wall P 1988 The challenge of pain. Penguin, London

Murphy D 2000 Conservative management of cervical spine syndromes. McGraw Hill, New York

Norris C 2000 The muscle debate. Journal of Bodywork and Movement Therapies 4(4): 232–235

Nsouli T M, Nsouli S M, Linde R E 1994 Role of food allergy in serous otitis media. Annals of Allergy 73: 215–219

Ogle K A, Bullock J D 1980 Children with allergic rhinitis and/or bronchial asthma treated with elimination diet: a five-year follow-up. Annals of Allergy 44: 273–278

Patterson M 1976 Model mechanism for spinal segmental facilitation. Academy of Applied Osteopathy Yearbook, Newark, Ohio

Richardson C, Jull G, Hodges P, Hides J 1999 Therapeutic exercise for spinal segmental stabilisation in low back pain. Churchill Livingstone, Edinburgh

Ringsdorf R, Cheraskin E 1980 Diet and disease. Keats, New Canaan, Connecticut

Rodbard S 1975 Pain associated with muscular activity. American Heart Journal 90: 84–92

Rosenthal E 1987 The Alexander technique and how it works. Medical Problems in the Performing Arts 2: 53–57

Schiable H 1993 Afferent and spinal mechanisms of joint pain. Pain 55: 5

Selye H 1980 The stress of life. McGraw Hill, New York

Simons D 1993 Referred phenomena of myofascial trigger points. In: Vecchiet L, Albe-Fessard D, Lindlom U. New trends in referred pain and hyperalgesia. Elsevier, Amsterdam

Simons D, Travell J, Simons L 1998 Myofascial pain and dysfunction: the trigger point manual, 2nd edn. Williams and Wilkins, Baltimore

Timmons B 1994 Behavioural and psychological approaches to breathing disorders. Plenum Press, New York

Travell J, Simons D 1983 Myofascial pain and dysfunction. Williams and Wilkins, Baltimore, vol 1

Travell J, Simons D 1992 Myofascial pain and dysfunction. Williams and Wilkins, Baltimore, vol 2

van Wingerden J-P, Vleeming A, Kleinrensink G-J, Stoeckart R 1997 The role of the hamstrings in pelvic and spinal function. In: Vleeming A et al (eds) Movement, stability and low back pain. Churchill Livingstone, Edinburgh

Vleeming A, van Wingerden J-P, Snijders S, Stoeckart R, Stijnen T 1989 Load application to the sacrotuberous ligament: influences on sacroiliac joint mechanics. Clinical Biomechanics 4: 204–209

Waersted M, Eken T, Westgaard R 1992 Single motor unit activity in psychogenic trapezius muscle tension. Arbete och Halsa 17: 319–321

Waersted M, Eken T, Westgaard R 1993 Psychogenic motor unit activity: a possible muscle injury mechanism studied in a healthy subject. Journal of Musculoskeletal Pain 1(3/4): 185–190

Ward R 1997 Foundation for osteopathic medicine. Williams and Wilkins, Baltimore

Wolfe F, Simons D 1992 Fibromyalgia and myofascial pain syndromes. Journal of Rheumatology 19(6): 944–951

Zink G, Lawson W 1979 Osteopathic structural examination and functional interpretation of the soma. Osteopathic Annals 7(12): 433–440

5

Interaction of psychological and emotional effects with breathing dysfunction

Christopher Gilbert

Breathing problems, from whatever source, cause stress in many systems. This stress includes an attempt to restore normal functioning, seeking a return to homeostasis. If a problem is forcing the patient (body or mind) to adapt in some way, then lightening the load by manipulation, increasing flexibility, suggesting exercises, providing hope, reducing overbreathing, treating trigger points, improving dietary habits, or changing attitudes all improve adaptation. This can only be helpful. The general payoff for an increased ability to adapt is less distress and less sense of threat, and this becomes a psychological matter. Regardless of the presence or absence of disease, transience or permanence, functional or organic, there is a person experiencing it all, and a person in distress can disrupt his breathing so much that other interventions are thwarted.

This chapter presents information about interactions between mind and body, which means essentially the organism communicating with different aspects of itself. Because of the close coupling of breathing with consciousness, many things can go wrong which have nothing to do with organic pathology. This resonating interface can also be used for improving the situation, if only by reducing the negative mental input which disrupts smooth functioning of the respiratory system.

THE DIAPHRAGM AND THE PHRENIC NERVE

The diaphragm is the muscular equivalent of an umbilical cord, linking us to the environment: it keeps us alive by pulling fresh air into the lungs and returning used air back out into the world. This process is not a mindless one, but is very responsive to our thinking. The word 'diaphragm' is related to the Greek word for mind: the diaphragm muscle is controlled by the phrenic nerve, and its Greek root, *phren*, designates the mind as well as the muscle. The Merriam-Webster dictionary (1991) definition of the word 'phrenic' is the following: '1. Of or relating to the diaphragm. 2. Of or relating to the mind.'

Considering such an odd dual meaning, one might conclude that the Greeks were confused, but the confusion is rather in the modern mind which attempts to separate mind and body into separate compartments. Ancient physicians had only their native senses for observing the action of breathing in themselves and others. This provided what no modern mechanical breathing monitor can offer – simultaneous registration of mental and breathing processes. With this opportunity for observation, parallels and correlations could be drawn between moments of emotion and changes in breathing rate, depth, regularity, and bodily placement. Interruption of attention, style of focusing, state of calmness or distress, degree of mental effort – such 'mental' variables can be observed in oneself and to a degree in others. These variables all interact with the breathing pattern via the phrenic nerve.

EMOTIONAL DISRUPTION OF OPTIMAL BREATHING

'Optimal breathing' can be defined first as a match between the amount of air exchange and the body's immediate needs. This applies not only to oxygen intake but also to carbon dioxide release. The metabolic demand for oxygen changes according to factors such as level of arousal, digestion, need for internal heat, and exercise. The need for excretion of carbon dioxide also changes according to exercise, digestion, and general metabolism as well as disease states that alter the pH of the blood, such as acidosis due to kidney disease.

Keeping the blood gases and pH closely balanced is very important physiologically. As expressed by Jennett (1994):

When there are not other overriding drives affecting breathing, the neural control system acts to maintain a constant arterial PCO_2. This must mean that the volume of CO_2 expired continually balances the volume produced by tissue metabolism. Measurements show that alveolar and arterial concentrations of CO_2 stay constant, which means that the volume of gas breathed out from the functional (alveolar) volume of the lungs must vary precisely with the rate of metabolic CO_2 production. In rest and activity, when the system is left to itself, it is so efficient that the matching occurs virtually breath-by-breath, even when metabolic activity is continually changing. (p. 73)

Optimal breathing, therefore, is what the body seeks continuously, with its various sensing systems and its ability quickly to adjust breathing depth and rate. This homeostatic stability is obviously important, yet it must sometimes yield to other priorities. Some, such as vocalizing, yawning, coughing, and breath-holding, are transient and easily terminated, but other conditions can affect this stability in more drastic and more long-term ways.

Of particular interest in this chapter are psychological factors which alter breathing. In texts about respiratory therapy, especially in descriptions of hyperventilation, statements such as 'Emotional stress can also affect breathing' or 'Psychogenic sources of hyperventilation should be considered' is usually offered, but details are usually lacking. This chapter presents these details, together with speculation as to why breathing is so sensitive to emotions.

The introduction of memory, associations, and the ability to imagine and anticipate all complicate the picture of breathing regulation. What may be optimal for the organism at a given moment, at a certain level of exercise and arousal, may not be so optimal in the next few moments if action is demanded. Action requires muscle contraction, which in turn calls for more oxygen. Prolonging the time during which the muscles can function well provides a survival advantage. Therefore, anticipating this need for action and preparing for it by increased breathing is a natural process in humans and animals. Other things happen also, such as muscle tensing, larger cardiac stroke volume, and adrenaline surge, but breathing affects the basic fuel supply without which nothing will work.

Anticipation of action may be very certain, as when falling out of a tree, or it may be a prediction based on odds. This betting is often unconscious, the result of fear conditioning creating a negatively charged image which is somehow coded as to intensity. If a person once fell out of a tree, this fact is remembered at many levels, and being in a tree again will activate those memories and their associated physical adaptations. Conscious recall is not necessary for these anticipatory preparations to occur. The system ends up adjusting the breathing and other survival-related variables because of a recognized sensory cue.

This mechanism predates the development of higher consciousness, and it triggers preparation faster than conscious awareness can decipher the meaning of a cue. This speed is of course an advantage; the disadvantage is that the conscious mind is removed from the decision circuit, in the same way that a nation's military, in an emergency, may act without consulting the chief executive.

Some specific ways in which breathing adjusts to differing conditions are described below:

Depth and rate of breathing

Both depth and frequency of breathing are adjustable depending on the body's need (or expected need) for air. These two are adjustable independently; in the case of pregnancy, for example, or a broken rib, depth of breathing will be reduced, but breathing faster will compensate for it. Some combination of the two factors is calculated by the brain to result in more or less air exchange.

Compared to increasing frequency, increasing the depth of respiration is more effective for boosting alveolar ventilation, but only up to a point. A central nervous system computation adjusts these two factors, depending on the body's fluctuating need for air. Increasing the depth of a breath is opposed by the elastic forces which bring about exhalation; breathing faster is opposed by the friction of moving air in and out of the airways. The relative importance of these two adjustments in the case of preparatory breathing is not known. Rapid breathing is common during anticipatory anxiety, and so are increased sighing and deep breaths. Complicating this picture is the role of emotion-based vocalization: incipient crying, screaming, or shouting. Either deeper or faster breathing could be part of preparing for vocalizing activity.

Breathing faster does not necessarily indicate hyperventilation. Hyperventilation is defined by the amount of air being exchanged rather than the rate of breathing – if more air passes through the system than the body needs, this qualifies as hyperventilation, which can be maintained with even three or four very deep breaths per minute. Breathing faster than normal, or panting, may happen in a variety of situations: for example in a person who is anxious, overheated (panting helps dissipate heat), or who has restricted abdominal and thoracic expansion. If fresh air is not exposed to the alveoli, however, it enters and leaves the body unchanged. A column of air can be moved up and down within the dead space of the system (mouth, trachea, and airways above the alveoli) by panting, with little actual air exchange.

Finally, rapid breathing increases turbulence within the airways. This aids the sense of smell, but smooth laminar airflow is compromised. This becomes more important in obstructive lung disease, including asthma, when the airways are narrowed.

Breath holding

Some life situations call for vigilant silence, a concealment response which may inhibit or suspend breathing altogether. Indecision about what action to take, or a decision to wait for more information, may be reflected in the breathing as the mind switches between action preparation, focused attention, and concealment. Each of these primary states calls for a particular modulation of breathing: focused attention on the environment benefits from smooth, steady breathing which stabilizes the 'sensory platform' – and in precise focusing of attention or in attempting to remain undetectable the breathing may be suspended for a few moments.

If the breathing is reduced or paused, oxygen reserve slowly falls and CO_2 rises, which stimulates more breathing (often a sigh) which pushes CO_2 down – and the cycle starts over again.

The human capacity for imagination allows us to create any scenario at any time, often in enough detail for our bodies to respond as though the scene were real. Therefore, the mere act of thinking about situations that would require action, concealment, vigilance, or emotional expression is likely to cause corresponding changes in the breathing.

LOCATION OF BREATHING

Chest vs. abdomen

Optimal breathing when we are awake makes use of the diaphragm, resulting in moderate abdominal expansion, with some involvement of intercostal muscles so that the lower rib cage expands, and minimal involvement of the pectoral, scalene, and other accessory breathing muscles. By contrast, chest breathing makes more use of the pectoral, scalene, trapezius, sternocleidomastoid, and upper intercostal muscles. These muscles are collectively termed accessory breathing muscles because they are used for back-up duty, either when it is difficult to breathe with the diaphragm or for extra-deep breathing. These two styles of breathing are end points on a continuum rather than discrete categories – one can breathe with any combination of chest and abdominal breathing.

Reasons for chest breathing

When asked either to take a deep breath or to breathe rapidly, almost everyone breathes into the chest, unless they actually intend to breathe abdominally (a trained singer, for instance). They also frequently take this voluntary breath through the mouth rather than the nostrils. Chest, or thoracic, breathing seems to be the preferred route for consciously mediated intentional breathing, while abdominal breathing is the main route for relaxed, automatic breathing.

Why should this be? Inquiring into this matter involves speculating about the differences between the types of breathing, what functions they may play, and what conditions might initiate each type.

ACTION PROJECTION

One major reason for an organism to override the automatic regulation of breathing is in order to prepare for sudden action. The word 'prepare' implies projecting oneself into, and predicting, the future. Ordinarily, breathing rate and volume closely follow immediate metabolic needs, with breathing changing at the moment when increased muscle activity demands more oxygen. But fuller breathing in advance of action confers a physiological advantage, not only by boosting oxygen saturation to the maximum, but also by lowering CO_2 which would help to balance the surge of CO_2, and acidity produced by sudden exercise. A familiar example is breathing deeply before lifting a heavy weight. This preparation is in the same category as postural adjustments; conscious mediation, if time allows, fine-tunes the preparation to the size of the expected effort.

As described by Taylor (1989), exercise physiologists have established that there is an instantaneous jump in ventilation at the onset of exercise. It is thought to be mediated by something other than simple metabolic demand, because the rise outstrips any current oxygen deficit. In Taylor's words: 'Phase I appears to be neurally mediated by a learned response related to an anticipation of exercise and/or an increased proprioceptor input from muscles and joints at the onset of exercise. Phase I is *load independent* and accompanied by increases in heart rate and sympathetic activity' (p. 214, italics added). Phase II and Phase III are determined more by current exercise load. This Phase I shift in breathing seems to be triggered by conscious anticipation of exercise, and represents a well-established route from the mind to the breathing muscles. This route would be the logical means by which more subtle action projection from emotional sources might influence the breathing.

Preparation for emergency action is generally more complex than preparing to run or to lift a heavy object. If a cerebral cortex is good for anything, it would be for times when a decision is required as to whether to freeze, attack, or flee, and when, and how. This moment-to-moment anticipatory planning in a perceived crisis depends on cognitive and perceptual processes, a judgment function based on close observation combined with experience. Even if seen as a situation of competing reflexes, some function must operate for choosing among them. Just as posture and balance will shift according to changes in anticipated movement, the breathing pattern will also be modulated according to what exactly is being predicted. Thus the breath holding typical of watchful observation increases the stability of the sense organs and also reduces breathing movement and sound which would work against concealment. This suppression of breathing is then normally balanced by a deep breath just before leaping into action.

Both respiratory suspension and overbreathing in preparation for action are actually unbalanced, because the individual is not living entirely in the present but partly in the future. The projection creates a discrepancy between actual metabolic needs and breathing pattern based on an imaginary projection. Consider a sprinter in an awkward starting position, waiting for the pistol, or a baseball pitcher just before delivering a pitch, one leg raised high. Such positions are not meant to be held for long. If the expected action is carried out as planned, the awkward position turns out to facilitate performance. But if the starting pistol does not fire or the baseball pitch is delayed, the posture becomes untenable.

This prolonged action projection can explain much about human breathing pattern problems: with their superior ability to predict, project, extrapolate, and imagine, people are well equipped to anticipate threats which might require action. When this occurs, the body obligingly prepares for such action with increased breathing or else erratic alternation between breath holding and overbreathing. The trouble comes when the threat is non-physical and not imminent; for instance, anxiety about planning a wedding 3 months hence, or anger over being insulted by something written in a letter. Situations like these do not require an immediate increase in breathing, but the body seems to take no chances when the mind is thinking about a threat; it prepares for action as if the event were just around the corner and includes a physical challenge. If such feelings become chronic, then the preparation will become chronic.

Action projection and accessory breathing muscles

There are several possible reasons why this preparation for action would be linked with overuse of the accessory breathing muscles:

1. The diaphragm is the main mechanism of automatic breathing, and does not need input from the conscious mind to operate well. Normal breathing at rest is primarily abdominal, reflecting diaphragm action with little or no activity of accessory breathing muscles. Thoracic breathing, on the other hand, is on call as a back-up system, especially for breathing preparatory to action. A good alternative term for the accessory breathing muscles might be discretionary breathing muscles, since they are the primary route for voluntary or emotional input.

An example of voluntary input to breath control would be preparing to blow up a balloon with an extra-deep breath; an example of emotional input would be perceiving an approaching person as hostile and threatening. In the first case the person consciously decides to take a deep breath in order to inflate the balloon. In the second case the person probably does not consciously decide to increase breathing, but it happens anyway because of the emotion of fear or anger. In either case, the possibility of a need for fast action is translated to activation of accessory breathing muscles. This breathing route seems responsive to any emotion which might lead to rapid action. Expanding thoracic volume can function either as a supplement to diaphragmatic breathing or as a substitute for it, depending on the circumstances.

2. Another reason for thoracic breathing is simply protective: during physical confrontation the abdomen is vulnerable to attack, and protection of this vital region would improve odds of survival. Tensing the abdominal muscles offers protection, but since such tensing flattens the abdomen and restricts expansion, it will interfere with diaphragmatic breathing. Switching to thoracic breathing solves this problem.

3. Thoracic breathing produces increases in cardiac output and heart rate – just the opposite of abdominal breathing (Hurwitz 1981). This would furnish an advantage during emergency action. It may be that some people like the cardiac boost and the feeling of enhanced readiness, and so this thoracic breathing becomes reinforced. The common military posture of flattened abdomen and chest expanded boosts activity of the cardiac system, working against relaxed economical breathing but maximizing preparation for action.

4. Rapid action also requires stabilizing the spine and trunk. Leaping into action, whether fleeing or attacking, involves close motor coordination of the trunk and the hips. This calls on the abdominal muscles such as rectus and transversus abdominis and external and internal obliques, which during abdominal breathing are normally relaxed. Richardson et al (1999) have published numerous studies that show which muscles are most involved in spinal postural stabilization. When these are recruited for action preparation, the auxiliary breathing mechanism must be brought into play. Many muscles have a dual involvement in postural control and breathing movements.

Even the diaphragm, specialized as it seems to be for breathing, contributes to spinal and pelvic stabilization. In a study which measured activity of both the costal and crural portions of the diaphragm as well as transversus abdominis, it was found that contraction occurred in all these areas when spinal stabilization was required (in this instance during shoulder flexion). The results provide evidence that the diaphragm contributes to spinal control and may do so by assisting with pressurization and displacement of the abdominal contents, allowing the transversus abdominis to increase tension in the thoracolumbar fascia or to generate intra-abdominal pressure.

Any gross body movement might interfere with abdominal breathing, leaving accessory muscle breathing as the back-up. Complex interactions take place whenever the need for core stability occurs. The involvement of the diaphragm in postural stabilization suggests that situations might easily occur where contradictory demands are evident – for example, where postural stabilizing control is required at the same time that respiratory functions create demands for movement.

5. Finally, there is a common association of mouth breathing with chest breathing (see below). The resistance to mouth breathing is far less than to nasal breathing (Barelli 1994), making it easier to draw air in through the mouth. Also, the air passage into the chest and upper lungs is shorter than to the abdomen and the base of the lungs. Together, these two facts give an advantage to the mouth/chest route for rapid air intake as preparation for action, including shouting or other vocalization.

Thus it makes sense that reliance on the accessory breathing muscles and the mouth would be more closely linked with voluntary breathing. The greater efficiency of using the diaphragm and relaxing the external abdominal muscles requires a context of safety and relative inactivity. At moments of urgency, greater respiratory efficiency may be sacrificed in favor of the mixed demands that the action orientation may take. A dichotomous distinction between abdominal and thoracic breathing is an oversimplification; these are polar opposites, and many degrees of blending between the two occur. Thus one may breathe in any ratio of abdominal to thoracic; among other factors, this may represent relative dominance of action orientation over a relaxed and safe orientation.

Nose breathing vs. mouth breathing

We can breathe through the mouth, the nose, or a combination of the two, and psychology enters even into this factor: 'Nasal breathing is *involuntary*. Mouth, or *voluntary*, breathing occurs when there is difficulty breathing through the nose, such as in exertion, under stress, and – in particular – when cardiac, pulmonary, or other illness hampers the supply of oxygen to the tissues' (Barelli 1994, p. 52). Significant anxiety triggers preparatory breathing, and since resistance is less through the mouth than through the nose, the lungs may be filled with less effort, and more quickly, by mouth breathing. A state of surprise or startle will cause the jaw to drop open.

One might think that lowered resistance to air flow is a good thing. When preparing for exertion it seems to be, because under such circumstances a large amount of air must be exchanged, and if the nostrils are bypassed the air can move more easily in and out. The nasal route adds at least 50% more resistance to air flow. This may seem undesirable, but there are reasons. The pressure rise during exhalation improves perfusion into the alveoli in the same way that lower altitude does: the higher pressure created within the lungs makes the air more dense, simulating a lower altitude where the air is richer in oxygen per unit volume.

The compliance and elasticity of the lungs are important for efficient air movement ('compliance' refers to the ability to stretch and expand; 'elasticity' refers to the ability to spring back after stretching). The increased resistance introduced into the system by nose breathing increases the vacuum in the lungs, resulting in a 10–20% increase in oxygen transported (Cottle 1972). Diaphragmatic movement also improves venous return to the heart, reducing its workload.

Cottle (1987), a renowned rhinologist, includes among the functions of nasal breathing:

... slowing down the expiratory phase of respiration and ventilation, and the interposing of resistance to both inspiration and expiration which in turn helps to maintain the normal elasticity of the lungs, thus assuring optimal conditions for providing oxygen and good heart function. Breathing through the mouth usually affords too little obstruction and could lead to areas of atelectasis and poor ventilation of the low spaces in the lung. (p. 146)

If a momentary state of alarm and action preparation becomes more chronic or habitual, then the physiological factors cited above become important. Mouth breathing often develops at a time of chronic nasal obstruction, such as sinus problems or injury to the nose. Once established, the habit may not subside, even after the obstruction is cleared.

CONDITIONED BREATHING RESPONSES

The preceding changes in breathing constitute most of the adaptations to stress of various sorts. They could be called generic in the sense that they are standard responses to common stimuli such as a loud, sudden noise, obvious physical threat, or a clear requirement to prepare for physical exertion. The breathing pattern of any individual will be altered by such experiences as hearing of the death of a loved one, experiencing an automobile accident, or being physically threatened by someone, but these are relatively rare events for most people while breathing disruptions are relatively common. Many stimuli capable of eliciting these breathing changes are unique to the individual as a result of personal experience; it is in this category that careful inquiry may be repaid by better understanding of what triggers this action preparation style of breathing.

Here the concept of psychophysiological time travel – memory and anticipation – may be useful. As discussed elsewhere (Gilbert 1998), an individual's significant emotional incidents become liable to time-shifting from the past to the present. The concept of memory is familiar enough, but when a memory causes body responses similar to the original experience, or flashbacks which include the body, then there is a confusion somewhere in the system between past and present reality.

Traumatic conditioning (also known as fear conditioning) has been extensively studied in both man and animals. The general principles derive from studies of conditioning dating back to Pavlov's work with salivating dogs, but the difference between that situation and a modern office worker hearing the approaching footsteps of a dreaded supervisor is conceptually very small. Classical conditioning is a ubiquitous learning mechanism which does not require conscious thought.

To understand how conditioning relates to breathing disorders in humans requires knowledge of several intermediate steps:

1. An autonomic response such as salivation can be elicited by an appropriate stimulus (e.g. food on the tongue). If a neutral stimulus such as a bell precedes the food by just a moment, the salivation will begin to occur in response to the bell because it gives more advance warning of the food. In time the salivation will occur to the bell alone, *without the food*, apparently because the bell has merged in some way with the food stimulus.

2. Salivation to food does not normally involve fear, but an electric foot shock does. If the experiment is done instead with shock delivery, an alarm/defense reaction will replace salivation as the normal, or unconditioned, response to the shock. This includes a jump in heart rate and blood pressure, freezing movement, a rise in adrenaline, and a change in breathing. This happens on the first trial; no learning is necessary. But if a bell, a change in lighting, a vibration in the floor, or any other neutral stimulus is made to precede the shock, the alarm response will soon be triggered by the neutral stimulus *whether or not the shock is delivered*. The neutral stimulus becomes a *conditioned* stimulus (synonyms are 'conditioning' or 'conditional'). This is how fear conditioning works – a formerly neutral stimulus acquires the power to set off the alarm response on its own.

3. Learning that involves fear is more rapid than learning involving things such as food and salivation because there is a potential threat to survival, and thus an urgency. The brain gets the connection sometimes after a single trial; there is obviously an advantage to learning certain connections quickly because Nature often does not provide a second chance. Imagine, for instance, that a hawk swoops down on a rabbit and grabs it with sharp talons. Suppose the rabbit gets away with only a wound, and remembers the sound of the approaching hawk's wings. It would be very useful for the rabbit to associate the sound with remembered pain and terror. The faster the rabbit's response to this warning stimulus the next time, the more likely it is that the rabbit will take effective evasive action.

The concept of evasive action introduces the variable of intention, which presupposes a kind of consciousness. The initial simple defense or escape response may be automatically conditioned, but the subsequent actions (knowing to jump into a narrow place where the hawk cannot follow) may call for more than the default blind leap or freezing response. In other words, the introduction of conscious control of the next move adds to the animal's advantage.

4. Many conditioning experiments are arranged so that the foot shock is terminated by the animal withdrawing its foot. A neutral stimulus such as a bell still precedes the shock, thus providing a warning. In this case foot withdrawal becomes conditioned by the neutral stimulus alone, and the experimenter can turn off the shock apparatus with confidence that the withdrawal response will not soon be extinguished. The bell alone will set off a leg muscle contraction. Since the shock can be avoided completely by the quick foot withdrawal, the subject may not even realize that the shock is no longer threatening. (This is now termed 'operant conditioning' rather than 'classical,' because the animal is operating on the environment rather than reacting passively, as with autonomic responses.)

5. Since leg withdrawal is in the realm of voluntary muscle control rather than strictly autonomic, the response is brought into the domain of choice: thinking about what to do next. This allows the use of memory in a less automatic way, and involves judgment. For instance, in the hawk–rabbit example, the automatic response may be to jump without regard to direction, on the chance that the swooping hawk will miss its target. But suppose the rabbit hole is a few inches away but in a particular direction. A simple jumping reflex would not be that specific; aiming toward the hole requires memory and judgment. Thus a reflex blends with directed action.

6. In human beings, breathing control moves in a broad zone between automatic and volun-

tary, although a person in a crisis will not be thinking about how to breathe appropriately for the situation. The mode of breathing seems to be selected automatically depending on what is anticipated in the next few seconds: breath holding may do for indecision or freezing; a deep gasp might prepare for major exertion or crying out; a sharp exhale might accompany anger, frustration, or aggression.

Behavioral research on man and animals has clarified the links by which breathing can be altered in the absence of an appropriate stimulus. The brain is doing its best to prepare for something based on projection from past experience, and consciousness is not necessarily part of this process. Since animals as low as snails have been successfully conditioned, the conditioning mechanism must have evolved before the development of a large cortex which allows a wide choice among possible actions. This means that certain breathing changes, difficult to explain otherwise, could represent conditioned responses to stimuli that either carry the signal of threat themselves, or were associated with a threat signal.

One advantage of bypassing consciousness is that of speed. The extra milliseconds resulting from more synaptic connections could be critical in avoiding danger. The term 'head start' refers to an advantage obtained in a race, but it can also refer to the advantage of anticipation by 'using the head' – whether through conscious anticipation or with an unconscious conditioned response. The disadvantage of being guided by conditioned responses is that the interpretation and response are not guided by consciousness, so a slammed door might, for example, be mistaken for a gunshot by a combat veteran with a conditioned phobia for gunshots.

Experimental conditioning of breathing changes

There is clear evidence that respiratory responses can be conditioned. Ley (1996, 1999) confirmed this by monitoring end-tidal CO_2 in college students while they coped with brief mental stressors such as doing calculations in their heads or counting backwards by sevens from 200. This was sufficient to increase their skin conductance (a measure of sympathetic nervous system activity), heart rate, and breathing rate, and also to shift CO_2 in the direction of hyperventilation. In this situation there was no clear threat which would justify activating the bodily stress response, so either a psychosocial threat (a blow to the ego) was present from the risk of failing the test, or else the effort involved in the mental tasks activated the body changes.

Ley presented a specific sound to the subjects along with the 'Start' instructions, linking the tone with the demand to perform. It took very few pairings before the two were firmly associated; in essence, the subjects identified a clue that would allow them to get a head start. However, sounding the tone alone without the 'Start' instructions was sufficient to set off the same stress responses of faster breathing and heart rate, skin conductance, and lower end-tidal CO_2. These responses were now conditioned to the tone, much like the rabbit hearing the faint sound of the hawk's wings.

It might be objected that this is a consciously-mediated common-sense association, that the subject simply looks for clues and responds to them. But this conscious process seems to be secondary or peripheral, not necessary for the conditioned responses to occur. Conditioning of this nature can be demonstrated in very primitive organisms such as earthworms, snails, and fruit flies. So it seems reasonable to conclude that disruption of breathing can occur because of associations to environmental stimuli, independent of conscious awareness.

Other conditioning experiments with breathing were carried out by Van den Bergh and colleagues (1997), and the findings have important implications for understanding the origins of certain breathing disorders. Subjects were exposed to low concentrations of particular smells along with either normal room air or a 7% concentration of CO_2. This procedure is often used to test for sensitivity to excess CO_2; the gas quickly stimulates an increase in breathing, but the degree of this effect varies from person to person. The test procedure is useful for studying panic disorder and predisposition to hyperventilation.

In essence, what Van den Bergh and colleagues found was that after a few pairings of a particular odor with the high-CO_2 air, the odor by itself would stimulate an increase in breathing, along with an increase in complaints of breathlessness, chest tightness, and other respiratory-related sensations. Ordinary air containing the conditioned odor was enough to create disturbances in the subjects' experience of their breathing. The way in which breathing increased varied: females tended to respond by breathing faster, and males responded by breathing more deeply. But either way, the fact that stimuli which were paired with 'bad air' (high CO_2 content) could later provoke an increase in breathing volume using normal air suggests a mechanism whereby dyspnea, uneasy breathing, and hyperventilation could seem to appear out of nowhere. Ley's findings with conditioned sounds show that the effect is not due only to the sense of smell, but also spans other senses.

In Van den Bergh et al's words (1997):

'patients with hyperventilation may be excessively attentive to typical respiratory complaints. Attentional direction may therefore prime both reporting more complaints of that type during acquisition and subsequently facilitate their conditioning. ...Occurrences of hyperventilation may be considered learning episodes in which subjects increasingly learn to attend to and anxiously interpret 'normal' somatic variations, which may produce complaints and cause altered breathing as well. Eventually, the relationship between hyperventilation and somatic complaints may become reversed over time within an individual'.

The authors also discuss the phenomenon of multiple chemical sensitivity in light of these findings, since many of the symptoms overlap with hyperventilation. It is possible that panic-like reactions to particular airborne chemical compounds, particularly irritant gases and strong odors, are in part classically conditioned responses rather than reflexive responses. If so, reduction of the response strength through a desensitizing procedure of graduated exposure might offer an alternative to rigid control of the environment.

FEAR CONDITIONING AND THE AMYGDALA

We have all experienced moments when a feeling of non-specific alarm seems to occur before we are consciously aware of the relevant stimulus. Examples are irrational avoidance of something, a flurry of rapid pulse, sweating, a feeling of dread, a freeze reaction, or a sudden disruption of breathing: a gasp or a pause. The time lag may be a few seconds or much longer, and the overall impression, on reflection, is that we are temporarily out of control of our behavior. A thoughtful person might wonder: do these moments represent intuition? Extrasensory perception? A warning from an angel?

The mechanism which probably explains such moments actually involves a dual, bi-level memory system. Neuroscientist Joseph LeDoux (1994, 1996) has been prominent in this area, and his book *The Emotional Brain* (LeDoux 1996) presents current research on the distinction between explicit and implicit memory. This difference corresponds physically to two somewhat independent memory systems based on the hippocampus and amygdala, respectively. These two structures, part of the limbic system deep within the temporal lobes of the cerebrum, are essential for memory storage. Memory is not a unitary phenomenon; our conscious, or 'explicit,' memories depend on the hippocampus, while our protective, survival-oriented memories are maintained by the amygdala. This second type of memory does not require conscious knowledge, and so this provides a mechanism for the previous observations about conditioned responses which may defy logic, yet are faster than our voluntary responses.

The amygdala has abundant chemical and neural outputs to body systems involved in the emergency action. On its command, blood pressure rises, muscles tense, and heart rate increases. Breathing may stop and then become more rapid as the brain attempts to prepare for an ambiguous threat.

To provide information for such commands, nerve pathways lead directly to the amygdala from the thalamus, where incoming sensory input is integrated and redirected. This means that sensory information can be fed directly to a brain nucleus responsible for initiating emergency action, bypassing the cortex and consciousness. This is comparable to a military system being authorized to sound an emergency alert before consulting the government. When the system works well, this power is usually limited to creating an initial state of readiness or reflexive defense; further actions would require instructions from higher decision centers. Freezing all current activities, even thinking, would be the first step in such a sequence; orienting all attention toward the threatening stimulus would be the second; avoiding a recognized situation (the edge of a cliff or a snake, for example) would be a third step. These are all simple procedures which can be initiated by the amygdala without immediate cortical input – and immediacy is often important.

Normally the stimulus in question goes to the cortex also and the two systems work together, but they are at some level separate. The explicit memory system, based in the hippocampus, is elaborate, extensive, and can access the rest of the cortex for fine-tuning decisions. The special nature of amygdala memories seems related to trouble of some kind, especially anything which has already caused a fear reaction. If memory traces and impressions stored in the amygdala match up with sensory input signifying danger, commands may go out to attack, hide, run, brace for action, or something more specific than a simple freeze or avoidance reaction. This can of course be a problem if conscious judgment and experience is bypassed. Mistakes can be made which imperil the organism from without (such as attacking, when running away would be better) or from within (such as issuing a reflex command for a rise in blood flow and pressure which the system cannot handle).

Thus the amygdala reigns over the body like an ever vigilant watchdog, with its permanent archive of stimuli associated with danger combined with its primitive repertoire of emergency actions. The conscious mind, like the watchdog's owner, gets the news more slowly; its compensating advantage is (supposedly) superior judgment

and broader access to experience, both personal and secondhand, and its ability to foresee consequences. Planning and carrying out a shifting, adaptive coping strategy requires the highest levels of the brain, but the more information is integrated, the more synaptic connections are needed, and these take time. Ideally, the differences between the two systems are smoothly coordinated as might occur between the military and legislative branches of a government, so that the strengths of each contribute to the final outcome.

Biological preparedness

The above system, however, originally evolved in a different environment from the one we live in now. Potential dangers were probably more direct and physical, for example danger from predatory animals, cliffs, falling rocks and branches, being lost in a cave or attacked by an aggressive rival. Our fear-warning systems are tuned to, and most sensitive to, such physical situations. This concept is called 'biological preparedness' (Seligman 1971). The assumption is that evolution has equipped humans with a heightened tendency to avoid situations which threatened the survival of our ancestors. Thus fear of confinement, snakes, insects, heights, strangers, and suddenly looming objects arose because they spelled danger in the distant past. We are especially likely to acquire fear responses of such things because fear triggers avoidance and avoidance reduces exposure, which on the average would improve survival. This general formulation has been supported by recent research showing, for example, that it is easier to create conditioned fear to snakes than to flowers, and that learned autonomic reactions to fear-relevant stimuli are harder to extinguish (Öhman 1992). Furthermore, fear conditioning in these experiments was possible from presenting these biologically prepared stimuli in a way that was not consciously perceived, so it seems that conscious perception is not necessary to acquire phobic responses.

In modern life we must contend with such things as televised plane crashes, glass-walled elevators, scary movies, loud highway and subway noises, crowded stadiums and cramped restaurants. These do not constitute immediate danger to us, even though they trigger alarm reactions because the 'watchdog' amygdala, in general, cannot tell the difference. The cortex must constantly damp down and cancel out the body responses, among which disrupted breathing is prominent. Breathing seems to be squarely in the midst of the turmoil between voluntary and automatic behavior (Fig. 5.1).

Incidental learning

Another factor which extends the influence of the amygdala is incidental learning, or conditioning to the entire context of a traumatic incident. Suppose a woman is assaulted in an elevator in which a particular song is playing. Fear conditioning would make it likely that she would become very uneasy about elevators in general, especially because they possess the biologically prepared factor of confinement. The assault would also boost her fear of strangers.

Suppose that months later she hears, somewhere else, the same music that was playing in the elevator, and she feels an unaccountable dread. Her breathing quickens, muscles tense, her heart starts to pound, and she sweats. Yet she may not know why. This is the result of the

brain's conditioning trying to warn her. The amygdala has stored a multisensory 'snapshot' of the context of the assault, and it is now activating the fear response, leaving the woman's conscious self bewildered as to why she is so uneasy. She may identify the music as the trigger, but she does not have to consciously recall that the music was playing in the elevator. Her amygdala memory system has already done that.

In this case the brain's protection system has gone woefully wrong; it is not only ineffective, it causes trouble. The woman may avoid the new context in which the song is heard or she may develop anxiety about what seems to be a surge of 'out of the blue' anxiety if she happens to believe that this reaction is dangerous to her. Yet if she were the rabbit instead, as in the previous example, with a hawk swooping down to grab her and the sound of the hawk's wings substituted for the elevator music, then the stimulus would be very relevant indeed, and reacting to it would save her life. It is probably beyond the capacity of the amygdala's memory system to designate certain details of a context as relevant and others as irrelevant. Indeed, there may be a biased rule built into the system to take account of the asymmetric payoffs: an error of overinclusion – reacting to a harmless stimulus from a traumatic context – means a brief flurry of

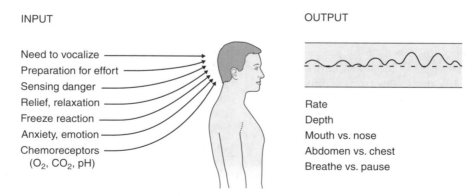

INPUT

Need to vocalize
Preparation for effort
Sensing danger
Relief, relaxation
Freeze reaction
Anxiety, emotion
Chemoreceptors
(O_2, CO_2, pH)

OUTPUT

Rate
Depth
Mouth vs. nose
Abdomen vs. chest
Breathe vs. pause

Figure 5.1 Final modulation of the breathing act includes input from many possible sources: the need for vocalization (a cry for help, a shouted warning, perhaps a growl), preparation for exertion, the need to freeze and become perhaps less noticeable, the need to maximize sensory acuity by stilling the body, the need to either remain calm or return to a baseline state of calmness. These inputs too often conflict with each other, but if there is the hint of a threat to survival, that seems to have priority over all other considerations.

anxiety and avoidance, a recoverable expenditure of energy. On the other hand, an error of underinclusion – ignoring a stimulus which actually signals the familiar danger returning – could be fatal.

Another discovery from this area of study is that there are many neural connections from the amygdala to higher cortical areas. There are far fewer connections, however, in the opposite direction (Amaral et al 1992). The system seems to be set up to deliver danger-relevant information to higher cortical areas so that the initial responses can be refined or controlled by judgment and experience. This downward-directed control is weaker, as judged by both the neural connections and the fact that phobias are more easily acquired than eradicated. Anxiety shifts priority to survival issues; at these times, loops of neurons in the amygdala perpetuate the connections between memory, perception, and alarm, and the cortex must struggle to oppose this process.

Worse yet, these conditioned fears may not be entirely erasable. In LeDoux's words:

Unconscious fear memories established through the amygdala appear to be indelibly burned into the brain. They are probably with us for life. This is often useful, especially in a stable, unchanging world, since we don't want to have to learn about the same kinds of dangers over and over again. The downside is that sometimes the things that are imprinted in the amygdala's circuits are maladaptive. In these instances, we pay dearly for the incredible efficiencies of the fear system. (LeDoux 1996, p. 252)

HYPNOTIC INVESTIGATIONS

Hyperventilation as a chronic syndrome or behavioral tendency is squarely in the category of disorders often called 'functional,' 'psychophysiological,' or 'psychosomatic.' But it is not always so clearly delineated; disruption of the optimal breathing pattern can happen in subtler ways. Increased variability from breath to breath is known to correlate with anxiety states (Han et al 1997, Beck et al 2000). Low $PaCO_2$ and increased frequency of sighing are typical of those with panic disorder, even when not panicking (Wilhelm 2001). These generalizations miss individuals who do not have a chronic breathing pattern disorder, but who do experience disrupted breathing under particular conditions. The conditions can provoke either an amygdala 'alarm' discharge or some specific, learned breathing response, as well as occasional panic.

Conway, Freeman, and colleagues (Conway et al 1988, Freeman et al 1986) have used hypnosis to investigate the sources of these hyperventilation episodes in a number of patients. Based on this research, they suggest that 'hyperventilators' is not a uniform category but consists of at least two groups: the chronic and the episodic. Many people are subject to hyperventilation episodes but breathe normally most of the time. They are susceptible to particular stimuli associated with some original event of intense emotion, and when reminded of this event are likely to breathe in a way that lowers CO_2 quickly, setting off many symptoms of hyperventilation, sometimes including panic:

It has been considered that emotional events, particularly involving loss, separation and impotent anger, are the precipitating factors that may initiate a trend to hyperventilation...

On some occasions the important initiating event, psychological strain or life event was evident from the history, but in others questioning under hypnosis revealed psychological triggers, not elucidated previously, which provoked marked falls in $PetCO_2$. Since it is a feature of many psychosomatic illnesses that the initiating factors are repressed and only the somatic symptoms remain, this technique may be of considerable help in some patients in whom therapy may not be progressing as well as might have been expected. (Freeman et al 1986, p. 80)

A test based on research by Hardonk & Beumer (1979; – see Ch. 8 for a fuller description) involves provoking a 3-minute period of forced hyperventilation followed by instructions to resume normal breathing. A delayed return to baseline after another 3 minutes is a positive diagnostic sign for hyperventilation syndrome, as based on symptom reports. Conway and colleagues (1988) found that those who showed slow return to baseline tended to be habitual overbreathers, and were usually most bothered by the physiological distress accompanying hyperventilation. This group would probably score higher on the Anxiety Sensitivity Index (see below), meaning they were hypersensitive to the sensations of anxiety. But another group of subjects were primarily sensitive instead to specific emotional triggers such as bereavement, anger, separation, loss, and grief. The onset of their hyperventilation episodes tended to come and go more quickly and did not turn into a habit.

This suggests that the emotion-triggered group may have more trouble dealing with such recalled experience, or perhaps that their respiratory systems are more closely tied to certain intense emotions. They did not appear to have the 'bad breathing habit' that Lum (1975) suggested is typical of hyperventilators; instead, their predisposition for plummeting CO_2 lay in wait to be released by certain reminders. These moments may be unpredictable and the trigger unknown. Hypnosis proved invaluable in uncovering triggers for hyperventilation attacks which were not easily apparent from either personal histories or the subjects' own awareness and recollection of events (Conway et al 1988, p. 303). These were not necessarily repressed memories; the hyperventilation was simply linked to the memory of certain experiences.

In another study (Freeman et al 1986), patients diagnosed as having the hyperventilation syndrome were studied during hypnotic recall of emotionally disturbing experiences, particularly those associated with the reported symptoms. Drops in $PetCO_2$ were measured and compared to a control group without symptoms of hyperventilation, during similar hypnotic recall of emotionally disturbing experiences. The average drop in 27 patients was 18.2 mmHg, while in 10 controls the mean drop was 5 mmHg. The range was also much larger in the patients, and overall the difference between the two groups was highly significant.

This study showed at least that individuals who reported several symptoms indicating hyperventilation (including chest pain and palpitations, dizziness, etc. – not exclusively respiratory symptoms) displayed rather strong hyperventilation in response to recalling emotionally disturbing events, whereas the control subjects did not. Bereavement, loss of control, grief, and anger were common topics associated with the symptoms.

Hypnosis is not essential for eliciting such symptoms, but the researchers chose it for its value in focusing attention on the memories. There is no guarantee with hypnosis that the recalled information is true, and there is clear evidence that hypnosis can blur the subject's distinction between real and imaginary. This has led to current controversy regarding whether recovered memories of childhood abuse are authentic or are products of inadvertent hypnotic suggestion. It is possible that hypnosis can provide a way of digging deeper into the memory systems, perhaps accessing impressions in the amygdala or overcoming inhibition within the hippocampal–cortical memory system. This is speculation, and far from being researched so far. But it seems valid to conclude at least that breathing can be easily disrupted in certain people when certain emotional traumas are recalled.

A large number of studies were carried out by Donald Dudley and colleagues investigating the effect of emotional states on variables of breathing. The model was similar to that used by Conway: obtain a baseline, engage the subject in discussion of emotionally meaningful and disturbing topics, and observe the effect on breathing. This was done sometimes with and sometimes without hypnosis, so the effect of hypnosis was probably to facilitate or enhance the emotional intensity rather than create a distinct new experimental situation.

In his book Dudley (1969) presents many instructive case studies as well as statistical summaries. Action orientation was seen as related to increased breathing, while inaction (such states as withdrawal, apathy, and depression) was related to decreased breathing. In general, other arousal-related variables such as pulse rate, skin temperature, and catecholamine secretion were not well correlated with the breathing changes. This suggests that adjustments to breathing signify a sensitive fine-tuning of oxygen delivery, directed by shifts in emotion and cognition.

Dudley's conclusions from study of a number of patients with asthma or other breathing-related disorders are quoted below:

1. In a pneumographic study of 22 subjects, respiratory patterns were found to vary closely with the emotional state.
2. Increased rate or depth or both and sighing were found chiefly with anxiety but sometimes during anger and resentment. Decreased rate or depth or both were found when the subjects felt tense and on guard with feelings of anxiety or anger and when feeling sad or dejected.
3. Irregularity of respiration was commonly associated with anger, particularly when the feeling was suppressed. It was also associated with feelings of guilt and occurred during weeping.
4. A prolongation of expiration during periods of emotional disturbance was found in a higher proportion of subjects with asthma than in those with anxiety. In three asthmatic subjects this change was associated with wheezing and dyspnea, and in one with dyspnea alone.
5. Discussions of attitudes and conflicts known to be associated with respiratory symptoms (dyspnea and chest discomfort) evoked such symptoms in more than half of the subjects, and the symptoms were related to changes in the respiratory pattern.
6. It is concluded that respiratory symptoms associated with emotional disturbances may arise from altered respiratory function in response to symbolic stimuli to action and often are related to conflict concerning such action. (Dudley 1969, pp. 98–99)

Dissociation

Hypnosis as a mode of investigation may be out of reach of most practitioners, but it is important to at least remember that an emotional memory can be triggered and can drastically disrupt breathing, either with or without conscious awareness. Breathing is not the only body reaction triggered; any organ system can be so conditioned. The phenomenon is consistent with

LeDoux's observations about implicit memory, contextual or incidental conditioning, and what is known about dissociation and repression. In victims of traumatic stress, evidence of dissociation at the time of the original trauma is considered a significant predictor for developing post-traumatic stress disorder (Van der Kolk et al 1996, p. 314). 'Dissociation' refers to compartmentalizing of experience, such that a traumatic experience is not properly integrated into a unitary sense of self. It is as if the person retreats either from the experience as it occurs or from the subsequent memory of the experience. This process manifests as disorientation, altered body image, tunnel vision, a sense of unreality, altered time sense, unusual detachment, and out-of-body experiences. Pierre Janet, at the end of the 19th century, proposed the concept of 'memory phobia' to explain instances of dissociation, and Sigmund Freud used Janet's ideas as a springboard for his own.

Dissociation seems to be an emergency maneuver for coping with something unbearable and still remaining conscious by achieving some psychological distance; it is the mental equivalent of running away. Though it may help endure what is happening at the moment, dissociation interferes with memory storage and creates a fragmentation of experience, so that later reminders of the incident may stimulate only isolated aspects of the memory. This explains the flashbacks of the traumatized combat veteran and the victim of rape. Hyperventilation triggered by reminders of bereavement of grief may fit in this same category.

THE ANXIETY SENSITIVITY INDEX

The Anxiety Sensitivity Index (ASI) is a 16-item scale developed to differentiate two kinds of anxiety: general apprehension about many things, and specific apprehension about the symptoms of anxiety itself (Box 5.1). It has been reported in research to distinguish panic patients and those displaying symptoms of hyperventilation syndrome from other anxiety disorders. A key trait in most panic patients is anxiety about the symptoms of being anxious. This is a self-referential problem that is often called a 'vicious circle' and is akin to 'fear of fear.' Whether the attention is focused on accelerated heart rate, sweating, dyspnea, light-headedness, or some other body sign of anxiety, some people react strongly to appearance of these symptoms. This response tendency makes them high scorers on the ASI.

Reiss et al (1986), originators of the ASI, suggested that anxiety sensitivity functions as an amplifier of anxiety. In their words:

…anxiety sensitivity may be a predisposing factor in the development of fears and other anxiety disorders. According to this view, people who believe that anxiety has few or no negative effects may be able to cope with a relatively high level of exposure to

anxiety-provoking stimuli. In contrast, people who believe that anxiety has terrible effects, such as heart attacks and mental illnesses, may tend to have anxiety reactions that grow in anticipation of severe consequences. Anxiety sensitivity implies a tendency to show exaggerated and prolonged reactions to anxiety-provoking stimuli.

Reported symptoms are not necessarily 'objective' data just because they are physical. Sturges et al (1998) gave female college students the ASI and then a hyperventilation challenge task consisting of eight 15-second intervals of hyperventilation, separated by 10-second periods in which they tried to estimate their heart rates. Skin conductance was also monitored. Subjects rated both the magnitude of their physiological sensations and their subjective degree of distress. Those who had high scores on the ASI judged their heart rate changes as larger, and their anxiety as higher, than those with low scores on the ASI. The physiological changes measured, however, did not differ between the two groups. This means that the group difference was due to biased perception alone. 'Anxiety sensitivity' somehow amplified the bodily changes in the minds of the subjects. Factor analysis has shown that simply having higher general anxiety is not responsible for high ASI scores; the questionnaire taps a specific kind of anxiety which might be termed a 'body phobia.'

The ASI is more specific to panic and to hyperventilation than a standard anxiety test such as the STAI or Hamilton Anxiety Inventory, which do not discriminate between panic and other anxiety disorders such as generalized anxiety disorder, obsessive-compulsive disorder, and simple phobias. According to some studies (e.g. Cox et al 1996, 1987), the ASI contains four somewhat separate factors:

1. Fear of cardiorespiratory distress and gastrointestinal symptoms
2. Fear of cognitive/psychological symptoms
3. Fear of symptoms visible to others (social fear)
4. Fear of fainting and trembling.

If, for example, a person is interpreting mental fogginess accompanying hyperventilation as an

---

Box 5.1 Items of the Anxiety Sensitivity Index

Instructions:
Rate according to 5 descriptions:
very little = 0
a little = 1
some = 2
much = 3
very much = 4

1. It is important to me not to appear nervous
2. When I cannot keep my mind on a task, I worry that I might be going crazy
3. It scares me when I feel 'shaky' (trembling)
4. It scares me when I feel faint
5. It is important to me to stay in control of my emotions
6. It scares me when my heart beats rapidly
7. It embarrasses me when my stomach growls
8. It scares me when I am nauseous
9. When I notice that my heart is beating rapidly, I worry that I might have a heart attack
10. It scares me when I become short of breath
11. When my stomach is upset, I worry that I might be seriously ill
12. It scares me when I am unable to keep my mind on a task
13. Other people notice when I feel shaky
14. Unusual body sensations scare me
15. When I am nervous, I worry that I might be mentally ill
16. It scares me when I am nervous

© Copyright 1985 IDS Publishing Corporation.
Reprinted with kind permission.
(Norms for college students are 15.4 for males and 20.4 for females)

indicator of losing his mind, this could be addressed with explanations and reassurance about the limits to the deficit. Another person may be unconcerned about the mental fogginess but may be quite anxious about the palpitations as possible warning signs of a heart attack. This could also be dealt with by education and reassurance. The test, ideally, directs the psychological treatment as surely as a blood test would direct treatment in another clinical realm.

Hyperventilation-related cognitive and performance deficits

Many authors have observed and collected data on transient mental deficits resulting from hyperventilation. Low CO_2 is known to cause cerebral vasoconstriction, which in turn causes brain hypoxia of variable degree. The EEG is generally slowed by this hypoxia. A surge of research occurred in the 1940s and 1950s, stimulated by study of Second World War combat pilots experiencing dangerous problems in performance (Hinshaw et al 1943; Balke & Lillehei 1956). $PaCO_2$ in student pilots during training flights was found to be as low as 15 mmHg (Wayne 1958). Various studies have found loss of concentration, memory, motor coordination, reaction time, judgment, and general intellectual functioning. Wyke (1963) summarized most of this early literature, which at times had poor experimental controls for such factors as possible distraction by other symptoms, and also impaired motor coordination interfering with manual rest responses.

More recently, Van Diest et al (2000) used a test of visual attention to measure the effect of overbreathing. The task was a challenging visual task which required subjects to alternate between naming numbers and making judgments about figure sizes. Trials were run under two conditions of normal breathing and deep breathing (30 breaths per minute for 3 minutes). In addition, $PaCO_2$ was allowed to fall naturally during one trial of hyperventilation, but in another trial the $PaCO_2$ was unobtrusively replaced in order to maintain normal $PaCO_2$ in the subject. Subjects were 42 'normal' women (those with signs of hyperventilation or panic were excluded). The

task was presented in the 3 minutes during recovery from the hyperventilation.

With these controls applied, there was a clear deficit in performance, both in slower reaction times and in more errors, in a subset of subjects during the 'true hyperventilation' trials in which PCO_2 was actually lowered (the 'sham hyperventilation' did not create deficits). Subjects whose performance suffered generally had brief apneas during the 3-minute recovery stage. The resulting performance deficits were tentatively explained as due to 'prolonged central hypoxia.' The authors describe other data showing that while $PaCO_2$ recovered faster in subjects with apneas, oxygen saturation stayed lower.

Breathing pauses during the recovery stage are common because the breathing drive is reduced by the lower $PaCO_2$ level. Recovery from brief hyperventilation poses a conflict for the brain's regulatory centers: CO_2 returns to normal in the blood more quickly after hyperventilation if there are apneas during recovery, but at those moments of suspended breathing there is no oxygen taken in, and because of the vasoconstriction the brain is in a more vulnerable state.

The most focused research on this matter was by Han et al (1997) with data gathered from 399 patients with either hyperventilation syndrome or anxiety disorders, as compared with 347 normal controls. The observations were brief, consisting of a 5-minute quiet breathing baseline period, then 3 minutes of hyperventilation followed by another 5 minutes of quiet breathing. The authors found that recovery to baseline $PaCO_2$ was slower in the patient group than in the control group, confirming the Hardonk & Beumer (1979) study. The incidence of pauses during recovery was clearly higher in the control subjects than in the patients, and this difference was especially obvious in younger subjects. Control subjects seemed to terminate the hyperventilation more definitively, whereas the patient group in effect kept on hyperventilating to some degree, at least by not pausing. If the conclusions of Van Diest's study described above can be generalized from the smaller number of subjects, it means that the slow-recovering hyperventilators *without* apneas are less prone to errors of performance and perception. The authors speculate that the resistance to pausing may indicate a higher level of vigilance, a quality which the patients presumably had in abundance.

Ley & Yelich (1998) reviewed several studies which found lower Pa_{CO_2} in naturally occurring stressful situations. They studied end-tidal Pa_{CO_2} levels of 32 boys and girls (12–14 years old) divided into high and low test-anxious, determined by a standard questionnaire. The students were given tests of mathematics and word recall, and questioned in a separate session about frequency of symptoms as listed in the Nijmegen Hyperventilation Questionnaire (see Chapter 7). High test-anxiety students did not perform more poorly than the low test-anxiety students, but they did average lower end-tidal CO_2 (36.6 mmHg vs. 38.3 mmHg) as well as a faster breath rate during the tasks. They also reported significantly more symptoms on the Nijmegen questionnaire. The authors concluded by proposing that: 'the propensity to hyperventilate may exist as a trait which requires stressful conditions for its expression as a negative emotional state. This suggests the possibility that hyperventilatory complaints may, to some extent, be state-dependent and thus contingent on the context in which hyperventilation appears.'

CONCLUSIONS

Aside from medical problems, there are still many factors in the psychological and behavioral realms competing for control of breathing (see Fig. 5.1). Successful regulation must take all factors into account, with special consideration for priorities of survival. The human brain adds a layer of complication with its power to imagine, project, and recall, often stimulating breathing reflexes without apparent reason. Chapter 8 presents some psychological techniques which engage the conscious mind to improve self-regulation, but all therapeutic approaches to disturbed breathing patterns must deal with the influence of perception, emotion, and consciousness.

REFERENCES

Amaral D G, Price J L, Pitkänan A, Carmichael S T 1992 Anatomical organization of the primate amygdaloid complex. In: Aggleton J P (ed) The amygdala: neurobiological aspects of emotion, memory, and mental dysfunction. Wiley-Liss, New York, pp. 1–66

Balke B, Lillehei J 1956 Effects of hyperventilation on performance. Journal of Applied Physiology 9: 371–374

Barelli P 1994 Nasopulmonary physiology. In: Timmons B H, Ley R (eds) Behavioral and psychological approaches to breathing disorders. Plenum, New York

Beck J G, Shipherd J C, Ohtake P 2000 Do panic symptom profiles influence response to a hypoxic challenge in patients with panic disorder? A preliminary report. Psychosomatic Medicine 62: 678–683

Conway A V, Freeman L J, Nixon P G F 1988 Hypnotic examination of trigger factors in the hyperventilation syndrome. American Journal of Clinical Hypnosis 30: 296–304

Cottle M H 1972 The work, ways, positions and patterns of nasal breathing (relevance in heart and lung illness). Proceedings of the American Rhinologic Society, Kansas City, Missouri

Cottle M H 1987 The work, ways, positions and patterns of nasal breathing (relevance in heart and lung illness). Reprinted in: Barelli P, Loch W E E, Kern E R, Steiner A (eds). Rhinology. The collected writings of Maurice H.

Cottle, MD. American Rhinologic Society, Kansas City, Missouri

Cox B J, Parker J D A, Swinson R P 1996 An examination of levels of agoraphobic anxiety sensitivity: confirmatory evidence for multidimensional construct. Behaviour Research and Therapy 34: 591–598

Dudley D L 1969 Psychophysiology of respiration in health and disease. Appleton-Century-Crofts, New York

Freeman L J, Conway A, Nixon P G F 1986 Physiological responses to psychological challenge under hypnosis in patients considered to have the hyperventilation syndrome: implications for diagnosis and therapy. Journal of the Royal Society of Medicine 79 (Feb): 76–83

Gilbert C 1998 Emotional sources of dysfunctional breathing. Journal of Bodywork & Movement Therapies 2: 224–230

Hardonk J, Beumer H 1979 Hyperventilation syndrome. In P Vinken, G Bruyn (eds) Handbook of clinical neurology. Amsterdam: North Holland, 309–360

Han J N, Stegen K, Simkens K et al 1997 Unsteadiness of breathing in patients with hyperventilation syndrome and anxiety disorders. European Respiratory Journal 10: 167–176

Hinshaw H C, Rushmer R F, Boothby W M 1943 The hyperventilation syndrome and its importance in aviation medicine. Journal of Aviation Medicine 14: 100–114

Hurwitz B E 1981 The effect of inspiration and posture on cardiac rate and T-wave amplitude during apneic breathholding in man. Psychophysiology 18: 179–180 (abstract)

Jennett S 1994 Control of breathing and its disorders. In: Timmons B H, Ley R (eds) Behavioral and psychological approaches to breathing disorders. Plenum, New York

Le Doux J 1994 Emotion, memory, and the brain. Scientific American (June): 50–57

LeDoux J 1996 The emotional brain. Simon and Schuster, New York

Ley R 1999 The modification of breathing behavior: Pavlovian and operant control in emotion and cognition. Behavior Modification 23: 441–479

Ley R, Ley J, Bassett C, Schleifer L 1996 End-tidal CO_2 as a conditioned response in a Pavlovian conditioning paradigm. Paper presented at the Annual Meeting of the International Society for the Advancement of Respiratory Psychophysiology, Nijmegen, The Netherlands

Lum L C 1975 Hyperventilation: the tip and the iceberg. Journal of Psychosomatic Research 19: 375–383

Merriam-Webster 1991 Random House Webster's college dictionary. Random House, New York

Öhman A 1992 Fear and anxiety as emotional phenomena: clinical, phenomenological, evolutionary perspectives, and information-processing mechanisms. In: Lewis M, Haviland J H (eds) Handbook of the Emotions. Guilford, New York, pp 511–536

Reiss S, Peterson R A, Gursky D M, McNally R J 1986 Anxiety sensitivity, anxiety frequency and the prediction of fearfulness. Behaviour Research and Therapy 24: 1–8

Richardson C, Jull G, Hodges P, Hides J 1999 Therapeutic exercise for spinal segmental stabilisation in low back pain. Churchill Livingstone, Edinburgh

Seligman MEP 1971 Phobias and preparedness. Behavior Therapy 2: 307–320

Sturges L V, Goetsch V L, Ridley J, Whittal M 1998 Anxiety sensitivity and response to hyperventilation challenge: physiologic arousal, interoceptive acuity, and subjective distress. Journal of Anxiety Disorders 12(2): 103–115

Taylor A, Rehder K, Hyatt R, Parker J 1989 Clinical respiratory physiology. W B Saunders, Philadelphia

Van den Bergh O, Stegen K, Van de Woestijne K P 1997 Learning to have psychosomatic complaints: conditioning of respiratory behavior and somatic complaints in psychosomatic patients. Psychosomatic Medicine 59: 13–23

Van der Kolk B, Van der Hart O, Marmar C R 1996 Dissociation and information processing in posttraumatic stress disorder. In: Van der Kolk B, McFarlane A, Weisaeth L (eds) Traumatic stress. Guilford Press, New York

Van Diest I, Stegen K, Van de Woestijne K P, Schippers N, Van den Bergh O 2000 Hyperventilation and attention: effects of hypocapnia on performance in a Stroop task. Biological Psychology 53: 233–252

Wayne H H 1958 Clinical differentiation between hypoxia and hyperventilation. Journal of Aviation Medicine 29: 307

Wilhelm F H, Trabert W, Roth W T 2001. Characteristics of sighing in panic disorder. Biological Psychiatry 49: 606–614

Wyke B 1963 Brain function and metabolic disorders: the neurological effects of hydrogen-ion concentration. Butterworth, London

6

Osteopathic assessment and treatment of thoracic and respiratory dysfunction

Leon Chaitow

The information in this chapter is designed to assist any practitioner who has been professionally trained in manual methods of treatment, whether based on osteopathic, chiropractic, physiotherapeutic, or massage therapy methodology, and who would therefore be equipped with a working knowledge of anatomy and physiology. (See precautionary note below.)

⚠ Caution

While the descriptions of assessment and treatment methods may be of interest to practitioners who are not trained in manual therapeutics (such as psychotherapists, physicians, etc.), there is no suggestion that the descriptions in this chapter should be used as a basis for application of the methods unless competency has first been achieved in soft tissue and osseous manipulation methods and the individual is appropriately licensed to perform the methods involved.

Why 'osteopathic'?

Many of the methods described in this chapter have their roots in osteopathy, although some have evolved in other disciplines. At times it may not be possible to give credit to a particular profession as a source of information or methodology because of the amount of modification and evolution that has occurred. Therefore the title of the chapter, 'Osteopathic assessment and treatment ...,' should be taken to refer to the author's (LC) professional background and philosophical bias rather than being seen as a claim that everything mentioned in the chapter is 'osteopathic' in origin.

The degree of cross-fertilization now evident in bodywork in general suggests that the historical barriers which previously divided, say, osteopathy, chiropractic, and physiotherapy are gradually vanishing. Methods and concepts are now freely borrowed and adapted by each profession from each of the others, to the extent that in recent years it has become difficult from observation of application of manipulative techniques alone to guess to which profession a practitioner belongs. Hopefully, evidence based medicine and therapy will, over time, ensure that this process continues, further blurring artificial professional boundaries.

RESTORATION OF 'THREE-DIMENSIONALLY PATTERNED FUNCTIONAL SYMMETRY' (Ward 1997)

A protocol for the restoration of normal function is suggested, in which there is:

1. Identification of patterns of ease/bind, loose/tight (short/weak, etc.; see Ch. 4) in a given body area, or the body as a whole, which can emerge from sequential assessment of muscle shortness and restriction, or palpation methods, or any comprehensive evaluation of the status of the soft tissues of the body.
2. Release of areas identified as tight, restricted, tethered, possibly involving myofascial release (MFR), muscle energy techniques (MET), neuromuscular technique (NMT), positional release technique (PRT), singly or in combination, plus other effective manual approaches. (Some of these methods will be detailed in this chapter.)
3. Identification and appropriate deactivation of myofascial trigger points contained within these structures (see Ch. 4).

4. Facilitation in tone of inhibited (weak) musculature.
5. Use of articulation/mobilization or high velocity thrust (HVT) methods, applied as appropriate to the status (age, structural integrity, inflammatory status, pain levels, etc.) of the individual, should restricted joints fail to respond adequately to soft tissue mobilization.

Whether step 2 precedes step 5, or vice versa, is a matter of clinical judgment (and debate). Reeducation and rehabilitation (including home work) should involve work on posture, breathing, and patterns of use in order to restore functional integrity and prevent recurrence, as far as is possible. Exercise (home work) has to be focused, time-efficient, and within the patient's easy comprehension and capabilities, if compliance is to be achieved.

Assessment

An osteopathic approach to the evaluation of respiratory function includes taking account of the following elements (Chila 1997):

- *Category*: does breathing involve the diaphragm? the lower rib cage? both? The pattern should be charted.
- *Locus of abdominal motion*: does it move as far as the umbilicus? as far as the pubic bone? The locus should be charted.
- *Rate*: rapid? slow? The rate should be recorded before and after treatment.
- *Duration of cycle*: are inhalation and exhalation phases equal? or is one longer than the other? This should be noted.

Additionally, a series of observations and palpation methods can usefully be combined into a sequence such as that outlined below. The patient's breathing function should be evaluated by palpation and observation, seated and supine, following on from a standard evaluation of posture in which head position, shoulder rounding, crossed syndromes (see Ch. 4) are noted.

The features listed above (category, locus, rate, and duration) should form part of this evaluation.

Seated

The patient is asked to place a hand on the upper abdomen and another on the upper chest (Fig. 6.1). The hands are observed as the individual inhales several times. If the upper hand (chest) moves first, and especially if it also moves superiorly rather than slightly anterosuperiorly, and moves significantly more than the hand on the abdomen, this should be noted as indicating a dysfunctional pattern of breathing.

The practitioner stands behind the seated patient and places his hands gently over the upper trapezius area. The patient is asked to inhale while the practitioner notes whether his hands move significantly toward the ceiling: If so, the upper fixators of the shoulder/accessory breathing muscles and the scalenes are overworking, and, as most of these are postural muscles (see Ch. 4), some degree of shortening is assumed. Specific muscles can subsequently be assessed individually (see later in this chapter).

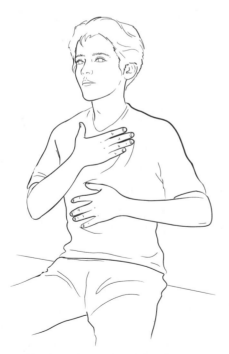

Figure 6.1 Hand positions for breathing function assessment. (Reproduced with kind permission from Chaitow & DeLany 2000.)

The practitioner kneels behind, or in front of, the patient and places his hands on the patient's lower ribs, laterally, and on inhalation notes the degree of lateral excursion (the hands pushed apart), and the degree of symmetry. (There should be a degree of lateral expansion and it should be equal.)

Supine

The patient's breathing pattern is observed, and the results recorded:

- Does abdomen move anteriorly on inhalation?
- How much of the abdomen is involved?
- Does the upper chest move forward on inhalation while the abdomen is seen to retract?
- Is there an observable lateral excursion of lower ribs?

Side-lying

Quadratus lumborum is assessed by palpation during hip abduction (see assessment method later in this chapter).

Prone

Observation is made of the 'breathing wave' (the movement of the spine from sacrum to base of neck on deep inhalation; see Ch. 4).

If appropriate (depending on the patient's degree of dysfunction), the patient is asked to perform a press-up, and to then slowly lower the body to the table, while the practitioner observes scapula stability. If winging occurs, or if either scapula moves significantly cephalad, the rhomboids and serratus anterior are considered to be inhibited (with a reasonable degree of certainty suggesting the upper fixators will be hypertonic and/or short). This imbalance will negatively impact on breathing function.

Accessory breathing muscles shortness assessment

The relative shortness of the following muscles should be assessed and charted: quadratus lumborum, psoas, pectoralis major, latissimus dorsi, upper trapezius, levator scapulae, scalenes, sternocleidomastoid, as well as thoracic and cervical paraspinal musculature (see individual assessment methods later in this chapter).

Functional assessments should be performed (involving firing sequences) in order to establish relative functional efficiency of scapulohumeral rhythm as well as hip extension and abduction (see functional tests later in this chapter).

Trigger point evaluation should be performed in muscles shown by previous assessments to be dysfunctional, using appropriate palpation methods (Boxes 6.1 and 6.2).

How well can the patient accept therapeutic intervention?

The concept of adaptation overload was discussed in Ch. 4.

Zink's work in particular suggested that rotational preferences could be ascertained via palpation assessment (Zink & Lawson 1979). Box 6.3

Box 6.1 Skin palpation methods (drag, etc.) for viscerosomatic and reflexive dysfunction

The skin overlying areas of reflexively active tissue has a heightened sympathetic tone and increased sweat activity (Lewit 1999). This increased hydrosis results in a sense of hesitation as a finger or thumb is very lightly passed across the skin. The degree of pressure required is minimal, with skin touching skin being all that is necessary (a 'feather-light' touch).

Movement of a single palpating digit should be purposeful, not too slow, and certainly not very rapid. Around 5–7 cm per second is a satisfactory speed.

A sense of 'drag' which suggests a resistance to the easy passage of the finger across the skin surface is felt for. This can be sensed as 'dryness', a 'sandpapery' feel, or a slightly harsh or rough texture. These may all indicate increased presence of sweat.

Once located, deeper pressure should elicit an area of discomfort, or, if over an active trigger point, an exquisitely sensitive area, which may refer pain elsewhere. Additional characteristics of skin overlying trigger points include the following (and see Fig. 6.2):

- Skin more adherent to underlying fascia, elicited by 'skin-rolling' or comparing bilateral skin 'pushes' which evaluate 'slideability' of local skin areas
- Skin loses local elasticity which is evaluated by introducing a sequential stretching of the skin, taking it to its elastic barrier and comparing with immediately adjacent area, and so on until an area is noted where elasticity is markedly reduced (this would also be an area of 'drag')
- There would be a variation in temperature compared with surrounding tissue, commonly warmer (indicating relative hypertonicity), but sometimes colder if tissues are ischemic (Barral 1996)
- A goose flesh appearance is observable in facilitated areas when the skin is exposed to cool air, the result of a facilitated pilomotor response
- A palpable sense of 'drag' is noticeable as a light touch contact is made across such areas, due to increased

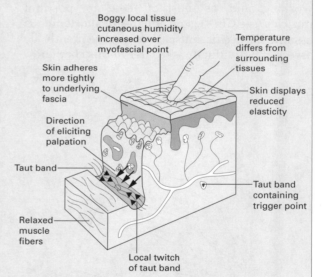

Figure 6.2 Altered physiology of tissues in region of myofascial trigger point. (Reproduced with kind permission from Chaitow & DeLany 2000.)

sweat production resulting from facilitation of the sudomotor reflexes
- There is likely to be cutaneous hyperesthesia in the related dermatome, as the sensitivity is increased (for example to a pin prick) due to facilitation
- An 'orange peel' appearance is noticeable in the subcutaneous tissues when the skin is rolled over the affected segment, due to subcutaneous trophedema.

Box 6.2 Red and white reaction

Many researchers and clinicians have described an assortment of responses in the form of 'lines', variously colored from red to white and even blue-black, after application of local skin dragging friction, with a finger or probe.

In the early days of osteopathy, in the 19th century, the phenomenon was already in use. Carl McConnell (1899) states:

I begin at the first dorsal and examine the spinal column down to the sacrum by placing my middle fingers over the spinous processes and standing directly back of the patient draw the flat surfaces of these two fingers over the spinous processes from the upper dorsal to the sacrum in such a manner that the spines of the vertebrae pass tightly between the two fingers, thus leaving a red streak where the cutaneous vessels press upon the spines of the vertebrae. In this manner slight deviations of the vertebrae laterally can be told with the greatest accuracy by observing the red line. When a vertebra or section of vertebrae are too posterior a heavy red streak is noticed and when a vertebra or section of vertebrae are too anterior the streak is not so noticeable.

More recently, Marshall Hoag (1969), writing on the examination of the spinal area using skin friction, observed:

With firm but moderate pressure the pads of the fingers are repeatedly rubbed over the surface of the skin, preferably with extensive longitudinal strokes along the paraspinal area. The blunt end of an instrument or of a pen may be used to apply friction, since the purpose is simply to detect colour change, but care must be taken to avoid abrading the skin. The appearance of less intense and rapidly fading colour in certain areas as compared with the general reaction is ascribed to increased vasoconstriction in that area, indicating a disturbance in autonomic reflex activity. The significance of this red reaction and other evidence of altered reflex activity in relation to (osteopathic) lesions has been examined in research. Others give significance to an increased degree of erythema or a prolonged lingering of the red line response.

Upledger & Vredevoogd (1983) write of this phenomenon:

Skin texture changes produced by a facilitated segment [localized areas of hyperirritability in the soft tissues involving neural sensitisation to long-term stress] are palpable as you lightly drag your fingers over the nearby paravertebral area of the back. I usually do skin drag evaluation moving from the top of the neck to the sacral area in one motion. Where your fingertips drag on the skin you will probably find a facilitated segment. After several repetitions, with increased force, the affected area will appear redder than nearby areas. This is the 'red reflex'. Muscles and connective tisues at this level will:

1) have a 'shotty' feel (like BBs under the skin);
2) be more tender to palpation;
3) be tight, and tend to restrict vertebral motion, and
4) exhibit tenderness of the spinous processes when tapped by fingers or a rubber hammer.

Irvin Korr (1970), writing of his years of osteopathic research, described how this red reflex phenomenon was shown to correspond well with areas of lowered electrical resistance, which themselves correspond accurately to regions of lowered pain threshold and areas of cutaneous and deep tenderness. He cautions:

You must not look for perfect correspondence between the skin resistance (or the red reflex) and the distribution of deeper pathologic disturbance, because an area of skin which is segmentally related to a particular muscle does not necessarily overlie that muscle. With the latissimus dorsi, for example, the myofascial disturbance might be over the hip but the reflex manifestations would be in much higher dermatomes because this muscle has its innervation from the cervical part of the cord.

By use of a mechanical instrument which quantified the pressure applied at a constant speed, followed by measurement of the duration of the redness resulting from the action of the frictional stimulator on the skin, Korr could detect areas of intense vasoconstriction which corresponded well with dysfunction elicited by manual clinical examination.

It could be said that the opportunity to 'feel' the tissues was being ignored during all these 'strokes' and 'drawing' of the fingers down the spinal musculature.

Osteopathic researchers Cox, Gorbis, Dick and Rogers (Cox et al 1983), regarding their work on identification of palpable musculoskeletal findings in coronary artery disease, describe their use of the 'red reflex' as part of their examination procedures (other methods included range of motion testing of spinal segments and ribs, assessment of local pain on palpation, and altered soft tissue texture). In this study the most sensitive parameters, which were found to be significant predictors for coronary stenosis, were limitation in range of motion and altered soft tissue texture.

'Red reflex' cutaneous stimulation was applied digitally in both paraspinal areas [T4 and T9–11] by simultaneously briskly stroking the skin in a caudad direction. Patients were divided arbitrarily into three groups.

a Grade 1 – erythema of the spinal tissues lasting less than 15 seconds after cutaneous stimulation.
b Grade 2 – erythema persisting for 15 to 30 seconds after stimulation.
3 Grade 3 – erythema persisting longer than 30 seconds after stimulation.

In this context grade 3 – maintained erythema – is seen to represent the most dysfunctional response.

Making sense of the red reaction

There appears to be a good deal to learn from the simple procedure of firmly stroking the paraspinal muscles to evoke the red reaction. The research of Cox and colleagues (1983) indicates that this one musculoskeletal assessment method alone is probably not sufficiently reliable to be diagnostic; however, when, for example, tissue texture, changes in range of motion of associated segments, pain, and the 'red reaction' are all used, a finding of the presence of several of these is a good indication of underlying dysfunction which may involve the process of viscerosomatic reflexive activity (segmental facilitation).

Box 6.2 (Continued)

Exercise

Perform the various 'strokes', as described, by running the fingers firmly down the tissues close to and parallel to the spine, on individuals with varying types of dysfunction. Observe the 'red reaction' and observe how it fades, looking for those areas which become more 'irritated' and those which become less 'irritated' when compared with surrounding tissues:

- Do tissues which seem hypertonic respond differently to normal or flaccid tissues?

- Is there increased sensitivity to pressure in areas which redden or which blanch when stroked in this way, or is there little difference?
- What is the degree of skin tightness over these different areas?
- What is the degree of skin adherence to underlying connective tissue (skin-rolling or lifting) in the different areas?

Is eliciting of the 'red reflex' likely to be of any clinical value to you?

Box 6.3 Postural patterns (Zink & Lawson 1979; Fig. 4.11)

Zink has described patterns of postural patterning determined by fascial compensation and decompensation:

- Fascial compensation is seen as a useful, beneficial and above all functional (i.e. no obvious symptoms result) response on the part of the musculoskeletal system, for example as compensation for anomalies such as a short leg, or overuse behavior.
- Decompensation describes the same phenomenon where adaptive changes are seen to be dysfunctional (to produce symptoms), evidencing a breakdown of homeostatic mechanisms.

By testing the tissue 'preferences' (loose/tight) in different areas it is possible to classify patterns in clinically useful ways:

- *Ideal* (minimal adaptive load transferred to other regions)
- *Compensated* patterns which alternate in direction from area to area (e.g. atlanto-occipital–cervicothoracic– thoracolumbar–lumbosacral) and which are commonly adaptive in nature
- *Uncompensated* patterns which do not alternate, and which are commonly the result of trauma.

It is well to keep in mind the discussion of 'tight/loose' assessments (Ch. 4) when these patterns are evaluated.
   Zink has described methods for testing tissue preference:

- There are four crossover sites where fascial tensions can be noted, occipitoatlantal (OA), cervicothoracic (CT), thoracolumbar (TL), and lumbosacral (LS).
- These sites are tested for rotation and side-bending preference.
- Zink's research showed that most people display alternating patterns of rotatory preference with about 80% of people showing a common pattern of L-R-L-R (termed the 'common compensatory pattern' or CCP).
- Zink observed that the 20% of people whose compensatory pattern did not alternate had poor health histories.

- Treatment of either CCP, or uncompensated fascial patterns, has the objective of trying, as far as is possible, to create a more symmetrical degree of rotatory motion at the key crossover sites.
- The methods used range from direct HVLA thrust, or muscle energy approaches, to indirect positional release techniques.

Assessment of tissue preference

Occipitoatlantal area

- Patient is supine
- Practitioner sits at head, slightly to one side so that he is facing the corner of the table
- One hand (caudal hand) cradles the occiput with opposed index finger and thumb controlling the atlas
- The neck is flexed so that rotatory motion is focused into the upper cervical area only
- The other hand is placed on patient's forehead
- The contacts on the occipitoatlantal joint evaluate the tissue preference as the area is slowly rotated left and right.

Cervicothoracic area

- Patient is supine in relaxed posture
- Practitioner sits at head of table and slides hands under the patient's scapulae
- Each hand independently assesses the area being palpated for its tightness/looseness preferences by easing first one and then the other scapula area towards the ceiling.

Thoracolumbar area

- Patient is supine; practitioner at waist level faces cephalad and places hands over lower thoracic structures, fingers along lower rib shafts laterally
- Treating the structure being palpated as a cylinder, the hands test the preference this has to rotate around its central axis. First one way and then the other.

Box 6.3 (Continued)

Lumbosacral area

- Patient is supine; practitioner stands below waist level, facing cephalad, and places hands on anterior pelvic structures, using the contact as a 'steering wheel' to evaluate tissue preference as the pelvis is rotated around its central axis seeking information as to its tightness/looseness preferences.

These general evaluation approaches, which seek evidence of compensation and of global adaptation patterns, involving loose and tight tissues, offer a broad means of commencing respiratory rehabilitation, by altering structural features associated with dysfunction.

---

gives details of Zink's functional evaluation approach.

OSTEOPATHIC APPROACHES TO BREATHING DYSFUNCTION

The treatment of respiratory dysfunction by means of osteopathic manipulative therapy (OMT) dates back to the beginning of the 20th century. It is logical that a therapeutic system which had normalization of the musculoskeletal system as a primary therapeutic goal should see breathing dysfunction as an appropriate focus for its work.

There is ample scope for biomechanical dysfunction to appear in the 'machinery' of breathing, involving as it does the thoracic cage acting as a pump, coordinated by complicated central controls, utilizing integrated muscular contractions and relaxations, together with fascial accommodations, all modulated by neural activity, and inducing movement in almost every joint in the body.

The viscerosomatic reflex and facilitation (Fig. 6.3)

The osteopathic profession's interest in viscerosomatic reflexes is strong, since these appear to create and maintain biomechanical changes. The rationale that structural compensation accompanies all functional change is at the heart of much osteopathic thinking. (See Ch. 4 for fuller discussion of this.)

The viscerosomatic reflex involves afferent stimuli, which arise from visceral disturbances, modifying somatic tissues, particularly the skel-

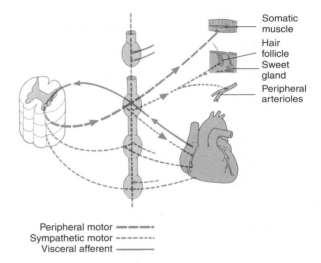

Peripheral motor ‒ ‒ ‒ ‒ ‒
Sympathetic motor ------------
Visceral afferent ─────

Figure 6.3 Schematic representation of viscerosomatic reflex. (Reproduced with kind permission from Chaitow & DeLany 2000.)

etal muscles and skin overlying the dorsal horn of the spinal cord at the level which supplies the organ involved. Palpable increased tone in skeletal muscle (including spasm and even paravertebral splinting) have been shown to derive from nociceptive visceral stimuli.

It is suggested that preclinical signs of visceral dysfunction may be noted in somatic tissues. The most obvious examples of this phenomenon are seen in cardiac conditions (Kolzumi & Brooks 1972; Beal 1984).

Since the segmental sites which display viscerosomatic responses relate directly to the levels of autonomic supply to the organ, pulmonary reflex changes are found at the levels of C3 and C4, as well as T2–T9 (D'Alonzo & Krachman 1997).

Viscerosomatic reflex studies

'In a 5-year, double-blind study of 5000 hospitalized patients who were examined for evidence of somatic dysfunction and its relationship to diagnosis, most visceral diseases appeared to have more than one region with an increased frequency of segmental findings' (Kelso 1971):

- Unpaired viscera demonstrated more one-sided segmental findings
- The number of segments involved seemed to correlate with the duration of the condition
- Subsequently, the same researcher reported that there was increased incidence of palpable dysfunctional findings (characterized by sensitivity, altered tissue feel, asymmetry, restricted mobility) in individuals with upper airway diseases, and in the upper thoracic spine in patients with lower respiratory illnesses (Kelso et al 1980).

Additional supportive research found the following:

- The majority of 40 patients with a diagnosis of pulmonary disease, predominantly chronic obstructive lung disease, demonstrated somatic dysfunction at two or more adjacent segments between T2 and T7, characterized by deep-muscle splinting and resistance to compression motion (see compression test description in Box 6.4) (Beal 1984).
- Paravertebral skin changes were evaluated in patients with chronic obstructive lung disease evaluating for skin 'drag' and 'red reaction' (see descriptions in Boxes 6.1 and 6.2). Additional evaluations involved tests for altered mobility. The greatest number of positive findings were noted at the levels of spinal segments T1–T9 (Miller 1975).

Box 6.4 Palpating facilitated spinal tissues (Beal 1983)

Somatic dysfunction is assessed most usually by use of palpatory investigation to evaluate four features: asymmetry (A), range of motion changes (R), tenderness (T), and tissue texture changes (T). Beal insists that investigation should also pay attention to the various soft-tissue layers: 'The skin for changes in texture, temperature and moisture: the subcutaneous tissue for changes in consistency and fluid; the superficial and deep musculature for tone, irritability, consistency, viscoelastic properties, and fluid content; and the deep fascial layers for textural changes.' He advises that, 'Special attention be given to the examination of the costotransverse area, where it is felt that autonomic nerve effects are predominant,' and he notes that tests for the quality and range of joints have not been found to differentiate between visceral reflexes and somatic changes, which confirms the importance of the soft tissue assessment in order to elicit such information.

Beal suggests the supine position is ideal for assessment of paraspinal tissues. The hand should be gently inserted under the region, and pressure or springing techniques applied (Fig. 6.4).

Beal suggests that the diagnosis of a paraspinal viscerosomatic reflex be based upon two or more adjacent spinal segments showing evidence of somatic dysfunction (ARTT), and being located within the specific autonomic reflex area. There should be deep confluent spinal muscle splinting, and resistance to segmental joint motion. Skin and subcutaneous tissue changes which are consistent with the acuteness or chronicity of the reflex should be noted.

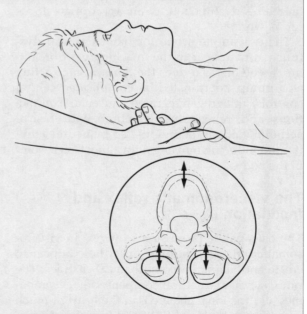

Figure 6.4 Springing assessment for tissue resistance associated with segmental facilitation. (Reproduced with kind permission from Chaitow & DeLany 2000.)

- It is generally accepted within osteopathic medicine that viscerosomatic reflexes involve afferent activity from the viscera, resulting in changes in paravertebral muscular status at the appropriate segmental level. It is suggested that viscerosomatic reflexes occur even in response to mild stimuli, a phenomenon known as facilitation. For reasons which are unclear, lung disease, irrespective of the side, produces changes paravertebrally/segmentally which are more obvious on the left side (Beal 1984).
- It is worth reemphasizing that any musculoskeletal changes which result from viscerosomatic reflex activity – i.e. the facilitation effects – are almost certain to restrict normal rib cage and spinal (including cervical) mobility, and so add to any existing respiratory dysfunction.
- D'Alonzo & Krachman (1997) also point out that, 'Spinal facilitation could interfere with appropriate diaphragmatic function.' Normal function of the diaphragm might be affected by rib and spinal restrictions resulting from viscerosomatic influences, leading to inappropriate recruitment of accessory breathing muscles such as the scalenes and sternocleidomastoid, with a further decline in respiratory function as a consequence.

Osteopathic benefits: supportive studies

The theoretical value of osteopathic methods in treating serious respiratory dysfunction are supported by studies which indicate significant benefit in some parameters. There exists some early evidence of the value of OMT in treating respiratory diseases such as whooping cough (Kurschner 1958). In that study the use of chloramphenicol alone was compared with chloramphenicol with OMT in treatment of children with whooping cough. This study was small and poorly controlled, but its general conclusion was that children receiving OMT had a shorter duration of illness and more rapid return to school, as well as having a lower daily cough average.

An 18-month study of over 250 hospitalized children with respiratory infections involved all children receiving various combinations of OMT and/or antibiotics. Those patients who received antibiotics, supportive therapy and manipulation recovered more rapidly than those who received either manipulation or antibiotics alone (Kline 1965).

Osteopathy and asthma

It is not suggested that osteopathic attention replace standard pharmacological asthma protocols, which should also attempt to identify and avoid environmental and psychological triggers. Osteopathic manipulative and rehabilitation approaches to assist the asthmatic patient include the following (Rowane & Rowane 1999):

- Explanation and reassurance (Paul & Buser 1996)
- Paravertebral thoracic soft tissue treatment with patient seated (D'Alonzo & Krachman 1997)
- Patient in same position, practitioner behind, rib mobilization ('rib raising') is carried out together with stretching and mobilizing of intercostal muscles from T1 to T6, as the patient carries out diaphragmatic breathing with pursed-lip breathing (PLB – see later in this chapter) (Beal 1985)
- Direct myofascial release with respiratory cooperation is employed to achieve doming of the diaphragm (DiGiovanna 1997)
- Controlled breath training is initiated (Faling 1995) involving PLB in order to relieve dyspnea, slow respiratory rate, reduce air trapping, and encourage diaphragmatic function (Muellen et al 1970).

Osteopathy and pneumonia

As for asthma, osteopathic adjunctive therapy in the treatment of pneumonia is not a replacement for standard pharmacological and medical care. Background research into the influence of osteopathic manipulative therapy (OMT) for these patients includes the following findings:

- Somatic dysfunction localized to the spinal areas of T2–T7 has been shown to be associated with pulmonary disease (Beal 1985, Beal 1984)

- Osteopathic thoracic lymphatic pump techniques (see later this chapter for description) has been shown to prevent lung atelectasis as effectively as incentive spirometry (Oppenheimer 1990)
- Adjunctive osteopathic OMT has been shown to be beneficial in treating patients with chronic obstructive lung disease, with significant improvement in $PaCO_2$, oxygen saturation, total lung capacity, and residual volume relative to baseline measures (Howell et al 1975).

D'Alonzo & Krachman (1997) list the main objectives of osteopathic adjunctive treatment of pneumonia as:

- Reduced parenchymal lung congestion
- Reduced sympathetic hyper-reactivity to the parenchyma of the lung
- Increased mechanical thoracic cage motion.'

A pilot study (Noll et al 1999) was conducted to evaluate the effectiveness of adjunctive OMT in treatment of pneumonia in elderly hospitalized patients. The criteria for inclusion were as follows:

- Age over 60
- New pulmonary infiltrate consistent with a radiological diagnosis of pneumonia, plus at least two other clinical findings
- fever, leukocytosis, new cough, or acute change in mental status.

Excluded were patients with lung abscess, tuberculosis, lung cancer, acute fractures, or metastatic bone disease.

After assignment to either the experimental or the control group, all patients received conventional medical treatment for pneumonia. The patients in the experimental group (eight women, three men) received a standardized OMT protocol which comprised:

- Bilateral paraspinal muscle inhibition (sustained digital pressure)
- Bilateral rib raising (see protocol for asthma OMT, above, and methodology, below)
- Diaphragmatic myofascial release

- Condylar decompression, cervical soft tissue technique
- Bilateral myofascial release to anterior thoracic inlet
- Thoracic osteopathic lymphatic pump technique (see later in this chapter).

All these procedures were performed by osteopathic physicians, with patients in their hospital beds, twice daily on weekdays and once a day at weekends, for 10–15 min. Specific somatic dysfunctions, assessed during structural examination, were also treated osteopathically in the treatment group.

Patients in the control group (seven women, three men) received light touch 'sham' treatments, in addition to their conventional medical care. The sham treatment comprised manual contact to the same physical areas, and for the same duration of time, as the treatment group, but with no joint articulation or movement of the soft tissues.

The attending physicians and the house staff were blind to patient group assignment. Neither patients nor their family members were informed as to the group to which they had been assigned.

During the study, two of the control group and none of the treatment group died.

The results showed that:

- There were no significant changes between the groups in X-ray status.
- Obtaining bedside pulmonary function test results was problematic in more than half the patients, due to inability to forcibly inhale and exhale (due to baseline dementia, acute delirium, or general physical weakness); therefore results from this test were not meaningful.
- There was no meaningful difference between the groups for mean duration or the number of febrile days.
- The mean duration of i.v. antibiotic therapy (8.2 days ± 5.2, as against 11.8 days ± 5.7), the duration of total antibiotic therapy, and the length of hospital stay (13.5 days ± 6.3 as against 15.8 days ± 6.4) were all significantly shorter in the treatment group.
- Of possible interest was the finding that those in the treatment group had a slightly greater duration of fever than the control group

(though not significantly). This hints at a more appropriate immune response in those receiving OMT treatment, something which has previously been suggested by Measel (1982).

- The most significant difference between the groups was the mean duration of oral antibiotic therapy, with the treatment group significantly longer (3.1 days ± 3) than the control group (0.8 days ± 1.3), due to removal from i.v. antibiotic therapy sooner than the control group, following more rapid clinical improvement.
- The shorter length of hospital stay and i.v. antibiotic use could have significant economic implications.

ADJUNCTIVE OSTEOPATHIC MANIPULATIVE THERAPY (OMT) METHODS FOR ENHANCING RESPIRATORY FUNCTION

Later in this chapter, assessment and treatment methods will be detailed for specific accessory breathing muscle dysfunction. Treatment methods for such dysfunction include muscle energy techniques (MET) and positional release (PR) techniques. In addition, protocols will be outlined for deactivation of trigger points which might be adding to the adaptive load of the patient.

The methods outlined immediately below are more broadly focused, and have a long and useful history of application in osteopathic medicine, some dating back to the late 19th century, having subsequently been validated in numerous studies.

1. Thoracic lymphatic pump techniques

Lymphatic pump techniques are indicated for conditions in which enhancement of thoracic range of motion and increased expiratory efficacy is desirable, particularly in cases of chronic obstructive pulmonary disease, upper and lower respiratory infections and for postsurgical reduction of respiratory volume.

Slesynski & Kelso (1993) demonstrated that when lymphatic pump technique was administered on the first day postoperatively in patients

who had undergone cholecystectomy there was a more rapid recovery and a quicker return towards preoperative values for FVC and FEV_1 than in patients treated with incentive spirometry.

D'Alonzo & Krachman (1997) report that this technique 'increases vital capacity, the mobility of the rib cage, improves diaphragmatic function, clears airway secretions and possibly enhances immune function.' Preliminary studies have indeed suggested enhanced immune function following use of lymphatic pump techniques (Measel 1982).

These osteopathic methods are designed to augment pressure gradients between thoracic and abdominal regions. Variations include methods which are rhythmic and those which are continuous. Contraindications include fractures, osteoporosis, dislocations, or malignancy of the lymphatic system.

⚠ Caution is advised in patients with reduced cough reflex.

Method

The patient is supine. It is important to ensure that the patient has no food, gum, or loose dentures in the mouth. The practitioner stands at the head of the table and places his hands on the patient's thoracic wall so that the thenar eminences cover the pectoral muscles just distal to the clavicle, with fingers spread towards the sides of the trunk. In this way the heels of the hands rest over ribs 2–4 (Fig. 6.5).

A rhythmic pumping action of the thorax is introduced by means of the practitioner lightly flexing and extending the elbows, with the forearms, wrists, and hands fixed, at a rate of approximately two per second. The patient is instructed to breathe normally during the process, which should continue for 2–5 minutes.

2. Doming of the diaphragm using indirect and direct approaches

This method is designed to relax the resting state of the diaphragm, enhancing its contraction and

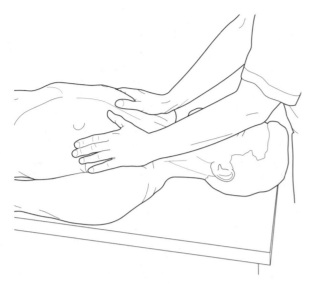

Figure 6.5 Thoracic pump. (From Ward 1997.)

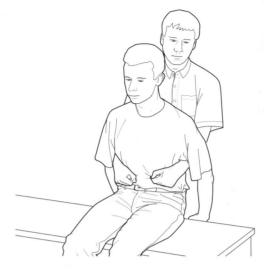

Figure 6.6 Doming of the diaphragm technique utilizes direct myofascial release with respiratory cooperation to improve diaphragmatic function. (From Rowane & Rowane 1999.)

relaxation functions, so creating a greater pressure gradient between the thorax and abdomen, thus improving venous and lymphatic circulation as well as augmenting expiration (Wallace et al 1997).

Indirect approach method (positional release)

The patient is seated erect, relaxed but not slumped. The practitioner stands behind the patient and passes his hands around the thoracic cage, carefully introducing fingers beneath the costal margins (Fig. 6.6).

The thorax should be carefully rotated left and then right to determine which direction offers the greatest degree of freedom and ease of motion. With the fingers remaining curled under the costal margins, so that the tips are close to the diaphragmatic attachment, the thorax is eased in the direction of greatest ease (the direction in which it rotates most freely).

This position is held, and the hands are used to support and follow the tissues as a slow releasing, 'unwinding', process ensues.

When the diaphragm resumes a free rhythmic vertical motion the rotational preference should be retested, and found to be more symmetrical.

Variation: direct approach

This uses the same starting position, with the practitioner standing behind the seated patient, fingers curled under costal margins (see Fig. 6.6). The patient slightly rounds the trunk in order to relax rectus abdominis, and breathes moderately deeply. During an exhalation the practitioner grasps the lower ribs and costal margin and eases the hands caudally.

This firm, but gentle, traction is maintained as the patient inhales, causing a doming effect of the diaphragm.

The pull toward the floor is maintained for several subsequent cycles of exhalation and inhalation, even if the finger/hand contact on the lower ribs and costal margin is lost (which it usually is), leaving only a soft tissue hold on the tissues.

The caudal traction on the soft tissues is sufficient to maintain the effect on the diaphragm.

3. Rib raising

The objective is to free restrictions in rib cage motion which impact on normal respiratory effort and retard venous blood and lymph movement.

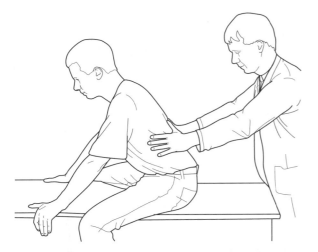

Figure 6.7 Rib raising. (From Rowane & Rowane 1999.)

The patient is seated, straddling the treatment table, back close to the end, hands placed on the table in front of the pelvis. The practitioner stands behind the seated patient and places his hands so that the fingers spread laterally as the thumbs lie parallel with, and inferior to, a pair of ribs (Fig. 6.7).

Pressure is applied anteriorly and slightly cephalad in order to stretch and release the intercostal and paravertebral musculature as the patient *inhales* and leans backward against the practitioner's contact hands. The patient is then asked to breathe slowly and deeply using diaphragmatic and pursed-lip breathing (see below). On *exhalation* the patient eases back to the start position and the practitioner either maintains contact or moves to a different pair of ribs, so that, sequentially, all ribs from T1 to the lower thoracics are 'raised' and released.

According to Rowane & Rowane (1999): 'This procedure is continued … especially on the left side, where the viscerosomatic reflex of the sympathetic nervous system to the lungs is located (Beal 1985).'

4. Pursed-lip breathing (PLB)

This form of breathing, when combined with diaphragmatic breathing, has been shown to enhance pulmonary mechanics and breathing efficiency.

The patient is seated or supine and places the dominant hand on the abdomen and the other hand on the chest. The patient is asked to breathe in through the nose and out through the mouth with pursed lips, ensuring diaphragmatic involvement, if possible, by means of movement against the hand on the abdomen at the outset of inhalation.

Exhalation through the pursed lips is performed slowly and has been shown to relieve dyspnea, slow the respiratory rate, increase tidal volume, and help to restore diaphragmatic function (Tisp et al 1986, Faling 1995).

NORMALIZING MUSCULAR AND JOINT RESTRICTIONS

The methods outlined below for normalizing muscular and joint restrictions are largely soft tissue focused. There is of course a place for high velocity, low amplitude (HVLA) thrust techniques, however, these are not described here (Gibbons & Teahy 2000).

In osteopathic methodology, assessment of spinal joint restrictions is made on the basis of a number of positive findings using, among other criteria, asymmetry (A), range of motion alteration (R), tissue texture changes (T) and, as a rule, reported tenderness (T). The 'ARTT' palpation sequence identifies areas of somatic dysfunction, and HVLA is one means of normalizing such dysfunction (see Box 6.4).

Alternatives to HVLA thrust approaches include MET, positional release (PR) methods, and physiotherapy approaches such as Mulligan's 'mobilization with movement' (MWM, e.g. SNAGs and NAGs) techniques (Mulligan 1992).

Practitioners trained in these methods (HVLA thrust, MWM, etc.) will know their relative clinical value. Those not so trained may wish to read more deeply about them: recommended texts are those by Greenman (1996), DiGiovanna (1997), Gibbons & Tehan (2000), and Mulligan (1992).

MUSCLE ENERGY TECHNIQUE (MET) PROCEDURES

A selection of MET treatment methods aimed at normalizing thoracic, spinal, rib, and short postural muscle dysfunctions are described below. First, the basic 'rules' of osteopathic MET are outlined:

MET methodology

- When the term 'restriction barrier' is used in relation to soft tissue structures, it is meant to indicate the first signs of resistance (as palpated by sense of 'bind', or sense of effort required to move the area, or by visual or other palpable evidence) and not the greatest pain free range of movement obtainable.
- In all treatment descriptions involving MET it will be assumed that the shorthand reference to 'acute' and 'chronic' will be adequate to indicate the variations in methodology which these terms call for, especially in relation to the starting position for contractions ('acute' starts at the barrier and 'chronic' just short of the barrier). Acute is defined as recent onset (under 3 weeks) following strain or trauma, or acutely painful (Moore 1980).
- Subsequent to an isometric contraction, the tissues are taken to the new barrier in an acute setting, and through the barrier into light stretch in a chronic setting. In treating fragile and/or pain-ridden individuals with MET, the acute mode is always adopted – i.e. no stretching!
- Assistance from the patient is valuable when movement is made to or through a barrier, providing the patient can be educated to gentle cooperation and not to use excessive effort.
- In most MET treatment guidelines the method described involves the isometric contraction of the agonist(s), the muscle(s) which require stretching. This employs the temporary release of tone (approximately 20 seconds) known as *post isometric relaxation* (PIR) (Lewit 1999).
- It is also possible to use the antagonists to achieve *reciprocal inhibition* (RI) before initiating stretch or movement to a new barrier. This alternative is used when appropriate (for

example if there is pain on use of the agonist or where there has been trauma to the agonist).
- Eccentric isotonic contractions, performed slowly, involving inhibited antagonists to shortened hypertonic structures, achieve the double benefit of both toning the weaker muscles and also releasing tone in the antagonists (Norris 2000).
- There should be *no pain* experienced during application of MET, although mild discomfort (stretching) is acceptable.
- The methods recommended provide a sound basis for the application of MET to specific muscles and areas. By developing the skills with which to apply the methods, as described, a repertoire of techniques can be acquired offering a wide base of choices appropriate in numerous clinical settings.
- Breathing cooperation may be used as part of the methodology of MET. A patient who is cooperative and capable of following instructions can be asked to inhale at the same time that an isometric contraction is slowly performed against resistance. The breath is held for approximately 7 seconds, and slowly released as the effort ceases. A further inhalation and exhalation is then performed, together with the instruction to 'let go completely.' As relaxation occurs, the new barrier is engaged, or the barrier is passed as the muscle is stretched.
- Eye movements are sometimes advocated during contractions and stretches, particularly by Lewit (1999), who uses these methods to great effect in treating muscles such as the scalenes and sternomastoid.
- Pulsed muscle energy technique (pulsed MET – see below), based on Ruddy's work, can be substituted for any of the methods described in the text below for treating shortened soft tissue structures, or increasing range of motion in joints (Ruddy 1962).

Ruddy's 'pulsed MET' variation

A promising addition to this sequence takes account of the potential offered by the methods developed by osteopathic physician T. J. Ruddy

(1962). The dysfunctional tissue or joint is held at its restriction barrier, at which time the patient (or the practitioner if the patient cannot adequately cooperate with the instructions), against the resistance of the practitioner, introduces a series of rapid (2 per second), *minute* contraction efforts towards the barrier. The barest initiation of effort is called for with, to use Ruddy's term, 'no wobble and no bounce.'

The application of this 'conditioning' approach involves contractions which are, 'short, rapid and rhythmic, gradually increasing the amplitude and degree of resistance, thus conditioning the proprioceptive system by rapid movements.' Ruddy suggests that the beneficial effects include improved oxygenation and enhanced venous and lymphatic circulation through the area being treated.

After a 10-second sequence of contractions, the patient relaxes and the tissues (or joint) are taken to a new barrier, and the process is repeated.

Pulsed facilitation of antagonists

In a context in which tense, hypertonic, possibly shortened musculature is treated by stretching following MET, it is important to begin facilitating and strengthening the inhibited antagonists. This is true whether the hypertonic muscles have been treated for reasons of shortness/hypertonicity alone or because they accommodate active trigger points within their fibers. The method has been termed *Ruddy's reciprocal antagonist facilitation* (RRAF). (An example of this is given at the end of the MET treatment of upper trapezius, below.)

The introduction of a pulsed muscle energy procedure (such as Ruddy's) involving these weak antagonists offers the opportunity for:

- Proprioceptive reeducation
- Strengthening facilitation of the weak antagonists
- Further inhibition of tense agonists
- Enhanced local circulation and drainage
- 'Reeducation of movement patterns on a reflex, subcortical basis' (Liebenson 1996).

MET for joint restrictions

Treatment of joint restrictions using MET involves the same preparatory steps as those required for a high velocity thrust – the barrier of resistance needs to be engaged. The difference is that, instead of a thrust, the MET procedure requires the patient to introduce a resisted isometric contraction to, or away from, the barrier, after which slack is taken out and the new barrier is engaged. No forceful movement through the restriction barrier is used: it either retreats or it does not.

As a general rule, soft tissue normalization should be encouraged prior to joint mobilization, with the degree of therapeutic input being tailored to the patient's conditions and vitality. There are sufficient variations and modulations available to allow for – extremely gentle – application of MET even to severely distressed and exhausted individuals, without overloading their adaptation potentials.

Some examples of the use of MET in treating joint restrictions are described below. The examples given are not intended to constitute a comprehensive list of all the possible MET joint applications available but rather a selection of specimen demonstrations. A wider range of MET applications can be found in osteopathic and other texts, including Ward (1997), Chaitow (2001) and Greenman (1996).

Evaluating and treating thoracic spine restrictions using MET
(Yates 1991)

In treating joint restriction with MET, Sandra Yates (1991) suggests the following simple criteria should be observed:

1. The joint should be positioned at its physiological barrier – specific in three planes.
2. When spinal segments are being treated, flexion–extension, side-bending, and rotation barriers should be engaged.
3. The patient should be asked to statically contract muscles toward their freedom of motion (i.e. away from the barrier(s) of

restriction) as the practitioner resists totally any movement of the part. The contraction, Yates suggests, should be held for about 3 seconds (many MET experts suggest longer – up to 10 seconds).

4. The amount of effort employed should be well short of total, and an instruction such as 'using only 25% of your strength, push toward the left,' or some such form of words, would be appropriate to achieve the postisometric effect.

5. Following the isometric effort, the patient is asked to relax for 2 seconds or so, at which time the practitioner reengages the joint at its new motion barrier(s).

This process is repeated until free movement is achieved or until no further gain is apparent following a contraction.

Harakal's cooperative isometric technique (Harakal 1975; Fig. 6.8)

This technique can be used when there is a specific or general restriction in a thoracic spinal articulation (for example). The area should be placed in neutral (patient seated usually). The permitted range of motion should be determined by noting the joint's resistance to further motion.

The patient should be rested for some seconds at a point just short of the resistance barrier, termed the 'point of balanced tension,' in order to 'permit anatomic and physiologic response' to occur. The patient is asked to reverse the movement toward the barrier by 'turning back toward where we started' (thus contracting any agonists which may be influencing the restriction).

The degree of patient participation at this stage can be at various levels, ranging from 'just think

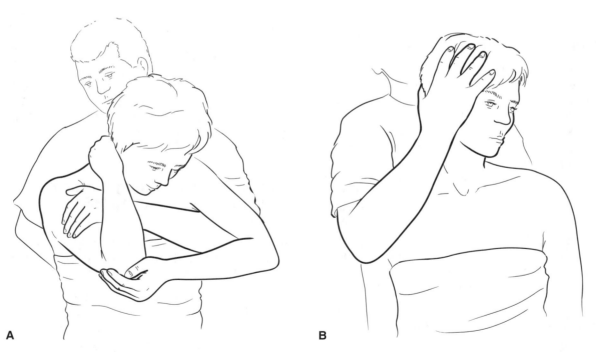

A   **B**

Figure 6.8 A Harakal's approach requires the restricted segment to be taken to a position just short of the assessed restriction barrier before isometric contraction is introduced as the patient attempts to return to neutral, after which slack is removed and the new barrier engaged. **B** Side-bending and rotation restriction of the cervical region is treated by holding the neck just short of the restriction barrier and having the patient attempt to return to neutral, after which slack is removed and the new barrier engaged. (Reproduced with kind permission from Chaitow & DeLany 2000.)

about turning' to 'turn as hard as you would like,' or by giving specific instructions.

Following a holding of this effort for a few seconds and then relaxing completely, the patient is taken further in the direction of the previous barrier, to a new point of restriction determined by the resistance to further motion as well as tissue response (feel for 'bind').

The procedure is repeated until no further gain is being achieved.

(It would also, of course, be appropriate to use the opposite direction of rotation, for example asking the patient to 'turn further toward the direction you are moving.')

MET for rib dysfunction
(Hruby & Goodridge 1997, Greenman 1996)

In order to use MET successfully to normalize rib dysfunction, the precise nature of the problem requires identification. In this segment of the chapter only a limited number of rib problems are considered in order to illustrate MET usefulness. Greenman (1996) and Ward (1997) offer a wider range of MET choices and repay further study.

Restrictions in the ability of a given rib to move fully (as compared with its pair) during inhalation indicates a depressed status, while an inability to move fully (as compared with its pair) into exhalation indicates an elevated status. As a rule, unless there has been direct trauma, rib restrictions of this sort are compensatory, and involve groups of ribs. Osteopathic clinical experience suggests that if a group of depressed ribs is located, the 'key' rib is likely to be the most superior of these: if successfully released, it will 'unlock' the remaining ribs in that group. Similarly, if a group of elevated ribs is located, the 'key' rib is likely to be the most inferior of these: if successfully released, this rib will 'unlock' the remaining ribs in that group.

If palpation commences at the most cephalad aspect of the thorax, the 2nd rib is the most easily palpated. The ribs are sequentially assessed, and if a depressed rib is noted this is clearly the most cephalad and is the one to be treated (see below). Similarly, if an elevated rib is identified the ribs continue to be evaluated until a normal pair is located and the dysfunctional rib cephalad to these is treated.

MET methods described below are one way of releasing such restrictions; however, there are also extremely useful positional release methods for treating such problems, based on Jones's Strain/counterstrain methods (Jones 1981).

As in all forms of somatic dysfunction, causes should be sought and addressed in addition to mobilization of restrictions using MET or other methods, as described in this text.

Rib palpation test: rib 1 (Fig. 6.9)

The patient is seated and the practitioner stands behind. The practitioner places his hands so that the fingers can draw posteriorly the upper trapezius fibers lying superior to the 1st rib. The tips of the practitioner's middle and index, or middle and ring fingers can then most easily be placed on the superior surface of the posterior shaft of the 1st rib.

Symmetry is evaluated as the patient breathes lightly.

The commonest dysfunction is for one of the pair of 1st ribs to be 'locked' in an elevated position ('exhalation restriction'). The superior aspect of this rib will palpate as tender, and attached scalene structures are likely to be short and tight (Greenman 1996).

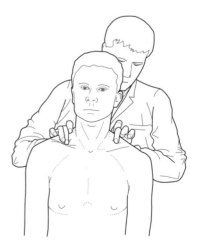

Figure 6.9 Rib palpation test. (From Greenman 1996.)

Or

The patient is seated and the practitioner stands behind. The practitioner places his hands so that the fingers can draw posteriorly the upper trapezius fibers lying superior to the 1st rib. The tips of the practitioner's middle and index, or middle and ring fingers can then most easily be placed on the superior surface of the posterior shaft of the 1st rib.

The patient exhales and shrugs his shoulders and the palpated 1st ribs behave asymmetrically (one moves superiorly more than the other), or:

The patient exhales fully and the palpated 1st ribs behave asymmetrically (one moves inferiorly more than the other).

The commonest restriction of the 1st rib is into elevation and the likeliest soft tissue involvement is of anterior and medial scalenes (Goodridge & Kuchera 1997).

Rib palpation test: ribs 2–10

The patient is supine. The practitioner stands at waist level, facing the patient's head, with a single finger contact on the superior aspect of one pair of ribs (Fig. 6.10). The practitioner's dominant eye determines the side of the table from which he is approaching the observation of rib function (right-eye dominant calls for standing on the patient's right side). The fingers are observed as the patient inhales and exhales fully (eye focus is on an area between the palpating fingers so that peripheral vision assesses symmetry of movement).

If one of a pair of ribs fails to rise as far as its pair on inhalation it is described as a depressed rib, unable to move fully to its end of range on inhalation ('exhalation restriction'). If one of a pair of ribs fails to fall as far as its pair on exhalation it is described as an elevated rib, unable to move fully to its end of range on exhalation ('inhalation restriction').

Rib palpation test: ribs 11 and 12

Assessment of ribs 11 and 12 is usually performed with the patient prone and palpation performed with a hand contact on the posterior shafts to evaluate full inhalation and exhalation motions (Fig. 6.11).

The 11th and 12th ribs usually operate as a pair, so that if any sense of reduction in posterior motion is noted on one side or the other, on inhalation, both are regarded as depressed, unable to fully inhale ('exhalation restriction'). If any sense of reduction in anterior motion is noted on one side or the other, on exhalation, the

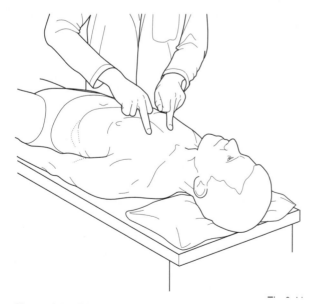

Figure 6.10 Rib palpation test. (From Greenman 1996.)

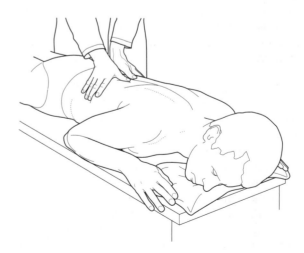

Figure 6.11 Rib palpation test. (From Greenman 1996.)

pair are regarded as elevated, unable to fully exhale ('inhalation restriction').

General principles of MET for rib dysfunction

Before using MET on rib restrictions identified in tests such as those summarized above, appropriate attention should be given to the attaching musculature, for example the scalenes for the upper ribs, and pectorals, latissimus, quadratus lumborum, and others for the lower ribs (see later in this chapter).

Additionally, evaluation and appropriate treatment should be given to any thoracic spine dysfunction which may be influencing the function of associated ribs, before specific attention is given to rib restrictions.

Attention should also be given to postural and breathing habits which may be contributing to thoracic spine and/or rib dysfunction, and appropriate reeducation and exercise protocols described.

MET treatment for restricted lst rib

The patient is seated. To treat a right elevated 1st rib, the practitioner's left foot is placed on the table and the patient's left arm is 'draped' over the practitioner's flexed knee (Fig. 6.12). The practitioner's left arm is flexed, with the elbow placed anterior to the patient's shoulder and the left hand supporting the patient's (side of) head.

The practitioner makes contact with the tubercle of the 1st rib with the fingers or thumb of his right hand, taking out available soft tissue slack as force is applied in an inferior direction. The practitioner eases his flexed leg to the left, and simultaneously uses his left hand to encourage the patient's neck into a side-flexion and rotation to the right, so unloading scalene tension on that side, and encouraging the 1st rib shaft to move anteriorly and inferiorly.

The contact thumb or fingers on the rib tubercle/shaft take out available slack, and the patient is then asked to 'inhale and hold your breath for a few seconds and at the same time gently press

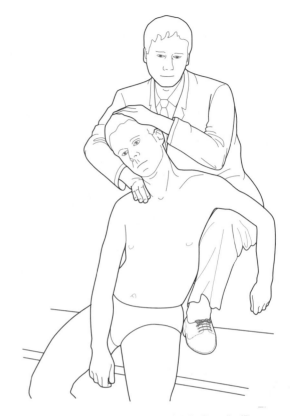

Figure 6.12 Treatment for elevated right first rib. (From Ward 1997.)

your head towards the left against my hand.' This 5–7 second effort will activate and isometrically contract the scalenes.

On releasing the breath, the slack is taken out of the soft tissues as all the movements which preceded the contraction are repeated.

Two to three repetitions usually result in greater rib symmetry and functional balance.

MET treatment for restricted 2nd to 10th ribs

For elevated ribs:

The most inferior of a group of elevated ribs is identified. The patient is supine and the practitioner stands at the head of the table, slightly to the left of the patient's head, with the right hand (for left-side rib dysfunction) supporting the patient's upper thoracic region, and the right forearm supporting neck and head (Fig. 6.13B).

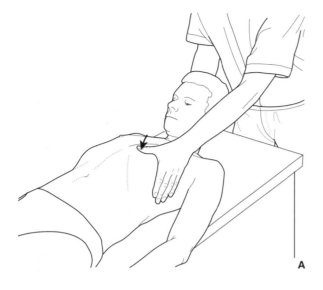

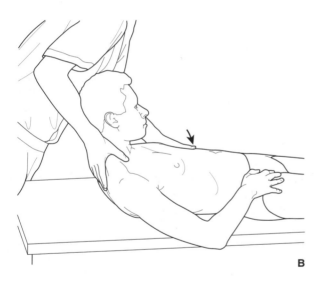

Figure 6.13 Treatment for elevated ribs, using MET. (From Greenman 1996.)

The left hand is placed so that the thenar eminence rests on the superior aspect of the costochondral junction of the designated rib, close to the midclavicular line (for upper ribs; for ribs 7–10 the contact would be more lateral, closer to the midaxillary line), directing the rib caudally (Fig. 6.13A).

The upper thoracic and cervical spine is eased into flexion, as well as side-flexion toward the treated side, until motion is sensed at the site of the rib stabilization. If the introduction of side-flexion is difficult, the patient should be asked to ease the left hand (in this example) toward the feet until motion is noted at the palpated rib.

The patient should then be asked to inhale fully and 'Hold your breath' (isometric contraction of intercostals as well as scalenes), and to attempt to return the back and head to the table, against the practitioner's resistance.

On release and full exhalation, the slack is removed from the local tissues (thenar eminence holding the rib toward its caudad position) as increased flexion and side-flexion is introduced.

This sequence is repeated once or twice only and usually results in release of the group of elevated ribs.

For depressed ribs:
Various muscles are used for different depressed rib restrictions (see method below), based on their attachments. Goodridge & Kuchera (1997) list (and recommended patient positioning to treat) these as:

Rib 1: anterior and middle scalenes. The patient's arm is flexed, forearm resting on forehead, head rotated away from the side to be treated (toward the right in this example); the patient is instructed to attempt to flex the neck and head further, against resistance, for 5–7 seconds.

Rib 2: posterior scalene. The patient's arm is flexed, forearm resting on forehead, head rotated away from the side to be treated (toward the right in this example); the patient is instructed to attempt to move the elbow and head anteriorly against resistance for 5–7 seconds.

Ribs 3–5: pectoralis minor. With the head in neutral, the arm flexed and placed along the side of head (Fig. 6.14) the patient is asked to bring the elbow toward the sternum against resistance for 5–7 seconds.

Ribs 6–9: serratus anterior. The patient's head is in neutral, the elbow is flexed, and the dorsum of the hand rests on the forehead. The patient is asked to bring the hand anteriorly against resistance for 5–7 seconds.

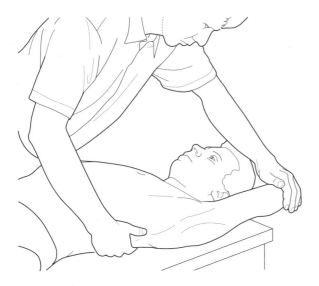

Figure 6.14 Treatment for depressed rib. (From Ward 1997.)

Ribs 10–12: latissimus dorsi. The patient is prone, the arm, elbow flexed, lies in abduction between 90° and 130°, depending on the localization of the forces to the rib being treated. The patient is asked to abduct the arm against resistance.

The most superior of an identified group of depressed ribs is treated.

The patient is supine and the practitioner stands on the contralateral side, and places his table-side arm across the patient's trunk, inserting the hand beneath the patient's torso so that he can engage, with fingertips, the superior aspect of the costal angle of the designated rib (the most superior of the group). The patient's head or arm is placed in the most suitable position so that an isometric contraction will engage the muscle(s) most likely to influence the key rib (see suggestions, above).

The patient is asked to move the head or arm as appropriate (see above), against practitioner resistance, while holding the breath (this is an isometric contraction of the intercostals), for 5–7 seconds.

On complete relaxation, the fingers draw the rib inferiorly to take out available slack and the process is repeated at least once more before reassessment of rib movement is carried out.

MET treatment for restricted (depressed rib) 11th and 12th ribs

The patient is prone, and the practitioner stands on the ipsilateral side, facing the patient. For a left side depressed 11th rib, the patient places the left arm above the head and the practitioner holds that elbow with his cephalad hand. The practitioner locates the depressed 11th rib and draws it superiorly to its barrier, with his fingerpads (Fig. 6.15).

The patient is asked to breathe in and hold the breath, while simultaneously attempting to bring the elevated and abducted left elbow sideways, back towards his side, against resistance.

After 5–7 seconds, and complete relaxation by the patient, the rib is drawn superiorly toward its new barrier via the finger contact.

A repetition of the procedure should then be carried out and the rib reassessed.

MET treatment for restricted (elevated rib) 11th and 12th ribs

The patient is prone, arms at his sides. The practitioner stands on the contralateral side to the

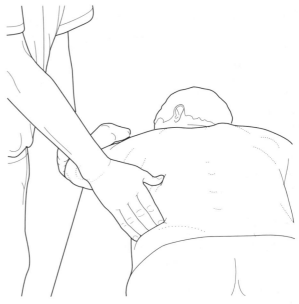

Figure 6.15 Treatment for depressed left eleventh rib. (From Ward 1997.)

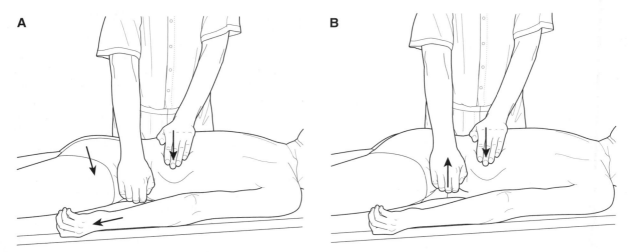

Figure 6.16 A, B Treatment for restricted (elevated rib) 11th and 12th ribs. (From Greenman 1996.)

dysfunctional ribs. For right-side 11th and 12th elevated ribs the practitioner places the thenar and hypothenar eminences of his cephalad hand on the medial aspects of the shafts of both the 11th and 12th ribs (these two ribs usually act in concert in the way they become dysfunctional). His caudad hand grasps the patient's right ASIS (Fig. 6.16).

The patient is asked to exhale fully, and hold this out, and to reach towards the right foot with the right hand, so introducing side-bending to the right, taking the elevated ribs toward their normal position.

At the end of the exhalation the patient is asked to bring the ASIS firmly into the practitioner's hand ('Push your pelvis toward the table').

After 5–7 seconds and complete relaxation by the patient, the practitioner takes out all slack with his contact hand and the process is repeated, before retesting.

General thoracic cage release using MET

The patient is supine, and the practitioner stands at waist level, facing cephalad, and places his hands over the middle and lower thoracic structures, with his fingers along the rib shafts. Treating the structure being palpated as a cylinder, the hands test the preference this cylinder

has to rotate around its central axis, first one way and then the other. (Does the lower thorax rotate with more difficulty to the right or to the left?)

Once the direction of greatest rotational restriction has been established, side-bending one way or the other is evaluated. (Does the lower thorax side-flex with more difficulty to the right or to the left?; Fig. 6.17.)

Once these two pieces of information have been established, the combined positions of restriction, so indicated, are introduced.

By side-bending and rotating *toward the tighter directions*, the combined directions of restriction are engaged, at which time the patient is asked to inhale and hold the breath, and to 'bear down' slightly (Valsalva maneuver).

These efforts introduce isometric contractions of the diaphragm and intercostal muscles.

On release and complete exhalation and relaxation, the diaphragm should be found to function more normally and there should be a relaxation of associated soft tissues, together with more symmetrical rotation and side-flexion potential of the previously restricted tissues.

Functional tests (Janda 1996)

The three functional tests described and illustrated below can be used to provide a rapid

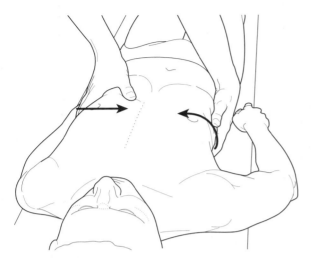

Figure 6.17 Treatment for fascias of thoracolumbar junction, rotated left, side-bent right. (From Ward 1997.)

screening serving to demonstrate firing sequence imbalances:

1. Seated scapulohumeral rhythm test (Fig. 6.18)

The test is positive if observable bunching in upper trapezius occurs, or if elevation of the shoulder, or winging of the scapula occurs, within the first 60° of shoulder abduction. This is evidence of poor scapular stabilization and suggests levator scapulae and upper trapezius tightness, and lower and middle trapezius inhibition.

2. Prone hip extension test (Fig. 6.19)

The normal activation sequence on prone hip extension is gluteus maximus and hamstrings followed by erector spinae (contralateral then ipsilateral). If the hamstrings and/or erectors fire first and take the role of gluteus maximus they are considered to be overactive and probably shortened, while gluteus is inhibited.

3. Hip abduction test: side-lying (Fig. 6.20)

Lewit (1986) has the patient side-lying. The practitioner stands facing the patient's front at hip level, simultaneously palpating gluteus medius, tensor fasciae latae (TFL), and quadratus lumbo-

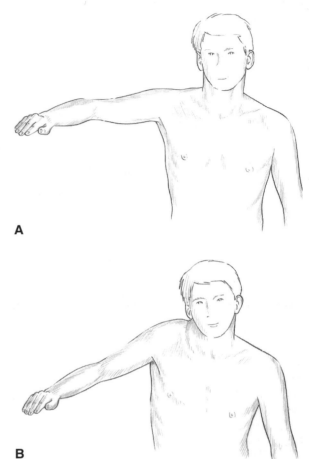

Figure 6.18 Scapulohumeral rhythm test. **A** Normal. **B** Imbalance due to elevation of the shoulder within first 60 degrees of abduction. (Reproduced with kind permission from Chaitow 1996c.)

rum (QL). The patient abducts the upper leg. In balanced abduction gluteus medius fires first, with TFL operating later in the pure abduction of the leg. QL should not become active until the leg has reached between 25° and 30° abduction. When it is overactive, QL will often fire first along with TFL. This evidence suggests shortness in QL (and therefore impacts on breathing as QL merges with the diaphragm as well as acting to stabilize the 12th rib on exhalation), and probable inhibition of gluteus medius.

Evidence from these tests, as well as from the palpation assessment and observation of breathing

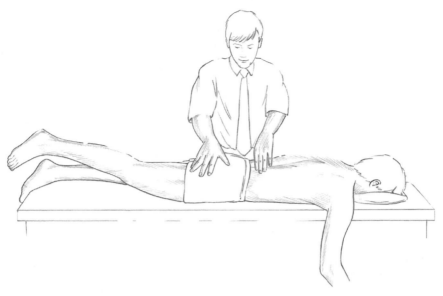

Figure 6.19 Hip extension test. (Reproduced with kind permission from Chaitow 1996c.)

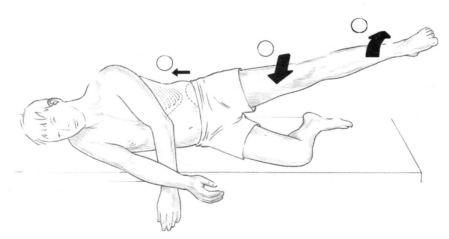

Figure 6.20 Hip abduction test which, if normal, occurs without hip hike, hip flexion or external rotation. (Reproduced with kind permission from Chaitow & DeLany 2000.)

function (see above), suggests which postural muscles are most likely to require normalization and stretching.

Assessment and MET treatment of shortened postural muscles associated with respiration

It is seldom necessary to treat all shortened muscles which may be identified as part of a dys-functional pattern. For example, Lewit (1999) and Simons (Simons et al 1998) assert that isometric relaxation of the suboccipital muscles will also relax the sternocleidomastoid muscles; release of the thoracolumbar muscles induces relaxation of iliopsoas, and vice versa; and treatment (MET) of the scalene and sternocleidomastoid muscles relaxes the pectorals.

The muscles described below are a selection of those most intimately involved with the biomechanical function of breathing. These muscles can become dysfunctional due to habitual overuse and misuse factors or due to trauma, as well as through the influence of emotions (see discussion of Latey's perspective in Ch. 2). Short, tight muscles predispose to the evolution of myofascial trigger points at both the motor end point (muscle belly, central points) and at the attachments (see notes on trigger point deactivation methods later in this chapter).

MET treatment of a shortened postural muscle has several effects:

- Release of hypertonicity
- Preparation for subsequent stretching
- Deactivation of trigger points (if the muscle can achieve normal resting length)
- Toning of antagonists if these have been inhibited
- Enhancement of associated joint function.

Assessing for shortness in pectoralis major (Fig. 6.21)

The patient lies supine, with the head approximately 40 cm from the top edge of the table, and is asked to rest the arms, extended above the head, on the treatment surface, palms upwards. If these muscles are normal the arms should be able easily to rest directly above the shoulders, in contact with the surface for almost all of their length, with no arching of the back or twisting of the thorax. If an arm cannot rest with the dorsum of the upper arm fully in contact with the table surface, without effort, then pectoral fibers are probably short.

Assessment of the subclavicular portion of pectoralis involves abduction of the arm to 90° from the body. In this position the tendon of pectoralis at the sternum should not be found to be unduly tense, even with maximum abduction of the arm.

MET treatment of pectoralis major (Fig. 6.22)

The patient adopts the test position, so that the arm is abducted in a direction which produces the most marked evidence of pectoral shortness assessed by palpation and visual evidence of the fibers involved:

- The more elevated the arm (i.e. the closer to the head) the more abdominal the attachments will be that are being treated
- The more lateral the arm, the more clavicular the fibers.

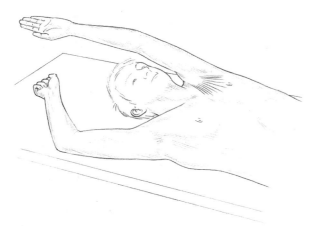

Figure 6.21 Assessment of shortness in pectoralis major and latissimus dorsi. Visual assessment is used: if the arm on the tested side is unable to rest along its full length, shortness of pectoralis major is probable; if there is obvious deviation of the elbow laterally, probable latissimus shortening is indicated. (Reproduced with kind permission from Chaitow 1996c.)

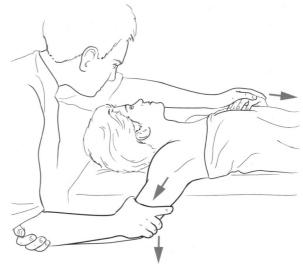

Figure 6.22 MET treatment of pectoralis major, supine position. (Reproduced with kind permission from Chaitow & DeLany 2000.)

Between these two extremes lies the position which involves the sternal fibers most directly.

The patient should be as close to the side of the table as possible so that the abducted arm can be brought below the horizontal in order to apply gravitational and passive stretch to the fibers, as appropriate. The operator stands on the side to be treated and grasps the humerus with one hand while the other hand contacts the thoracic attachment of the shortened fibers (attaching to ribs, or sternum or clavicle). The long axis of the patient's upper arm should be in line with the fibers being treated. The contact hand stabilizes the attachment site during the contraction and stretch, preventing its movement, but not exerting pressure. Placement of the patient's hand on the contact area (with practitioner's hand superimposed) allows this to act as a 'cushion,' as well as preventing physical contact with sensitive areas (see Fig. 6.22).

All stretch is via the positioning and leverage of the arm, the contact hand on the thorax.

The practitioner grasps the anterior aspect of the patient's flexed upper arm, just proximal to the elbow, while the patient cups the practitioner's elbow and maintains this contact throughout the procedure.

The patient introduces adduction and/or elevation, against resistance, for 7–10 seconds, using no more than a quarter of available strength. On complete release of the contraction effort, a stretch is introduced, either up to or (a short way) through the new barrier. The stretch needs to be one in which the arm is distracted from the thoracic/clavicular attachment, as well as being taken below the horizontal (i.e. eased away from the trunk and extended at the shoulder). The thoracic insertion of the muscle is constantly stabilized to prevent any movement.

The stretch is held for not less than 30 seconds and then repeated following a further isometric contraction.

Assessment for shortness of upper trapezius

Lewit simplifies the need to assess for shortness by stating. 'The upper trapezius should be treated if tender and taut.' Since this is an almost universal state in modern life, it seems that *everyone* requires MET application to this muscle. Lewit also notes that a characteristic mounding of the muscle can often be observed when it is very short, producing the effect of 'Gothic shoulders,' similar to the architectural supports of a Gothic church tower (see Fig. 7.1).

The patient is seated, and the practitioner stands behind the patient, with a hand resting on the patient's shoulder on the side to be assessed. The patient is asked to extend the shoulder, bringing the flexed arm/elbow backwards. If the upper trapezius is stressed/short on that side, it will inappropriately activate during this arm movement. This suggests hypertonicity and probable shortness.

The patient is supine, with the head/neck fully rotated and laterally flexed away from the tested side. The practitioner stands at the head of the table and assesses the ease with which the shoulder can be depressed (moved distally). There should be an easy springing sensation as the shoulder is pushed toward the feet, with a soft end-feel. If there is a 'solid' end-feel, the posterior fibers of upper trapezius are probably short. Rotation of the head toward the side being tested allows assessment of the anterior fibers, using the same shoulder springing evaluation.

With the neck fully flexed, side-flexed, and rotated away from the tested side, the same springing of the shoulder evaluates levator scapulae.

MET treatment of shortened upper trapezius
(Fig. 6.23)

The patient lies supine, head/neck side-flexed away from the side to be treated, with the practitioner stabilizing the shoulder with one hand and cupping the ear/mastoid area of the same side of the head with the other.

In order to bring into play all the various fibers of upper trapezius, the neck is held in three different positions of rotation, coupled with side-bending as described below:

1. Full side-flexion and full rotation *away from* the side being treated involves the posterior fibers of upper trapezius

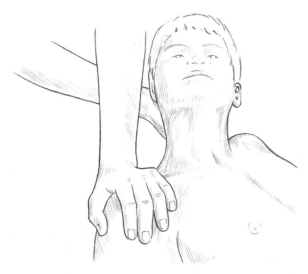

Figure 6.23 MET treatment of right side upper trapezius muscle. The head is in the upright position, with no rotation in this example, which indicates that the anterior fibres are being treated. Note that stretching in this (or any of the alternative positions which access the middle and posterior fiber) is achieved following the isometric contraction by means of an easing of the shoulder away from the stabilized head with no force being applied to the neck and head themselves. (Reproduced with kind permission from Chaitow 1996c.)

2. Full side-flexion and half-rotation *away from* the side being treated involves the middle fibers of upper trapezius
3. Full side-flexion away from and rotation *toward* the side being treated involves the posterior fibers of upper trapezius.

NOTE: The MET description below is applied to the upper trapezius with the head/neck in all three positions listed above, in order to access all fibers efficiently.

Treatment details:

Using no more than small degree of effort (under 20% of available strength), the patient introduces a resisted effort to take the stabilized shoulder toward the ear (a shrug movement) and the ear toward the shoulder. This introduces a contraction of the muscle from both ends. No pain should be felt.

After a 7-second (or so) contraction, and complete relaxation of effort, the practitioner gently eases the head/neck into an increased degree of side-flexion and rotation, before – *with the patient's assistance* – easing the shoulder away

from the ear while stabilizing the head, to achieve a light degree of stretch.

⚠ No stretch is introduced from the head end of the muscle as this could stress the neck unduly (see Fig. 6.23).

This stretch is held for not less than 30 seconds and the entire procedure is then repeated.

Eye movement alternative

As an alternative to an active contraction, particularly in cases where pain is a feature, Lewit (1999) suggests the use of eye movements to facilitate initiation of postisometric relaxation before stretching:

The patient is supine, while the practitioner fixes the shoulder and the side-flexed head and neck (as in the methodology described above) at the restriction barrier and asks the patient to look, with the eyes only (i.e. not to turn the head) toward the side away from which the neck is flexed. This eye movement is maintained, while the practitioner resists the slight isometric contraction that it creates. Simultaneously, the shoulder should attempt to lightly push into a shrug against practitioner resistance.

On an exhalation, and complete relaxation, the head/neck is taken to a new barrier and the process repeated.

Ruddy's reciprocal antagonist facilitation (RRAF)

In treatment of a shortened, hypertonic upper trapezius, whether this contains active trigger points or not (according to Simons & Travell (1983), this is the second most common trigger point site in the body after quadratus lumborum), a form of stretching (MET or other) might form part of a treatment approach to normalizing the dysfunctional pattern with which it is associated.

It is suggested that in order to commence a rehabilitation and proprioceptive reeducation program, following appropriate stretching procedures, pulsed MET could be introduced as follows:

The patient is seated and the operator places a single digit contact very lightly against the lower medial scapula border, on the side of the treated upper trapezius. The practitioner offers a sensory cue to the patient by lightly pushing against the medial scapula border with the digit for a brief moment.

The request is made: 'Press back against my finger with your shoulder blade, toward your spine, just as hard (i.e. very lightly) as I pressed against it, for less than a second.'

Once the patient has managed to establish control over the particular muscular action required to achieve this subtle movement (which can take a significant number of attempts), and can do so for a second at a time, repetitively, the pulsing sequence can begin.

The patient is told something such as the following: 'Now that you know how to activate the muscles which pushed your shoulder blade lightly against my finger, I want you to try to do this 20 times in 10 seconds, starting and stopping, so that no actual movement takes place, just a contraction and a stopping, repetitively.'

This repetitive, 'pulsing' contraction will activate the rhomboids, and the middle and lower trapezii, producing an automatic reciprocal inhibition of upper trapezius.

The patient can then be taught to place a light finger or thumb contact against the medial scapula so that self-application of this method can be performed.

A degree of creativity can be brought to bear when designing similar applications of Ruddy's reciprocal antagonist facilitation (RRAF) for use elsewhere in the body in order to complement stretching procedures and trigger point deactivation, in the knowledge that the treatment process then expands into an educational and rehabilitation phase. The patient should be encouraged to use the method described as home work.

Assessment of shortness in levator scapulae

See the scapulohumeral rhythm test and the modified upper trapezius test, which are used to assess shortness in levator scapula, both described above.

MET treatment of levator scapulae (Fig. 6.24)

The patient lies supine, with the arm of the side to be tested stretched out with the hand and lower arm tucked under the buttocks, palm upward, to help restrain movement of the shoulder/scapula. The practitioner's arm is passed across and under the neck to rest on the shoulder of the side to be treated. The other hand supports the head.

The neck is lifted into full flexion by the forearm (aided by the other hand) and is turned toward full side-flexion and rotation, away from the side to be treated.

The patient is asked (using very small amounts of force) to return the head toward the table, and slightly to the side from which it has turned, against the practitioner's unyielding resistance. At the same time a slight shoulder shrug is also resisted.

Following a 7-second isometric contraction and complete relaxation, slack is taken out as the shoulder is depressed further and the neck is taken to or through (acute or chronic) further flexion, side-flexion, and rotation.

⚠ Caution is required not to overstretch this sensitive area.

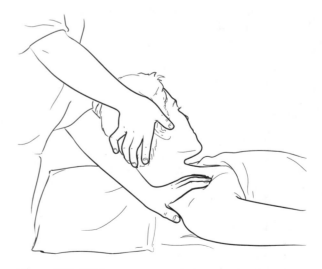

Figure 6.24 MET assessment and treatment of right levator scapula. (Reproduced with kind permission from Chaitow & DeLany 2000.)

Assessment of shortness in scalenes

The scalenes, which are prone to trigger point activity, are a controversial muscle since they seem to be both postural and phasic in nature, their status being modified by the type(s) of stress to which they are exposed (Lin 1994). Janda (1996) reports that, 'spasm and/or trigger points are commonly present in the scalenes as also are weakness and/or inhibition.'

There is no easy test for shortness of the scalenes apart from observation, palpation, and assessment of trigger point activity/tautness and a functional observation as follows:

In most people who have marked scalene shortness there is a tendency to overuse them (and other upper fixators of the shoulder and neck) as accessory breathing muscles. Clinical experience suggests that the scalenes are commonly excessively tense in people with chronic fatigue symptoms.

The observation assessment consists of the practitioner placing his relaxed hands over the patient's shoulders so that the fingertips rest on the clavicles, at which time the seated patient is asked to inhale moderately deeply. If the practitioner's hands noticeably rise toward the patient's ears during inhalation, then there exists inappropriate use of scalenes, suggesting that they will have become shortened and would benefit from stretching.

Active trigger points in the scalenes refer pain, and sometimes paresthesia symptoms, into the ipsilateral arm (Fig. 6.25).

MET treatment of short scalenes (Fig. 6.26)

The patient lies with a thin cushion under the shoulders to enable the neck to rest in slight extension on the treatment table surface. The head/neck is supported by the practitioner, in a neutral (i.e. not extended) position and turned away from the side to be treated.

There are three positions of rotation required in scalene treatment:

1. Full rotation produces involvement of the more posterior fibers of the scalenes on the side from which the turn is being made
2. A half rotation recruits the middle fibers

3. A position of only slight turn involves the more anterior fibers.

The *patient's* non-treatment side hand is placed on the area just below the lateral end of the clavicle on the affected side, to act as a 'cushion' for the practitioner to push against when introducing stretch (see Fig. 6.26). The patient is instructed to inhale and hold the breath and to attempt to lift the forehead a fraction while turning the head toward the affected side. Resistance from the practitioner's hand prevents both movements ('lift and turn').

The effort, and therefore the counterpressure, should be modest and painless at all times.

After a 7-second contraction, the head is eased into extension and the practitioner's contact hand, covering the patient's hand, which is resting inferior to the clavicle, lightly pushes obliquely, caudally, to follow the ribs into their exhalation position.

This scalene stretch is held for up to 30 seconds to encourage lengthening.

This whole procedure should be performed several times, in each of the three positions of the head, for each side, as necessary.

A degree of eye movement can assist scalene treatment. If the patient looks downwards, towards the feet and toward the affected side, during the isometric contraction, this will induce a degree of contraction in the muscles.

If during the resting phase, when stretch is being introduced, the patient looks away from the treated side with eyes focused upward, toward the top of the head, this will enhance the stretch of the muscle (Lewit 1999).

⚠ **CAUTION:** It is important not to allow unsafe degrees of neck extension during any phase of this treatment: *15° is suggested as the upper limit, or less in patients over 45 years of age.*

Assessment for shortness of sternocleidomastoid

As for the scalenes, there is no absolute test for shortness of sternocleidomastoid (SCM), but

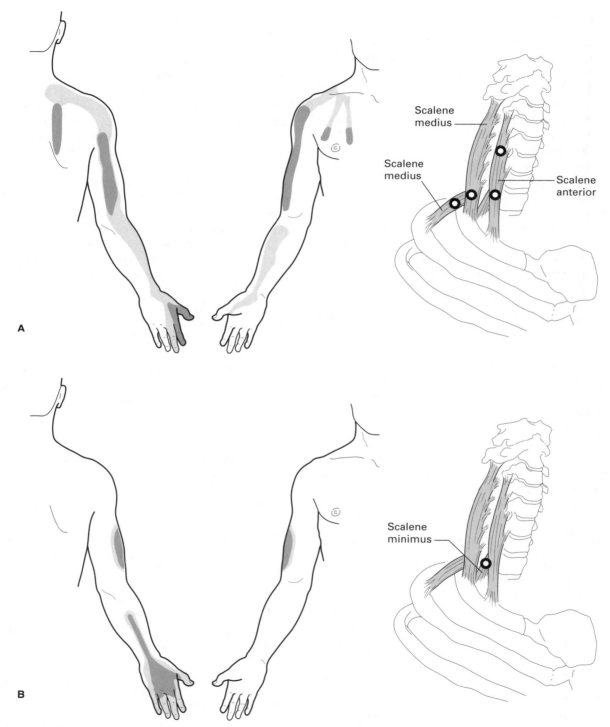

Figure 6.25 A,B Scalene trigger points produce patterns of common complaint which may come from any of the scalene muscles. (Reproduced with kind permission from Chaitow & DeLany 2000.)

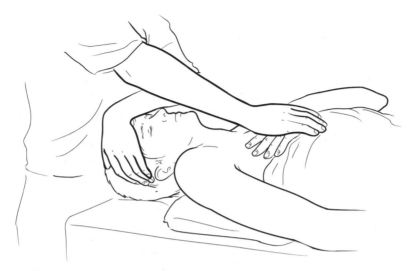

Figure 6.26 MET treatment of scalene anticus. (Reproduced with kind permission from Chaitow & DeLany 2000.)

observation of posture (hyperextended neck, chin poked forward) and palpation of the degree of induration, fibrosis, and trigger point activity can all alert to probable shortness. This is a postural, accessory breathing muscle which, like the scalenes, will be shortened by inappropriate breathing patterns which have become habitual.

Observation is an accurate assessment tool. Since SCM is only just observable when normal, if the clavicular insertion is easily visible, or any part of the muscle is prominent, this can be taken as a clear sign of tightness of the muscle.

If the patient's posture involves the head being held forward of the body, often accompanied by cervical lordosis and dorsal kyphosis (see Ch. 4, notes on upper crossed syndrome), weakness of the deep neck flexors and tightness of SCM can be suspected.

MET treatment of shortened sternocleidomastoid

The patient is supine, in the same position as that described for scalene treatment above, with a thin cushion under the shoulders.

Whereas in scalene treatment the instruction to the patient was to 'lift and turn' the rotated head/neck against resistance, in treating SCM the instruction is simply to 'slightly lift the head.' When the head is raised there is no need to apply resistance, as gravity effectively does this.

After 7 seconds of isometric contraction, the patient is asked to release the effort and to allow the head/neck to return to a resting position involving a small degree of extension.

The practitioner applies oblique pressure/ stretch to the sternum, with his hand resting on the patient's 'cushion' hand (on the sternum), easing the sternum away from the head toward the feet. The practitioner's other hand restrains the tendency the head will have to follow this stretch by holding at the mastoid area.

⚠ *Under no circumstances apply pressure* to stretch the head/neck while it is in this vulnerable position of slight extension. The degree of extension of the neck should be slight, 10–15° at most. Maintain this stretch for some seconds to achieve release/stretch of hypertonic and fibrotic structures. Repeat as necessary.

Other muscles

In addition to the muscles described above, quadratus lumborum and psoas should be assessed and treated if shortened, since they both merge with the diaphragm and are involved in breathing function. Descriptions of the treatment of these muscles using MET have not been included in this text since they are readily available in texts by Ward (1997), Greenman (1996), Chaitow (2001), and others.

POSITIONAL RELEASE TECHNIQUES

Strain/counterstrain (Jones 1981, Chaitow 1996a)

There are many different methods involving the positioning of an area, or the whole body, in such a way as to evoke a physiological response which helps to resolve musculoskeletal dysfunction. The means by which the beneficial changes occur seems to involve a combination of neurological and circulatory changes which come about when a distressed area is placed in its most comfortable, most 'easy', most pain-free position (Deig 2001).

All areas which palpate as inappropriately painful are responding to, or are associated with, some degree of imbalance, dysfunction, or reflexive activity which may well involve acute or chronic strain. Jones (1981) identified positions of tender points relating to particular strain positions. However, it makes just as much sense to work the other way round: any painful point found during soft tissue evaluation could be treated by positional release, whether the strain pattern (acute or chronically adaptive) which produced or maintains it can be identified or not.

Common basis

All positional release techniques (PRT) methods move the patient, or the affected tissues, away from any resistance barriers and toward positions of ease – 'tissue comfort.' The shorthand terms used for these two extremes are 'bind' and 'ease' (see discussion of 'tight–loose' concepts in Ch. 4).

Strain counterstrain (Jones's method), SCS, involves monitoring the reported pain level in a tender point (not necessarily a trigger point, but an area of unusual sensitivity to which digital pressure is applied) while the area is carefully and slowly repositioned until the level of reported pain reduces from an initial level of '10' to '3' or less.

This position of ease is then held for not less than 90 seconds. During this period (it is hypothesized), spindle resetting and circulatory changes take place to beneficially modify the status of the tissues involved and calm neural reactivity.

If the tender area is an active trigger point, then the positional release process commonly deactivates it or reduces trigger point referral activity significantly.

It is possible to imagine a situation in which the use of Jones's 'tender points as a monitor' method would be inappropriate, for example, in an individual who has lost the ability to communicate verbally, or in someone who is too young to verbalize. In such a case there is a need for a method which allows achievement of the same ends without verbal communication. This is possible using 'functional' approaches. These involve finding a position of maximum ease by means of palpation alone, assessing for a state of 'ease' in the tissues.

Method

SCS involves maintaining pressure on the monitored tender point, or periodically probing it, as a position is achieved in which:

1. There is no additional pain in whatever area is symptomatic, and
2. The monitor point pain has reduced by at least 70%.

This is then held for an appropriate length of time (90 seconds or more).

Strain/counterstrain rules of treatment

The following 'rules' are based on clinical experience and should be kept in mind when using positional release (SCS, etc.) methods in treating pain and dysfunction, especially where the patient is fatigued, sensitive and/or distressed:

● Never treat more than five 'tender' points at any one session, and treat fewer than this in sensitive individuals in order to avoid adaptation overload.

- Forewarn patients that, just as in any other form of bodywork which produces altered function, a period of physiological adaptation is inevitable, and that there will therefore be a 'reaction' on the day(s) following even this extremely light form of treatment. Soreness and stiffness are therefore to be anticipated.
- If there are multiple tender points, select those most proximal and most medial for primary attention (i.e. those closest to the head and the centre of the body, rather than distal and lateral pain points).
- Of these tender points, select those that are most painful for initial attention/treatment.

Strain/counterstrain guidelines

The general guidelines which Jones (1981) gives for relief of the dysfunction with which such tender points are related involves directing the movement of these tissues toward ease, which commonly involves the following elements:

- For tender points on the anterior surface of the body, flexion, side-bending, and rotation should be toward the palpated point, followed by fine-tuning to reduce sensitivity by at least 70%.
- For tender points on the posterior surface of the body, extension, side-bending, and rotation should be away from the palpated point, followed by fine-tuning to reduce sensitivity by 70%.
- The closer the tender point is to the midline, the less side-bending and rotation should be required, and the further from the midline, the more side-bending and rotation should be required to effect ease and comfort in the tender point (without any additional pain or discomfort being produced anywhere else).
- The direction toward which side-bending is introduced when trying to find a position of ease often needs to be away from the side of the palpated pain point, especially in relation to tender points found on the posterior aspect of the body.

Strain/counterstrain treatment of elevated and depressed ribs (Fig. 6.27)

Depressed rib strains produce points of tenderness at the anterior axillary line in the space above or below the affected rib. Elevated ribs have tender points in the intercostal space above or below the affected rib, at the angle of the ribs posteriorly.

In order to gain access to these, the scapula requires distraction or lifting to allow for palpation of the particular point. This is done by the arm of the affected side of the patient being pulled across the chest, or the shoulder being raised by a pillow with the patient supine. The practitioner stands on the side of the disorder, and palpation of the tender point, once identified, is continuous (although pressure may be intermittent in order to assess pain reduction as repositioning/fine-tuning is carried out, see SCS notes).

The patient's knees should be flexed during treatment of elevated ribs, and should be allowed to move to the side of the dysfunction. If this fails to achieve ease, the knees are taken toward the opposite side to evaluate the effect on palpated pain. As a rule pain will reduce by around 50% as the knees fall to one side or the other. The head may be turned toward or away from the affected side, to further fine-tune and release the stress in the palpated tissues.

Additional fine-tuning for elevated ribs may then be accomplished by raising the arm or shoulder cephalad, in effect exaggerating the positional deformity, as well as by introducing deep breathing so that the patient can evaluate which phase of the cycle reduces pain most, this phase being maintained as long as is comfortable during the 'holding' of the position of ease.

The tender point for a depressed rib, lying as it does in the intercostal space above or below the affected rib on the anterior axillary line, is easily palpated by the patient.

For treatment of depressed ribs, the patient should be supine with knees flexed and falling to one side or the other, whichever produces greatest release in the tissues being palpated at the anterior axillary line. The head is turned

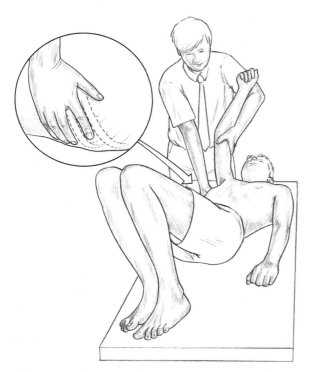

Figure 6.27A Positional release of an elevated rib involves the monitoring of a tender point on the posterior surface close to the angle of the ribs in an interspace above or below the affected rib. Ease is achieved by means of taking the flexed knees to one side or the other, with fine-tuning involving positioning of the head, neck and/or arms. Assessment of the influence of respiratory function on the tender point pain may also be used. (Reproduced with kind permission from Chaitow 1996a.)

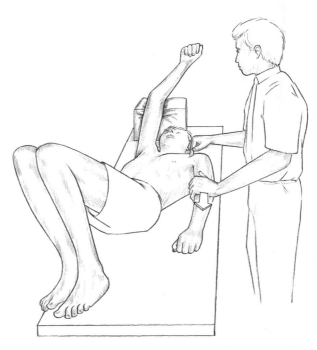

Figure 6.27B Positional release of a depressed rib involves the monitoring of a tender point on the anterior axillary line in an interspace above or below the affected rib. Ease is achieved by positioning of flexed legs, head and/or arms as well as use of the respiratory cycle, until a position is found in which the palpated pain eases markedly or vanishes from the tender point. (Reproduced with kind permission from Chaitow 1996a.)

toward or away from the affected side to further fine-tune and release the stress in the palpated tissues.

For additional fine-tuning, the practitioner stands on the side of dysfunction and draws the patient's arm, on the side of dysfunction, caudad until release is noted. In some cases the other arm may need to be elevated to enhance release of tender point discomfort.

Breathing can be used to increase the degree of 'ease' and release.

A notable improvement in rib range of motion is commonly felt after this simple treatment method, with an obvious increase in the excursion of the thoracic cage and subjective feelings of 'ease of breathing' being reported.

Strain/counterstrain interspace dysfunction

Tender points used as monitors for treatment of dysfunction involving the intercostal tissues lie between the insertions of the contiguous ribs into the cartilages of the sternum. Dysfunction and discomfort in the intercostals seems to relate to non-specific stress of the thorax, sometimes following trauma, or a recent stressful coughing or asthmatic episode. Ribs may be overapproximated, and the pain reported when the tender points are palpated may be severe.

In chronic conditions, pressure on the intercostal and attachment soft tissues may produce a reactivation of the extreme tenderness noted in more acute situations. Jones (1981) reports that 'strains' such as these are noted in costochondritis. Painful points are common in these tissues in people with asthma, those with chronic bronchitis, and in patients with upper-chest breathing/hyperventilation breathing patterns.

Treatment of intercostal dysfunction points involves placing the patient supine while the tender point is contacted by the practitioner or the patient. The practitioner should be on the side of dysfunction, with the caudad hand providing contact on the point (unless the patient is performing this function). The cephalad hand cradles the patient's head/neck and the upper thorax. Flexion is introduced toward the side of dysfunction at an angle of approximately 45° until pain reduces by at least 70%.

If fine-tuning is adequate (minor adjustments of the degree of flexion, with some side-flexion added if this helps reduce the reported pain score), the palpation-induced pain will ease. This position should be maintained for at least 90 seconds.

This same procedure for release of interspace dysfunction tender points can be achieved in a seated position, and the patient can be taught to use it as a home treatment. The point is located and the patient, alone or with assistance, flexes gently toward the painful side until it reduces or vanishes. This position is held for 90 seconds and another point located and treated.

The methodology of positional release variations can be more fully explored in a number of texts, including Jones (1981), D'Ambrogio & Roth (1997), Deig (2001), and Chaitow (2002).

DEACTIVATING MYOFASCIAL TRIGGER POINTS

The trigger point phenomenon was discussed fully in Chapter 4. This chapter suggests a protocol in which a combination of modalities is used in an integrated sequence to deactivate active trigger points. An alternative approach would be to use the trigger point as a marker, so that the degree of sensitivity noted on pressure is seen to reduce as rehabilitation processes (such as postural or breathing reeducation) reduce the stress on the tissues housing it.

Trigger point deactivation possibilities

These include:
- Inhibitory soft tissue techniques including neuromuscular therapy/massage (Hong et al 1993)
- Chilling techniques (cold spray, ice) (Simons et al 1998)
- Acupuncture, injection (procaine, xylocaine) (Hong 1994)
- Positional release methods (Deig 2001)
- Muscle energy (stretch) techniques (see above) (Kuchera 1997, Chaitow & DeLany 2000)
- Myofascial release methods
- Combination sequences such as INIT (see below) (Chaitow 1994, Chaitow 1996b)
- Correction of associated somatic dysfunction possibly involving HVT adjustments and/or osteopathic or chiropractic mobilization methods (see Ch. 4)
- Education and correction of contributory and perpetuating factors including posture, diet,

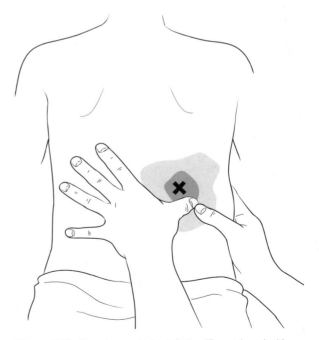

Figure 6.28 Serratus posterior inferior. (Reproduced with kind permission from Chaitow & DeLany 2000.)

stress, habits of use, etc. (see Chs 5, 6, 7, 8, 9, 10) (Bradley 1999)

- Self-help strategies (see Ch. 10).

Why is ischemic pressure technique effective?

Research suggests that: 'Deep pressure massage, if done appropriately, [may] offer better stretching of the taut bands of muscle fibers than manual stretching because it applies stronger pressure to a relatively small area compared to the gross stretching of the whole muscle. Deep pressure may also offer ischemic compression which [has been shown to be] effective for myofascial pain therapy' (Simons 1989).

The use of algometrics in treating trigger points

An area of concern in trigger point evaluation lies in the non-standard degree of pressure being applied to tissues when they are being tested manually. In order to standardize pressure and to establish the patient's 'myofascial-pain index' (MPI), a small pressure gauge (algometer) may be used (Jonkheere & Pattyn 1998, Hong et al 1993).

The 18 sites used in assessing for fibromyalgia are tested to assess the pressure required before a report of pain is noted (or any group of currently active trigger points). Based on the results of this a 'myofascial pain index' is calculated. The calculation of the MPI is made by averaging the total amount of pressure needed to evoke pain in the tested points and calculating an average by dividing this by the number of points tested. The purpose is to create an objective base (the MPI), which emerges initially from the patient's subjective pain reports, when pressure is applied to the test points. This process is repeated periodically to evaluate the current poundage required to evoke pain, on average, and becomes a means of evaluating a rise in pain threshold, or a decline in sensitivity.

Integrated neuromuscular inhibition technique (Chaitow 1994, Chaitow & DeLany 2000)

The integrated neuromuscular inhibition technique (INIT) involves using a sequence which commences with the location of a tender/pain/trigger point, followed by application of ischemic compression (this is optional – it is avoided if pain is too intense or the patient too sensitive), followed by the introduction of positional release (see above) to ease sensitivity by at least 70%.

After the tissues have been held in 'ease' for at least 90 seconds, the patient introduces an isometric contraction into the affected tissues, involving precisely the tissues surrounding the trigger point, for 7–10 seconds, after which these are stretched (or they may be stretched at the same time as the contraction, if fibrotic tissue calls for such attention). Subsequently, antagonists to the muscle housing the trigger point should be facilitated to enhance their tone and to further inhibit the agonist (see Ruddy's reciprocal antagonist facilitation, RRAF, above).

INIT method

Ischemic compression ('inhibition') is applied to an active trigger point by means of direct finger or thumb pressure until local or referred pain begins to modify (Fig. 6.28). Following this, the tissues in which the trigger point lies are positioned in such a way as to modify the pain (by at least 70%). After 90 seconds the patient is asked to introduce an isometric contraction into the tissues and to hold this for 7–10 seconds. This recruits the precise fibers which had been repositioned to obtain the positional release.

These previously hypertonic or fibrotic tissues are then stretched so that the specifically targeted fibers are lengthened.

A rhythmic activation of antagonist muscles in a series of 'pulsed' contractions is a useful final stage of this sequence (see notes on the methods of Ruddy, above).

CRANIAL AND FACIAL BONE ASSESSMENT EXERCISES
(Chaitow 1999) (Fig. 6.29)

⚠️ This brief summary of the facial structures associated with breathing function is accompanied by palpation exercises. Treatment using

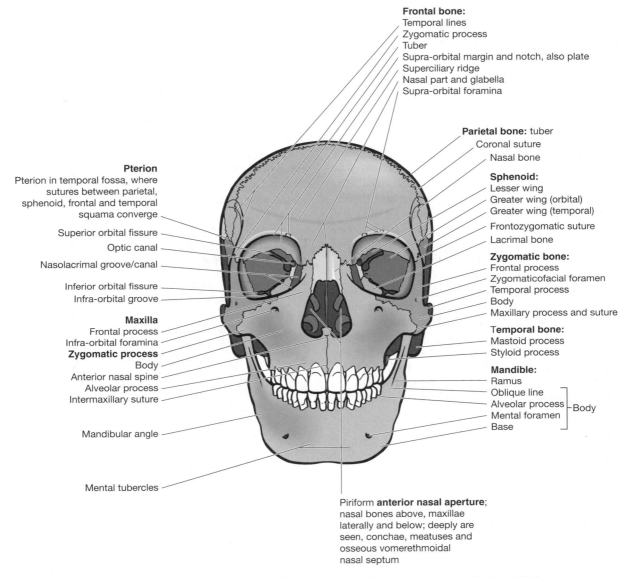

Frontal bone:
Temporal lines
Zygomatic process
Tuber
Supra-orbital margin and notch, also plate
Superciliary ridge
Nasal part and glabella
Supra-orbital foramina

Parietal bone: tuber
Coronal suture
Nasal bone

Sphenoid:
Lesser wing
Greater wing (orbital)
Greater wing (temporal)
Frontozygomatic suture
Lacrimal bone

Zygomatic bone:
Frontal process
Zygomaticofacial foramen
Temporal process
Body
Maxillary process and suture

Temporal bone:
Mastoid process
Styloid process

Mandible:
Ramus
Oblique line
Alveolar process ⎤
Mental foramen ⎥ Body
Base ⎦

Pterion
Pterion in temporal fossa, where
sutures between parietal,
sphenoid, frontal and temporal
squama converge

Superior orbital fissure
Optic canal
Nasolacrimal groove/canal

Inferior orbital fissure
Infra-orbital groove

Maxilla
Frontal process
Infra-orbital foramina
Zygomatic process
Body
Anterior nasal spine
Alveolar process
Intermaxillary suture

Mandibular angle

Mental tubercles

Piriform **anterior nasal aperture;**
nasal bones above, maxillae
laterally and below; deeply are
seen, conchae, meatuses and
osseous vomerethmoidal
nasal septum

Figure 6.29 Anterior view of skull with major features. (Reproduced with kind permission from Chaitow 1999.)

these requires the skills which evolve through cranial manipulation training (craniosacral technique, sacro-occipital technique, cranial osteopathy, etc). See also the precautionary note at the end of this section (end of the chapter).

Dysfunctional patterns associated with the ethmoid (see Ch. 1)

- When sinus inflammation exists, the ethmoid is likely to be swollen and painful.
- Because of its role as a shock-absorber, the ethmoid is potentially vulnerable to blows of

a direct nature and to absorbing stresses from any of its neighbors.

- There is no direct access for contacting the ethmoid, but it can be easily influenced via contacts on the frontal bone or the vomer.

Nasal (ethmoid) palpation (Fig. 6.30)

The patient's forehead (frontal bone) is gently cupped by the practitioner's caudad hand as he stands to the side facing the supine patient. The practitioner's cephalad hand is crossed over the caudad hand so that the index finger and thumb can gently grasp the superior aspects of the maxillae, inferior to the frontomaxillary suture. The unused fingers of the previously cephalad and now caudad hand should be folded and resting on the dorsum of the other hand.

The practitioner introduces a slow rhythmical separation of the two contacts so that the hand on the forehead is applying gentle pressure towards the floor, so pushing the falx cerebri away from the ethmoid, dragging on it, at the same time as the finger and thumb ease the maxillae anteriorly. This slight movement should be easily sensed without any force being used.

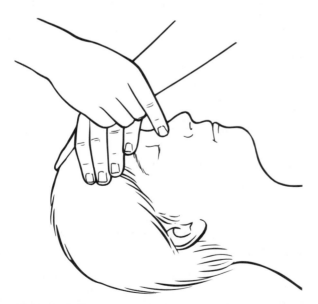

Figure 6.30 Treatment of ethmoid utilizing pincer contact. (Reproduced with kind permission from Chaitow 1999.)

In treatment of the ethmoid, these 'pumping', repetitive separation and release applications continue for at least a minute to achieve a local drainage effect, enhanced air and blood flow through the ethmoid, and (it is assumed) release of sutural restrictions. Alternatively the separation hold, using ounces of force or less, can be maintained until a sense of 'release' is palpated.

The separation action (pulsed or constant) eases sutural impaction which may exist between the ethmoid as it is moved away from the frontal, nasal, and maxillary bones.

Dysfunctional patterns associated with the vomer

- In rare cases, the vomer can penetrate the palatine suture, producing an enlargement/swelling of the central portion of the roof of the hard palate, a condition known as torus palatinus.
- As with the ethmoid, inflammation of the vomer may occur in association with sinusitis.
- Direct trauma can cause deviation of the vomer and so interfere with normal nasal breathing.

Vomer palpation (Fig. 6.31)

The practitioner cups the supine patient's occiput with one hand. The (gloved) thumb of the other hand is placed into the patient's mouth in such a way that the pad rests on the hard palate just behind the upper incisors. The index and middle fingers of that hand should be placed either side of the patient's nose, so that they rest on the superior aspects of the maxillae, inferior to the suture.

It is possible for the practitioner to utilize these contacts to *gently* separate the vomer in an anteroinferior direction as the hand holding the head offers simultaneous gentle separation force to the occiput. Motion of the vomer should be sensed by the thumb if alternating separation and release forces are applied (using under an ounce of pressure from the thumb).

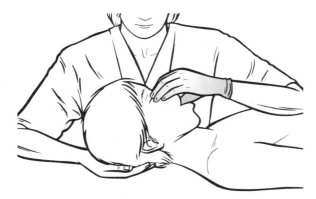

Figure 6.31 Intra-oral thumb approach to treatment of vomer. (Reproduced with kind permission from Chaitow 1999.)

Dysfunctional patterns associated with the zygomata (Fig. 6.32)

- Clinical experience suggests that sinus problems can benefit from increased freedom of the zygomata.
- One or both zygomata may require attention after dental trauma, especially upper tooth extractions, as well as trauma to the face of any sort, as they may have absorbed the effects of the stresses involved.

- Habits such as supporting the face/cheekbone on a hand when writing should be discouraged as the persistent pressure can traumatize the zygoma.

Palpation exercises for the zygoma

The patient is supine and the practitioner is seated at the head. The practitioner rests the tips of the middle, index and ring fingers just below the inferior surface of the anteroinferior border of each zygoma, with the thumbs resting on the forehead, facing each other above the eyebrows. The practitioner should make absolutely sure that contacts are anterior to the zygomaticotemporal suture, and should *gently* (grams only), rhythmically encourage 'flexion' and 'extension' of the bones, easing them superiorly and then inferiorly together with extremely light pressure (ounce or less) laterally.

Decompression can be introduced in any direction from this contact, bilaterally or unilaterally, as appropriate.

Dysfunctional patterns associated with the maxillae (Fig. 6.33)

- The maxillae house the air sinuses and are associated with almost all the small facial bones associated with breathing.

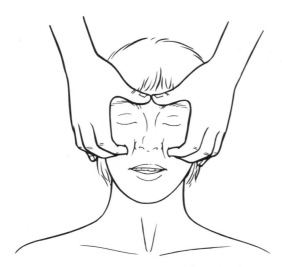

Figure 6.32A Palpation of the zygoma utilizing three fingers. (Reproduced with kind permission from Chaitow 1999.)

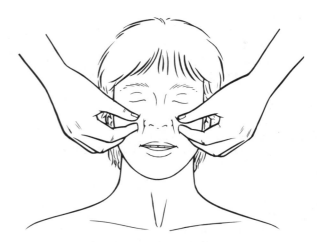

Figure 6.32B Testing for directions of freedom of zygomatic motion utilizing fingers and thumb. (Reproduced with kind permission from Chaitow 1999.)

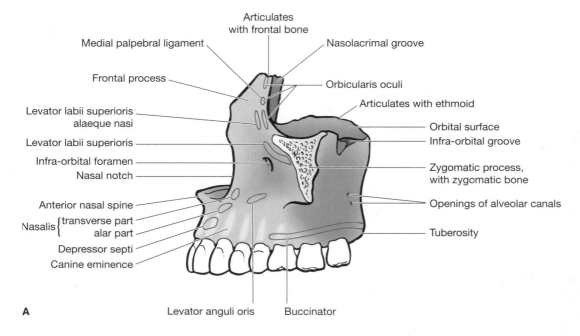

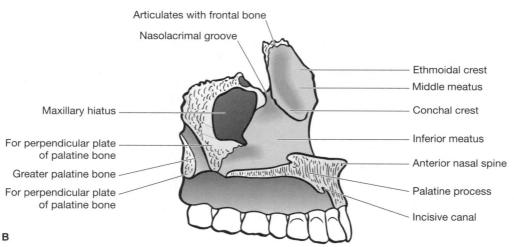

Figure 6.33A Left maxilla, lateral aspect showing major features, articulations and muscular attachment sites. (Reproduced with kind permission from Chaitow 1999.) **B** Left maxilla, medial aspect showing major features and articulations. (Reproduced with kind permission from Chaitow 1999.)

- Headaches, facial pain, and sinus problems, plus a host of mouth and throat connections (including 'unspoken' emotional ones), mean that this is seen in craniosacral work to be an interface between purely biomechanical and mind–body problems (Milne 1995).

Palpation of inferior maxillary decompression

The practitioner is seated at the head of the supine patient. Absorbent paper should be used to dry saliva from the upper incisors. Surgical gloves should be worn. The practitioner places his elbows to rest alongside the patient's face, with wrists markedly flexed, and grasps each of the upper incisors between a finger (index is best) and thumb.

Using very light traction, the practitioner introduces a pull caudally to distract the maxillae from their superior attachments, and to initiate a caudad movement of the vomer, ethmoid, and, ultimately, the falx cerebri.

There should be a sense of pliable distraction if the force used remains under an ounce. Holding the distracting pull for several minutes can ensure

a release of these structures if they are crowded as a result of trauma (dental for example).

⚠ In a report on iatrogenic effects from inappropriately applied cranial treatment, Professor John McPartland (1996) presented nine illustrative cases, of which two involved intraoral treatment. All cases seemed to involve excessive force being used, but these cases nevertheless highlight the need for extreme care when working cranially, and especially when working inside the mouth.

REFERENCES

Barral J-P 1996 Manual thermal diagnosis. Eastland Press, Seattle

Beal M 1983 Palpatory testing of somatic dysfunction in patients with cardiovascular disease. Journal of the American Osteopathic Association 82: 822–831

Beal M 1984 Somatic dysfunction associated with pulmonary disease. Journal of the American Osteopathic Association 84: 179–183

Beal M 1985 Viscerosomatic reflexes. Journal of the American Osteopathic Association 85: 786–800

Bradley D 1999 In: Gilbert C (ed) Breathing retraining advice from three therapists. Journal of Bodywork and Movement Therapies 3, 159–167

Chaitow L 1994 Integrated neuromuscular inhibition technique. British Journal of Osteopathy 13: 17–20

Chaitow L 1996a Positional release techniques, 1st edn. Churchill Livingstone, Edinburgh

Chaitow L 1996b Modern neuromuscular techniques. Churchill Livingstone, Edinburgh

Chaitow L 1996c Muscle energy techniques. Churchill Livingstone, Edinburgh

Chaitow L 1999 Cranial manipulation: theory and practice. Churchill Livingstone, Edinburgh

Chaitow L 2001 Muscle energy techniques, 2nd edn. Churchill Livingstone, Edinburgh

Chaitow L 2002 Positional release techniques, 2nd edn. Churchill Livingstone, Edinburgh

Chaitow L, DeLany J 2000 Clinical applications of neuromuscular techniques. Vol 1. The upper body. Churchill Livingstone, Edinburgh

Chila A 1997 Fascial-ligamentous release. In: Ward R (ed) Foundations for osteopathic medicine. Williams and Wilkins, Baltimore

Cox, Gorbis, Dick, Rogers 1983 Journal of the American Osteopathic Association 82: 11

D'Alonzo G, Krachman S 1997 Respiratory system. In: Ward R (ed) Foundations for osteopathic medicine. Williams and Wilkins, Baltimore

D'Ambrogio K, Roth G 1997 Positional release therapy. Mosby, St Louis

Deig D 2001 Positional release technique. Butterworth, Heinemann, Boston

DiGiovanna E 1997 An osteopathic approach to diagnosis and treatment. Lippincott-Raven, Philadelphia

Faling L 1995 Controlled breathing techniques and chest physical therapy in chronic obstructive pulmonary disease. In: Casabur R (ed) Principles and practices of pulmonary therapy. W B Saunders, Philadelphia

Gibbons P, Tehan P 2000 Manipulation of the spine, thorax and pelvis. Churchill Livingstone, Edinburgh

Goodridge J, Kuchera W 1997 Muscle energy techniques for specific areas. In: Ward R (ed) Foundations for osteopathic medicine. Williams & Wilkins, Baltimore

Greenman P 1996 Principles of manual medicine, 2nd edn. Williams and Wilkins, Baltimore

Harakal J 1975 An osteopathically integrated approach to whiplash complex. Journal of the American Osteopathic Association 74: 941–956

Hoag M 1969 Osteopathic medicine. McGraw Hill, New York

Hong C-Z 1994 Considerations and recommendations regarding myofascial trigger point injection. Journal of Musculoskeletal Pain 2(1): 29–59

Hong C-Z, Chen Y-C, Pon C, Yu J 1993 Immediate effects of various physical medicine modalities on pain threshold of an active myofascial trigger point. Journal of Musculoskeletal Pain 1(2)

Howell R, Allen R, Kapper R 1975 Influence of OMT in management of patients with chronic obstructive lung disease. Journal of the American Osteopathic Association 74: 757–760

Hruby R, Goodridge J 1997 Thoracic region and rib cage. In: Ward R (ed) Foundations of osteopathic medicine. Williams and Wilkins, Baltimore

Janda V 1996 Evaluation of muscular imbalance. In: Liebenson C (ed) Rehabilitation of the spine. Williams and Wilkins, Baltimore

Jones L 1981 Strain and counterstrain. Academy of Applied Osteopathy, Colorado Springs

Jonkheere P, Pattyn J 1998 Myofascial muscle chains. Trigger vzw, Brugge, Belgium

Kelso A 1971 A double-blind clinical study of osteopathic findings in hospital patients. Journal of the American Osteopathic Association 70: 570–592

Kelso A, Larson N, Kappler R 1980 A clinical investigation of the osteopathic examination. Journal of the American Osteopathic Association 79: 460–467

Kline C 1965 Osteopathic manipulative therapy, antibiotics and supportive therapy in respiratory infections in children. Journal of the American Osteopathic Association 65: 278–281

Kolzumi K, Brooks McC C 1972 Integration of autonomic system reactions. In: Ergebnisseder physiologic. Springer-Verlag, Berlin

Korr I 1970 The physiological basis of osteopathic medicine. Postgraduate Institute of Osteopathic Medicine and Surgery, New York

Kuchera M 1997 Travell and Simons myofascial trigger points. In: Ward R (ed) Foundations for osteopathic medicine. Williams and Wilkins, Baltimore

Kurschner O A 1958 Comparative clinical investigation of chloramphenicol and OMT of whooping cough. Journal of the American Osteopathic Association 57: 559–561

Lewit K 1986 Muscular patterns in thoraco-lumber lesions. Manual Medicine 2: 105

Lewit K 1999 Manipulative therapy in rehabilitation of the locomotor system, 3rd edn. Butterworths, London

Liebenson C 1996 Rehabilitation of the spine. Williams and Wilkins, Baltimore

Lin J-P 1994 Physiological maturation of muscles in childhood. Lancet (June 4): 1386–1389

McConnell C 1899 The practice of osteopathy.

McPartland J 1996 Craniosacral iatrogenesis. Journal of Bodywork and Movement Therapies 1(1): 2–5

Measel J 1982 Effect of lymphatic pump on immune response: preliminary studies on the antibody response to pneumonococcal polysaccharide assayed by bacterial agglutination and passive hemagglutination. Journal of the American Osteopathic Association 82(1): 28–31

Miller W 1975 Treatment of visceral disorders by manipulative therapy. In: The research status of manipulative therapy. US Department of Health Education and Welfare. Bethesda, Maryland

Milne H 1995 The heart of listening. North Atlantic Books, Berkeley, CA

Moore M 1980 Electromyographic investigation manual of muscle stretching techniques. Medical Science and Sports Exercise 12: 322–329

Muellen R, Petty T, Filley G 1970 Ventilators and arterial blood gas changes induced by pursed lip breathing. Journal of Applied Physiology 28: 784–789

Mulligan B 1992 Manual therapy. Plane View Services. Wellington, New Zealand

Noll D, Shores J, Bryman P, Masterson E 1999 Adjunctive osteopathic manipulative treatment in the elderly hospitalized with pneumonia: a pilot study. Journal of the American Osteopathic Association 3: 143–152

Norris C 2000 Back stability. Human Kinetics, Leeds

Oppenheimer S 1990 Comparison of thoracic lymphatic pump and incentive spirometry. Journal of the American Osteopathic Association 90: 839–840

Paul F, Buser B 1996 Osteopathic manipulative treatment applications for the emergency department patient. Journal of the American Osteopathic Association 96: 403–409

Rowane W, Rowane M 1999 An osteopathic approach to asthma. Journal of the American Osteopathic Association 99(5): 259–264

Ruddy T 1962 Osteopathic rapid rhythmic resistive technic. Academy of Applied Osteopathy Yearbook, pp 23–31. Carmel, California

Simons D 1989 Myofascial pain syndromes. Current Therapy of Pain. B. C. Decker, pp 251–266

Simons D, Travell J 1983 Low back pain, part 2. Post Graduate Medicine 73(2): 81–92

Simons D, Travell J, Simons L 1998 Myofascial pain and dysfunction: the trigger point manual. Vol 1: Upper half of body. 2nd edn. Williams and Wilkins, Baltimore

Sleszynski S, Kelso A 1993 Comparison of thoracic manipulation with incentive spirometry in the prevention of post-operative atelectasis. Journal of the American Osteopathic Association 93: 834–845

Tisp B, Burns M, Kro D, Kao D, Madison R, Herrera J 1986 Pursed lip breathing using ear oximetry. Chest 90: 218–221

Upledger J, Vredevoogd W 1983 Craniosacral therapy. Eastland Press, Seattle

Wallace E, McPartland J, Jones J, Kuchera W 1997 Lymphatic system. In: Ward R (ed) Foundations for osteopathic medicine. Williams and Wilkins, Baltimore

Ward R (ed) 1997 Foundations for osteopathic medicine. Williams and Wilkins, Baltimore

Yates S 1991 Muscle energy techniques. In: DiGiovanna E (ed) Principles of osteopathic manipulative techniques. Lippincott, Philadelphia

Zink G, Lawson W 1979 An osteopathic structural examination and functional interpretation of the soma. Osteopathic Annals 12(7): 433–440

7

Physiotherapy breathing rehabilitation strategies

Dinah Bradley

INTRODUCTION

Hyperventilation syndromes/breathing pattern disorders (HVS/BPDs) are still alive and thriving in the early 21st century. They have a very long history, dating back at least as far as Hippocrates, who in the 5th century BC observed that breathing is the balancing force in maintaining mental and physical health: his words, 'The brain exercises the greatest power in human-kind – but the air supplies sense to it,' are as relevant today as they were 2500 years ago. More recently called 'a diagnosis begging for recognition' (Magarian 1982), these disorders are increasingly being recognized as major causes of ill health, though still remaining widely underdiagnosed and undertreated.

Patients seeking a diagnosis have faced the paradox of being told by their doctors, often after exhaustive tests showing that nothing is clinically wrong with them to 'go away, have counseling, join a yoga class, relax.' But the symptoms continue, fueled by habitual breathing dysfunction, and their bodies continue to signal distress. What can they do? Who can help?

Self-confidence evaporates and secondary problems emerge. Avoidance behaviors and phobias may flourish along with feelings of extreme anxiety. Sighing and breathing discomfort are seen as signs of these understandable fears, when in fact habitual overbreathing is in and of itself a major cause of stress and anxiety (Lum 1975). Unravelling sometimes

---

Box 7.1 Cascade of symptoms

Original cause (emotional or physical)
↓
Tension and anxiety
↓
Hyperventilation
↓
Acute hyperventilation attack
↓
Anticipation anxiety
↓
Avoidance behaviors/phobias

---

years of suffering takes time and patience, as well as a good deal of detective work in identifying the source and effects of the original trigger. The cascade of symptoms is shown in Box 7.1.

Breathing dysfunction affects emotions. While there are prescribed rituals to deal with well understood major upheavals such as death, divorce, or trauma, those who experience the frightening and worrying symptoms of chronically disordered breathing are often poorly understood. They suffer without the automatic social support given to more tangible life events, or, sadly, are pigeon-holed as 'highly strung,' hypochondriacs, or malingerers. It is time to make this disorder 'acceptable' – one that people are able to talk freely about and for which they are able to find effective help and treatment.

The acclaimed British actress Imogen Stubbs speaks eloquently of her personal experience of HVS, which threatened to ruin her career (Pitman 1996), as follows:

When I was 22, on a plane in Mexico, I experienced tingling in my lips and fingers, and a heaviness in my limbs. I suddenly and terrifyingly found myself completely paralysed for a few hours. I flew back to England and I was treated by many doctors who gave me pills – Valium – and things like that but who didn't really know what was wrong with me. Finally I was referred to a physiotherapist, and within a few months I no longer had symptoms of hyperventilation. I was completely cured and have never had any problems again. I feel sure if I hadn't had physiotherapy treatment I wouldn't have had an acting career.

Stubbs's story introduces an excellent video put out in 1996 by the UK organization Physiotherapy for Hyperventilation (Pitman 1996), and she is to be congratulated for telling her story and in so doing helping other 'overbreathers.'

PHYSIOTHERAPY REHABILITATION STRATEGIES

The physiotherapy approach to treating people with breathing pattern disorders can be summarized as 'maximum involvement with minimum intervention' (Hough 1998, p. 278). Many patients have already been tested exhaustively – sometimes by painful or invasive tests – and often arrive with nervous expectations of yet more. The 'low-tech' approach makes a refreshing change for most.

Management includes assessment and treatment involving detailed explanations of breathing pattern disorders, and building an individual integrated recovery program based on:

- Breathing retraining
- Tension release through talk and relaxation
- Stress perception and management
- Enjoyable graduated exercise prescriptions
- Rest/sleep guides (Bradley 1998).

Musculoskeletal protocols for particular problems are covered in Chapter 6, which represents interdisciplinary manual therapy methods. As many new patients present in a state of hyperarousal, the initial assessment and treatment programs suggested in this chapter highlight this. Emphasis on desensitizing through breathing retraining and relaxation is presented as one starting point.

THE ENVIRONMENT

An airy, quiet room with a relaxed atmosphere is recommended for assessment and treatment. This may be difficult to find in busy hospital outpatient departments. A welcoming sense of safety, confidentiality, and privacy is essential, with comfortable chairs and treatment bed. Space for extra family members or friends should be provided if requested, and a box of tissues and drinking water should be on hand. Allow an hour for the first appointment.

PHYSIOTHERAPY ASSESSMENT

Patient referrals may arrive from many sources: a variety of consultants, general practitioners, psychologists, practice nurses, community health workers, speech therapists or dentists, or patients may refer themselves. Some provide a detailed picture, while others offer only scant information with little or no background data. Clear communications with referral agents are essential.

When patients self-refer to physiotherapists and present with no records of previous tests or health problems, it is recommended that physiotherapists should seek permission from these individuals to liaise with their general practitioners/physicians.

⚠ **CAUTION:** If these patients have unexplained chest pain, breathlessness, or dizziness, the physiotherapist must check with the patient's doctor before starting treatment, in order to rule out more sinister causes.

Detailed history

Prescribed medications should be recorded to establish current treatments and conditions, and possible side-effects. For example, beta-blockers may have been prescribed to patients experiencing stress/adrenalin-induced cardiac arrhythmias. These medications may cause bronchospasm, exacerbating hyperventilation.

Past medical history

Past health problems may provide clues and should be listed, for example 'chesty' as a child, sinus problems, history of allergy, anemia, migraine, emotional or physical trauma, 'panic' attacks, past surgery, or other health problems such as irritable bowel, premenstrual or menopausal hormone difficulties, chronic fatigue or occupational overuse syndromes (OOS).

Socially acceptable drug use (e.g. tobacco, caffeine) and alcohol intake should be noted. Recreational drug use or past or present history

---

Box 7.2 Smokers

Inhalations from cigarettes, cigars, and pipes reinforce upper-chest breathing patterns. While not wanting to encourage smokers to breathe abdominally (drawing smoke into the depths of the lung):

- Smokers can be offered smoking cessation programs
- Marijuana smokers, who tend to prolong hyperinflation, must be discouraged from doing this
- Those who choose to continue can be encouraged to breathe in lightly and very shallowly.

---

of addiction as possible contributing factors to present health status should be discussed. Referral on to appropriate agencies may be offered if the patient requests help (Box 7.2).

Where the patient was born may also provide clues: 'People born at high altitude have a diminished ventilatory response to hypoxia that is only slowly corrected by subsequent residence at sea level. Conversely, those born at sea level who move to high altitudes retain their hypoxic response intact for a long time. Apparently, therefore, ventilatory response is determined very early in life' (West 2000).

A chance to talk about symptoms and give a subjective view to an empathetic ear will help establish rapport and trust: for some patients it may the first time they have really been listened to – a case of literally 'getting it off one's chest.'

History taking is also an excellent time to note autonomic disturbances (e.g. clammy hands, sweating, postural tension/restlessness, rapid speech, indicating sympathetic dominance) (Nixon 1989).

Social history

Inquiries will help reveal stress-related events/triggers. Occupation, job satisfaction, redundancy issues, marital status, whether the patient's domestic life is calm, complicated, or isolated should be covered. Record how many days off work or school the patient has had in the last 6 months – this is also a useful statistic to keep for long-term outcome measures.

Sensitive topics may surface such as abuse, emotional, or sexual problems. If the patient wishes, further expert help can be offered from appropriate specialist counselors.

History of tests/investigations

An inventory of tests and investigations gives a clear picture to the physiotherapist of the number of interventions the patient has endured, and what coexisting problems may have been revealed (e.g. anemia), or ruled out (e.g. brain tumor). Possible interventions include blood tests, X-rays, lung function, tests, scans, neurology or cardiology tests (see Ch. 2).

Alternative therapies

Natural remedies or dietary changes which may currently be impacting on the patient's health profile need to be recorded. Encourage openness in discussing these. Orthodox medicine's failure to recognize and offer treatment to people with chronic breathing pattern disorders often drives sufferers to seek alternatives – sometimes drastic,

and often very expensive alternatives, which may have no accountability or research to back up claims. There is also the risk of harm caused by dangerous combinations of prescribed medication with herbal remedies.

⚠ **CAUTION:** As with all drugs, whether prescription or naturopathic, make sure that your patients understand exactly what they are swallowing, and why.

Questionnaire

As yet there is no 'gold standard' laboratory test to clinch the diagnosis of chronic HVS. However, the Nijmegen questionnaire (Box 7.3) provides a noninvasive test of high sensitivity (up to 91%) and specificity up to 95% (Van Dixhoorn & Duivenvoorden 1985). This easily administered, internationally validated (Vansteenkiste et al 1991) diagnostic questionnaire is the simplest, kindest, and, to date, most accurate indicator of acute/

Box 7.3 Nijmegen questionnaire					
	Never 0	Rare 1	Sometimes 2	Often 3	Very often 4
Chest pain					
Feeling tense					
Blurred vision					
Dizzy spells					
Feeling confused					
Faster or deeper breathing					
Short of breath					
Tight feelings in chest					
Bloated feeling in stomach					
Tingling fingers					
Unable to breathe deeply					
Stiff fingers or arms					
Tight feelings round mouth					
Cold hands or feet					
Palpitations					
Feelings of anxiety					
Total: /64*					

* Nijmegen. Patients mark with a tick how often they suffer from the symptoms listed. A score above 23/64 is diagnostic of hyperventilation syndrome.

chronic hyperventilation. It also has great educative value as patients often for the first time appreciate the widespread nature of their symptoms.

Retesting at a later date is helpful in showing patients their progress as their symptoms decrease or vanish. It is common for chronic hyperventilators to concentrate on the most worrying symptom (i.e. chest pain) and ignore other discomforts. Retesting may help patients to accept that faulty breathing affects all systems and in fact they have 'a welter of bodily symptoms' (Lum 1985). The results also help establish:

- Whether the initiating trigger causing the HVS/BPD has been resolved; the patient will then only have to deal with the 'bad breathing' habit and the musculoskeletal and motor pattern changes they have been left with.
- Whether the initiating trigger(s) are ongoing or unresolved; the patient may need further cognitive help. Shared care with a psychiatrist, psychologist, or psychotherapist may be offered to this group of patients.
- An appreciation by the physiotherapist as to what the patient is struggling against.

Clinical observation of rate and patterns of breathing

Note should be taken of the following:

1. Resting respiratory rate (normal adult range is 10–14 per minute) (West 1995).
2. Nose or mouth breather?
3. Resting breathing pattern:
   — Effortless upper chest/hyperinflation?
   — Accessory muscle use?
   — Frequent sighs/yawns?
   — Breath holding ('statue breathing')?
   — Abdominal splinting?
   — Chaotic/combinations of the above?
   — Repeated throat clearing/air gulping?

These observations can be made unobtrusively while taking the patient's radial pulse.

Nasal problems

Patients with chronic uni- or bilateral nasal airflow restriction or obstruction need further investigation. Discuss with the patient's doctor the option of scheduling a mini series CT scan to establish the source of the problem. Referral on to an otorhinolaryngeal (ORL) specialist may be required to sort out these problems before starting effective breathing retraining.

Some chronic mouth breathers simply have 'soggy' noses through disuse which respond well to saline/bicarbonate nasal washes. This aids the mucociliary linings to slough off excess mucus build-up and restore normal function. The addition of bicarbonate of soda adds to the effectiveness by acting rather like Teflon (non-stick), coating the nasal linings to aid drainage (see recipe in Ch. 10, p. 261).

Breath-hold tests

While no standardized test yet exists, breath-hold times are recorded by many clinicians as a part of HVS/BPD assessment. Failure to hold beyond 30 seconds is considered by some a positive diagnostic sign of chronic hyperventilation (Gardner 1996). In practice, chronic hyperventilators seldom hold beyond 10–12 seconds before gasping. It makes a useful marker to test at regular intervals, and note improved breath-holding times.

Musculoskeletal inspection/ observation

Observe:

1. The jaw, facial and general postural tension, tremor, tics, twitches, bitten nails
2. Chest wall abnormalities, such as:
   — pectus carinatum (anterior sternal protrusion)
   — pectus excavatum (depression or hollowing of the sternum)
   — kyphosis (abnormal forward anteroposterior spinal curvature)
   — scoliosis (lateral spinal curvature)
   — kyphoscoliosis (a combination of the former two).
3. Adaptive upper thoracic and shoulder-girdle muscle changes (e.g. raised shoulders, protracted scapulae) (Fig. 7.1).

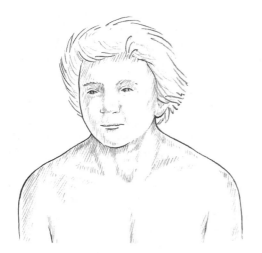

Figure 7.1 A typical pattern of upper thoracic and cervical stress as described by Janda would involve a degree of TMJ stress. Note the 'gothic shoulders' which result from upper trapezius hypertonicity and shortening. (Reproduced with kind permission from Chaitow 1996.)

Box 7.4 describes some of the factors thought to contribute to occupational overuse syndrome and repetitive strain injury.

Upper thoracic trigger points (Figs 7.3–7.5)

Selection of three ventral upper chest trigger points (e.g. Figs 7.3, 7.4, 7.5), and recording the subjective response by the patient on the Numeric Pain Scale (Jensen et al 1986; Box 7.5) to palpation of these points provides a repeatable objective measure of:

- The intensity of chest wall pain at assessment
- Reduction in chest wall pain in response to breathing retraining and employment of relaxation techniques.

For research purposes, an algometer (pressure threshold device) would be required to standardize the intensity of palpation. The American College of Rheumatology guide (1990) suggests a pressure of 4 kilograms (10 lb) over selected trigger points. For non-research clinical purposes, digital pressure is sufficient. (Practice on a set of scales to establish the right 'feel'.)

So while no move to deactivate trigger point pain by compression is part of the treatment

plan, rechecking at regular intervals monitors progress and motivates patients to perservere with breathing retraining, body awareness of tension, and relaxation. It also serves as a useful marker for the patients themselves to check as part of symptom recognition (Chaitow 2000).

Oximetry

An oximeter is a small battery-operated hand-held device allowing for noninvasive instant feedback of arterial oxygen saturations. A sensor which may be attached to a finger, toe, or ear lobe pulses alternately red and infrared light through the vascular bed, and a microprocessor determines the oxygen saturation value, displayed as a digital readout. It is recorded as SpO_2 to differentiate from arterial blood gas (ABG) saturations of haemoglobin with oxygen (SaO_2) analyses obtained from arterial puncture (Hanning & Alexander-Williams 1995). Measured as a percentage, pulse oximetry is reasonably accurate at values above 75%. Desaturation is indicated at values below 95% in black people, 92% in white people, or a drop of 4% (Durbin 1994). Oximeters may be fooled by the presence of anemia, hypotension, hypovolemia, peripheral vascular disease, or vasopressor drugs. Nicotine stains and nail varnish both compromise finger sensor readings (Hough 1998).

Normal resting SpO_2 levels are between 95% and 98% (West 1995) (Box 7.6).

With patients who demonstrate breathing pattern disorders, there are two purposes in using an oximeter:

1. First, as a safety measure to check patients with concurrent cardiac or respiratory disease. For example, unexplained chest pain, breathlessness with hypoxemia may indicate pulmonary embolus.
2. Second, its use as a teaching aid is a positive way of showing patients in otherwise good health they have plenty of available O_2 and can easily afford to reduce their respiratory rate and volume. Chronic overbreathers tend to be well above 95%, the minimum normal level. A high proportion are 100% saturated, much to their surprise.

Box 7.4 Work-related breathing problems (Fig. 7.2)

Thoracic outlet nerve and blood vessel compression due to musculoskeletal changes from persistent upper-chest breathing has been implicated in the development of occupational overuse syndrome (OOS)/repetitive strain injury (RSI) – the blight of the electronic age. Schleifer & Ley (1994) have presented a hyperventilatory model of psychological stress as a contributing factor to the current epidemic of musculoskeletal problems in repetitive VDU/computer work.

They found that under stressful conditions (high workload demands, long hours, boredom, and fatigue), sedentary breathing exceeds metabolic requirements for oxygen, and hypocapnia results. At the cellular level, relatively mild reductions in arterial CO_2 result in a rise in pH (alkalosis). Under such conditions, heightened neuronal activity, increased muscle tension and spasming, paresthesias, and a suppression of parasympathetic activity, and consequent sympathetic dominance of the autonomic nervous system, result in amplified responses to catecholamines. These hyperventilatory-induced stress reactions have been implicated as an important factor in work-related overuse and stress injuries.

While there are excellent OOS prevention schemes, with on-site ergonomic checks and strategies, few include breathing awareness/retraining as part of overall stress reduction. Schleifer & Ley's findings indicate a positive correlation between work-related hyperventilation and onset of symptoms, and reveal an important area requiring further research.

In addition to breathing retraining, mobilizing exercises to reduce thoracic outlet restrictions and neural stretches can be taught, in liaison with occupational safety and health officers and GPs.

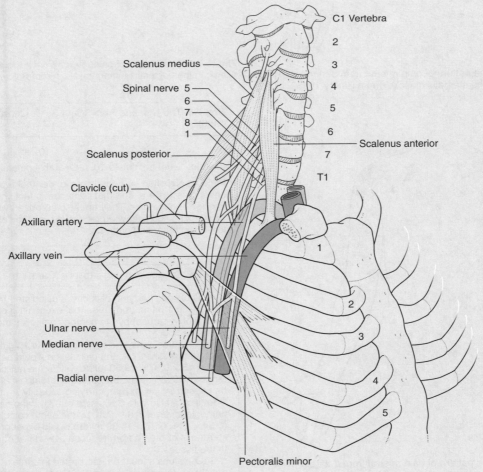

Figure 7.2 Thoracic outlet.

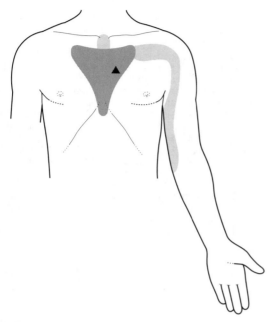

Figure 7.3 The pattern of pain referral from a trigger point (or points) in the sternalis muscle. (From Baldry 1993.)

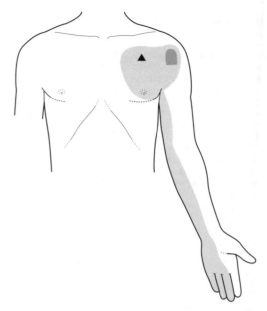

Figure 7.5 The pattern of pain referral from a trigger point (or points) in the pectoralis minor muscle. (From Baldry 1993.)

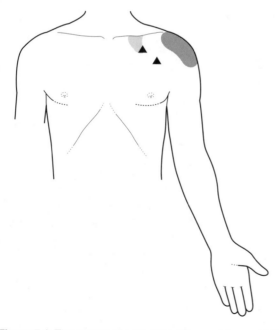

Figure 7.4 The pattern of pain referral from a trigger point or points in the clavicular section of the pectoralis major muscle.

Box 7.5 The Numeric Pain Rating Scale (Jensen et al 1986)

1 − − − − − − − − − 10

(Range: 1, not painful; to 10, unbearably painful.)

Patients are often surprised how tender their upper chest muscles are, and that pains are in fact chest wall in origin, not cardiac. They are also surprised when chest pains subside when rechecked, as they adopt low-chest breathing patterns.

Box 7.6 Oxygen carrying capacity (Carroll 1997)

Overall oxygen carrying capacity is calculated by multiplying 1.34 ml (the amount of oxygen 1 g of hemoglobin carries) by the hemoglobin level and the SpO_2 reading.

For instance, patient X's hemoglobin is 15 g/dL, SpO_2 saturations 97%, the calculation would be: $1.34 \times 15 \times 0.97 = 19.50$ ml/dL, within the normal range of 19–20 ml/dL. Shortness of breath would not be caused by low oxygen carrying capacity.

Patient Y, also with SpO_2 sats of 97%, who has a low hemoglobin level of 11 g/dL, by the same calculation ($1.34 \times 11 \times 0.97 = 14.30$ ml/dL) would experience shortness of breath from reduced availability of oxygen to the tissues.

SpO_2 values should be interpreted in context with the patient's total hemoglobin levels where possible.

Capnography (see also Ch. 5)

Hospital physiotherapists may have access to capnography. This device measures end tidal CO_2 levels from exhaled air (collected via nasal prongs), which resembles those of arterial values. Fluctuating CO_2 levels, or those below 32 mmHg (4.3 kPa) would suggest chronic hyperventilation (Timmons & Ley 1994).

It makes a positive biofeedback tool (Conway 1994) for patients who can see their CO_2 levels normalize as they practice 'low slow nose' breathing. Outcome measures are also provided (Hough 1996).

Peak expiratory flow rate (PEFR)

A peak flow meter is a simple, inexpensive device which measures the highest flow of air out of the lungs, from peak inspiration, in a fast single forced breath out. This reflects airflow resistance, the elasticity of the supporting lung tissues, and ease of breathing. Its uses are those listed below:

- As a kinder and less risky alternative to the hyperventilation provocation test (HVPT) (see Ch. 2).
- The best of three blows in quick succession may elicit light-headedness or familiar tingling, linking the relationship between overbreathing and symptoms to the patient.
- Revealing 'normal lung power' often surprises those who frequently feel 'air hunger' or chest tightness.
- Reductions in normal expected flows would indicate the need for spirometry/further investigations for more accurate measures.
- Establishing a baseline for people with asthma, or chronic airflow limitation at the start of treatment.

Another use is for patients who have been on repeated or prolonged courses of oral steroids, for whatever reason, and who may therefore have reduced skeletal muscle strength. The diaphragm is not exempt.

Breathing retraining with diaphragm strengthening and inspiratory muscle training (IMT) (Weiner 1995) may show an improvement within 2–6 weeks. A simply measured outcome is a repeat PEFR after a month of retraining.

Education

The time spent on history taking and data gathering is an excellent opportunity for explanations of the consequences of breathing dysfunction. At the summing up of findings, complete a fuller teaching session with the help of visual aids (e.g. diagrams of the chest walls, lungs, diaphragm, nasopharynx, typical and atypical breathing patterns (Fig. 7.6).

Discretion as to how much detail to go into at first should be considered, since too much information may sail in one ear and out the other. Highly stressed patients often have poor concentration. Getting straight to physical coping skills, with physiological explanations being left until later, may be the better option.

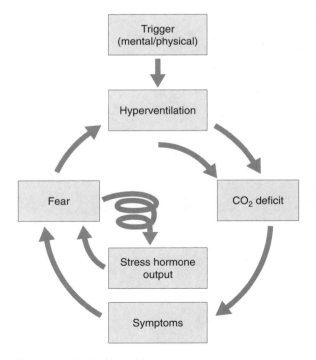

Figure 7.6 Atypical breathing patterns.

GETTING STARTED

The following six-part approach, using the acronym BETTER*, helps establish priorities and step-by-step planning of physiotherapy treatment.

*B = breathing retraining, E = esteem/self-image, T = total body relaxation, T = talk/breath control, E = exercise prescription, R = rest/sleep (Bradley 1998).

After collating all the findings, an individual treatment plan can be drawn up with patient involvement. Find out what your patient's expectations are as well as their commitment to schedule time for retraining and possible lifestyle changes (i.e. reduce caffeine intake, prioritize obligations, etc.). A pact with clear, measureable, attainable goals should be drawn up.

BREATHING RETRAINING

Four basic principles in restoring normal energy-efficient and physiologically balanced breathing are:

1. Awareness of faulty breathing patterns
2. Relaxation of the upper chest, shoulders, and accessory muscles
3. Abdominal/low-chest breathing pattern retraining
4. Awareness of normal breathing rates and rhythms, both at rest and during activity.

1. The patient is half lying (Fig. 7.7). Ask the patient to place one relaxed hand on the stomach, above the navel, and the other on the upper chest and clavicle. The patient is asked to take a 'deep' breath. The chances are they will take a 'big' breath instead, through the mouth, inflating the upper chest first with little or no low-chest

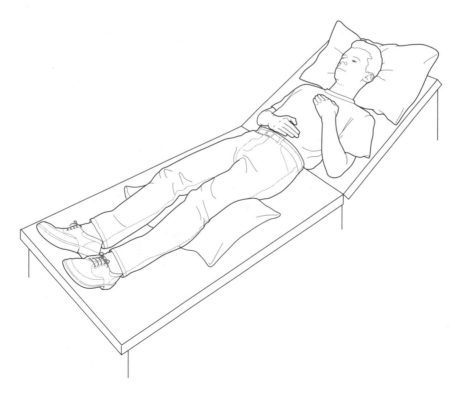

Figure 7.7 Half-lying. Hand-check test (Bradley 1998).

involvement, or even drawing in the stomach at the peak of inspiration. Using their own hands as guides, patients can appreciate the difference between vigorous 'big' and gentle 'deep' breathing. They can also feel the movement of their habitual upper chest – or 'reverse breathing' – pattern, along with little or no diaphragmatic excursion/abdominal movement. Switch from mouth to nose breathing so the patient can feel the difference in both resistance and patterning.

⚠ **CAUTION:** It is also a good idea to issue a warning at this stage that being aware of breathing is both unnatural and uncomfortable, and to be prepared for transient feelings of discomfort and 'air hunger' (Pitman 1996).

2. Once patients can identify their faulty patterns, the second step is for them to learn how to relax the upper chest and accessory muscles. A simple way of helping achieve this is to have them clasp their hands on top of their head. This helps put the upper chest muscles into 'neutral' and patients can usually immediately feel their diaphragm recruited into action. The diaphragm descends as they breathe in and their stomach gently rises, then relaxes down as they exhale.

Bending the knees helps loosen tense abdominal muscles (beach pose) (Fig. 7.8).

Patients often describe feelings of 'air hunger' or upper-chest tension as they try to relax their shoulders and upper chest. (Rechecking SpO_2 saturations will help convince doubting patients they are *not* hypoxic.) Swallowing and *concentrating on the exhale* usually helps the patient to overcome this discomfort (Innocenti 1988). As progress is made the patient is encouraged to practice with the arms down and legs out straight and loose, shoulders relaxed. Some patients respond well to placing a 1 kilogram wheatbag on their upper chest, helping focus on upper-chest stillness and relaxation, and switching off trigger-happy accessory and jaw muscles.

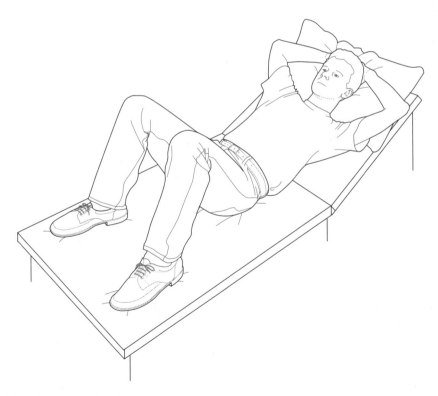

Figure 7.8 Beach pose (Bradley 1998).

3. Having felt abdominal breathing while in the beach pose, concentration can be switched to low-chest breathing with quiet in-breaths dissolving into the out-breath without pause, until the end of the out-breath is reached. (Habitual 'reverse breathers' will have been doing the exact opposite. Pausing instead at the top of the inhalation (tense) driven by their upper-thoracic breathing patterns they lose the natural relaxed pause or neutral point at the end of exhalation.)

A 1 or 2 kilogram wheatbag (depending on the size of the patient) placed over the navel provides an excellent and inexpensive biofeedback mechanism. The patient can feel, see, and control the rise, fall, and relaxation of the abdominal wall by focusing on the weight. Patients often remark how hard it is at first, and how intensely they have to concentrate (followed by how intensely relaxing it feels when they 'get it').

4. Restoring an energy-efficient, low-chest, nose-breathing pattern, with a *relaxed pause at the end of the exhale* often restores normal breathing rates at the same time. Counting out loud while timing helps at the beginning, with positive reinforcement from the physiotherapist. It is important that the patient be encouraged to relearn the *feeling* of 'low slow nose breathing.' Mentally repeating the phrases, 'When in doubt, breathe out' and 'Lips together, jaw relaxed, breathing low and slow' helps cement the normal rate and pattern back in place.

After practicing while lying down, the patient may then be checked while sitting. Clasping hands together behind the chair (Fig. 7.9) helps relax upper-chest muscles (a modification of hands on head). The patient is asked to 'breathe into the belt' and relax the stomach wall. As progress is made, the patient is encouraged to sit with the arms forward, hands resting on thighs, palms up, and continue energy efficient (EE) breathing.

After covering these points the patient is asked to duplicate practice at home and:

- To commit to, and schedule, two 10-minute sessions each day in lying. It must be emphasized that the breathing retraining–relaxation – 'time out' regimen is a three-way assault on

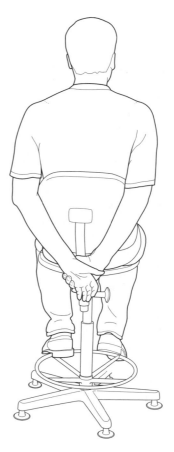

Figure 7.9 Arms behind (Bradley 1998).

the problem, and is far from 'lying about doing nothing' as many hypervigilant overbreathers perceive it to be.

- To try the beach pose in bed for 2 minutes, 'low slow nose' breathing on waking, and for 2 minutes before going to sleep.
- During the day, in sitting or standing, *on the hour every hour*, the following 'stop, drop flop' maneuver needs be practiced:

STOP: check chest
DROP: drop and relax shoulders and jaw
FLOP: relax/go loose all over

- Patients need to be reminded to forget about their breathing in between times, as it is both unnatural and uncomfortable to be aware of breathing all the time. Short effective practice is to be encouraged.

- A workbook may be given to patients to fill in to help adhere to the schedule (see Ch. 10 for an example).
- Discretion should be used; for the very distressed, filling in charts would be adding to their immediate stress levels and be counterproductive. A personalized handwritten *brief* check-list may be more acceptable.
- Timers (Hough 1996) or coloured stickers (Clifton-Smith 1999) as visual cues give non-verbal reminders to 'stop, drop, flop.' (The patient is advised to place a dot on the dashboard of the car, or on the TV, computer, refrigerator, telephone, etc.)
- The patient should be reminded that breathing retraining may feel very uncomfortable at first, and to be prepared for this. Feelings of 'air hunger' are an expected and normal reaction to changes in breathing rates and volumes.
- Changing any behavior takes time and a realistic estimate is, with consistent practice, between 6 and 8 weeks before habitual 'low and slow' breathing becomes re-established.

Follow-up

A follow-up appointment should be scheduled within a week to review retraining, in order to sort out any difficulties encountered and re-evaluate. The patient should be checked in lying, sitting, and standing positions.

During this session, a 'sniff' test should be performed in sitting to check diaphragm action (Box 7.7). This tests bilateral diaphragm function and is useful in checking dominance of upper or lower chest patterns. Placing the hand against the patient's upper abdominal wall three fingers below the xiphoid process, ask the patient to take a quick sniff in. A firm outward movement of the abdominal wall should be felt, showing both hemi-diaphragms are working (Kumar & Clarke 1998).

Sitting

Entrenched upper-chest breathers invariably 'sniff' into their dominant upper-chest pattern, with no diaphragmatic excursion at all, or even

---

> **Box 7.7** 'Sniff' test
>
> Unilateral paralysis can be detected in sitting by a sniff, which causes the paralysed side to rise and the unaffected diaphragm to descend. Causes include phrenic nerve injury from surgery, trauma, or carcinoma of the bronchus; neurological, including herpes zoster or poliomyelitis; or infection such as tuberculosis, or pneumonia.
>
> Bilateral diaphragm weakness or paralysis: paradoxical indrawing of the abdominal wall is best checked in supine. Patients with, for example, multiple sclerosis, postviral infections, exacerbations of COPD (Kumar & Clarke 1998) may demonstrate weakness.
>
> Where appropriate it may be useful to add inspiratory muscle training to increase strength and endurance (Weiner et al 1992, Caine & McConnell 1998).

---

indrawing of their abdominal wall. Most are easily able to 'lead with the diaphragm' when shown. Those who find it difficult will be helped by trying with hands on head. It's useful at this follow-up session to check this, to reinforce that in breathing retraining it takes time to reestablish the diaphragm as the dominant pattern.

The sniff test should be repeated at subsequent sessions to monitor progress.

Standing

For patients, to feel abdominal breathing in standing, have them clasp the hands behind the back to reduce upper-chest involvement. Alternatively, have them clasp hands on top of the head to establish low-chest breathing.

Awareness of this, and being able to breathe abdominally in standing with arms relaxed at the sides, should be noted.

Reinforce the need to schedule time to practice breathing retraining effectively and regularly between treatment sessions.

Subsequent treatment sessions, once abdominal nose breathing is restored, can include breathing and speech, exercise, or other problem areas the patient may have integrating energy efficient breathing into daily life, sleeping and awake (see below). Box 7.8 gives some techniques which can be used in situations in which symptoms are likely to be triggered.

Box 7.8 Rescue breathing techniques

Rescue breathing techniques for risk situations which are likely to trigger symptoms (such as laughing, crying, high intensity exercise, prolonged speech, humid or hot conditions, flying) include:

- Short breath-holds (to allow CO_2 levels to rise) followed by low chest/low volume breathing. Great care must be taken to teach patients to breath-hold only to the point of slight discomfort and to avoid deep respirations on letting go (Pitman 1996).
- Rest positions – i.e. arms forward, resting on a table or chair back, to reduce upper-chest effort and concentrate on nose/abdominal breathing.
- Hands on head, or thumbs forward hands on hips helps with breathlessness during exercise.
- Breathing into hands cupped over the nose and mouth for a minute or two helps patients effectively identify and separate symptoms from triggers.
- Use of a fan, with the sensation of moving air over the trigeminal nerve outlet on each side of the face, helps deepen and calm respiration.

Four common coexisting problems

Asthma (see Ch. 2)

Patients who have asthma, children and adults, usually experience chaotic patterns of breathing during an attack. This is a normal response to cope with fatigue as the work of breathing increases, alternating between upper-chest/accessory and diaphragmatic/abdominal effort. Using rest positions (see Ch. 8) and the 'stop, flop, drop' maneuver helps reduce distress while waiting for asthma medications to work. Reestablishing abdominal nose breathing patterns and normalized CO_2 levels are top priorities once the attack is over. Inspiratory muscle training (IMT) has been shown to be of benefit in abdominal/diaphragmatic pattern strengthening and in reducing exertional dyspnea in mild to moderate asthmatics (Weiner et al 1992), (McConnell 1998).

Chronic obstructive airways disease (COAD) (see Ch. 2)

Patients with chronic obstructive airways disease (COAD) benefit from breathing assessments, as they may experience disproportionate breathlessness in relation to their level of lung impairment (Howell 1990). This may be in part due to anxiety and/or depression over symptoms, as well as associated poor patterns of breathing (i.e. upper chest/mouth/increased repiratory rates). IMT has been found useful in combating the sensation of breathlessness (Weiner 1995, Lisboa 1997).

Chronic pain

Chronic pain is invariably accompanied by chronic hyperventilation, which is a perfectly reasonable reaction to it. Abdominal or pelvic pain frequently involves splinting of the abdominal muscles leading to upper-chest breathing patterns, while pain sited elsewhere may simply increase resting respiratory rates (Glynn et al 1981).

Breathing retraining and relaxation are useful additions to the chronic pain patient's repertoire of pain management techniques, and assists in the reduction of hyperarousal associated with intractable pain.

Hormonal influences

Women between menarche and menopause are affected by progesterone level changes during their menstrual cycle. A respiratory stimulant, its influence in the postovulatory phase may drive Pa_{CO_2} levels down as far as 25% below normal (Damas-Mora et al 1980) and lower during pregnancy (Novy & Edwards 1967). Patients with premenstrual syndrome (PMS) benefit from awareness of breathing rate changes and breathing retraining to prevent excessive CO_2 depletion and consequent HVS symptoms. Perimenopausal and menopausal hormone levels may fluctuate dramatically and women unable or unwilling to take hormone replacement therapies (HRT) have benefited from breathing retraining to reduce hot flashes and improve sleep (Freedman & Woodward 1992).

ESTEEM, OF SELF AND OTHERS

Psychosocial measurement is an important part of physiotherapy assessment in chronic disorders including HVS/BPDs. Structured recording of the patient's own view of their emotional and social health and how improvements from physiotherapy interventions have helped in these areas have equal validity, along with traditional biophysical outcome measures (Chesson 1998). There are many commonly used scales to record these findings. One simply administered example is the Hospital Anxiety and Depression (HAD) scale (Zigmond & Snaith 1983; see Ch. 10, p. 262).

This simple type of scale is recommended in those patients who express persistent anxiety or depression as their most disabling symptoms. As with the Nijmegen scale, it makes a useful educative tool as well. Referral on to and cotreatment by a psychologist, psychiatrist, or psychotherapist would be recommended as an additional option for patients with positive scores, if they wish (Tweedale et al 1994).

Physiotherapists tend to underestimate their value as good listeners. Literally being able to get fears, frustrations, and anxieties off their chests, and being able to put frightening symptoms into a physiological context can be a turning point for many patients. Chronic hyperventilation, whether a primary disorder or secondary to other physical or mental health problems, is in and of itself a major stress. Equipping patients with physical coping skills to deal with this is an essential ingredient in rebuilding self-reliance and esteem.

TOTAL BODY RELAXATION

Patients may have been struggling for weeks, months, even years with worrying symptoms and consequent tension brought on by breathing pattern disturbances. Ensuring patients have an understanding of the stress response is the first step. This physically-based defense mechanism preparing the body for 'fright, flight, do battle' is mediated through the sympathetic branch of the autonomic nervous system. While this response is a major part of the human defense system, life-saving in some instances, the sequel to prolonged bouts of hyperarousal (Nixon 1986) is exhausting, and detrimental to health (Selye 1956).

Those in the grip of ongoing or unresolved fear or mental tension, however, may experience anxiety and/or panic episodes which in turn may lead to avoidance behaviors/phobias (Gilbert

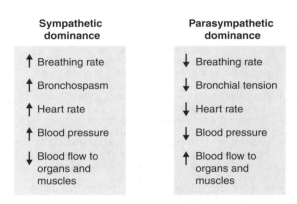

Figure 7.10 Simplified ANS chart, indicating effects of stress/relaxation.

1999). This group of patients tend to be hypervigilant, deriving as much stress from having to control their 'fright, flight' reactions as from experiencing the initiating stressors themselves. The notion of 'letting go' is tantamount to losing control, and might at first heighten anxiety levels. Anxiety sufferers are often the first to agree that they have been dominated by their thoughts (busy brain), with poor body awareness.

A simple explanation of these reactions helps the patient understand the process and possible initial discomforts of releasing tension (Fig. 7.10).

The next step is understanding the relaxation response (Benson 1975) where the patient learns how to identify and switch *off* anxiety or stress responses (mediated by the parasympathetic branch of the autonomic nervous system) (p. 27).

Just as the stress reponse is greatly influenced by fear, pain, or negative thoughts and emotions, so the reverse is found in eliciting the relaxation response. Described as 'non-doing' (Kabat-Zinn 1995), patients learn how to replace negative thoughts and physical tension with regular practice of 'calm stillness of mind and body.'

Mastering low volume, low chest 'minimalist' breathing is an integral part of this. Understanding both sides of the stress/relaxation equation helps equip the patient with powerful self-help skills along with awareness of the effects of CO_2 depletion from overbreathing, onset of symptoms, and consequent systems derangements (Box 7.9).

Box 7.9 Panic attacks

- Identifying triggers and using 'rescue breathing' techniques (Box 7.8) helps patients alter their perception of fear of losing control, to being 'in the driving seat'
- A discussion on the phrases 'out of control,' 'under control,' and 'in control' is useful
- The majority of panickers agree they spend most of their time swinging between the first two
- Learning physical coping skills and understanding the physiological consequences of overbreathing can be immensely empowering in remaining 'in control' in high risk circumstances
- A telephone back-up service to the therapist may be offered to help panic patients regain confidence in self-managing their symptoms
- A specific 'panic cycle' information sheet is helpful, such as the one shown in Chapter 10

The third step is scheduling regular daily practice:

- Teaching a variety of mental and physical relaxation techniques helps address both physical and mental approaches to stress (see Ch 8). Variety also helps prevent boredom.
- Lying comfortably supported by pillows, with anti-gravity reflexes switched off, the patient can initially concentrate on the relaxed pause at the end of each exhalation before practicing, for instance, progressive muscle relaxation (Mitchell 1988; see also Ch. 8).
- Biofeedback machines, where available, make a useful therapeutic adjunct, especially when treating adolescents, notoriously resistant to relaxation.
- Hotpacks, aromatherapy, massage, acupressure and/or gentle stretches may be a useful prelude to practice.
- Prone lying is an alternative for those who at first feel vulnerable relaxing while lying on their backs.
- Survivors of torture or abuse need specialist care. Required reading is Alexandra Hough's well-documented paper on this topic (Hough 1992).
- Progress to teaching relaxation in sitting once a positive outcome has been achieved in lying. Mini-relaxes using 'stop, drop, flop' as a guide may then be used hourly by patients – at work, in the car at traffic lights, on bus, train, or aircraft.

- A discussion about ergonomics at work may be included in this session to review posture and breathing patterns on the job, with perhaps a worksite visit, liasing with the patient's occupational safety and health officer.
- It is important to ensure that patients understand that relaxation only helps eliminate the symptoms, not the causes of stress; examination of achievable lifestyle changes is encouraged. (There is further discussion of this topic in Ch. 8)

TALK

Coordinating breathing and talking is a common problem in HVS/BPDs where speech interferes with the background rhythm of breathing (Timmons & Ley 1994). Restoring respiratory confidence during speech is an important part of the treatment program. Patients may fall into one, or a combination of the following groups:

1. Patients with chronic breathing pattern problems whose jobs require them to use their voices: teachers, courtroom lawyers, actors, singers, telephonists, and sales people for instance. They relate difficulties with breath control and vocal tone. Secondary loss of confidence and 'performance anxiety' are common additions to their repertoire of symptoms.

2. Mouth breathers with chronic sinus problems or postnasal drip with coexisting problems of throat dryness and soreness.

3. Patients suffering anxiety, stress, or depressive disorders, with concurrent increased sympathetic arousal, upper thoracic tension, and sighing respirations often report excessive jaw and throat tightness or pain. This group often speak in a monotone. Help with voicing problems may require the additional help of a skilled counselor.

4. Patients with a history of hiatus hernia, gastroesophageal reflux disease (GORD) or laryngopharyngeal reflux disease (LPRD) frequently complain of irritated throat, chronic throat clearing, shoulder tension, and vocal fold impairment. In response to gut discomfort, upper-chest breathing becomes the norm. Abdominal bracing leads to ineffective breath control while speaking – commonly petering out

before the end of a sentence is reached (it is important to check medication compliance).

Common to all groups is reduced diaphragmatic strength/usage.

Assess speaking and breath control in sitting and standing, once an abdominal pattern is reestablished, perhaps at the second or third session. The most common problems are:

- Hyperinflating the upper chest when starting to speak
- Forgetting to pause for breath during speech
- Speaking to the very end of the out breath, followed by a gasping inhalation.

Having the patient read from a simple text, or recite the alphabet out loud if they have reading difficulties, is an effective way of identifying problems and correcting them. Steps include:

- Relaxed breath out before speaking
- Breathe in softly through the nose to start
- Light, low-chest mouth-breaths between sentences
- Speak slowly.

Any continuing voice/speech problems should be referred on to a speech pathologist or speech therapist.

EXERCISE

The ability to exercise depends on the capacity of the cardiovascular and respiratory systems to increase delivery of oxygen to the tissues and remove excess carbon dioxide and metabolites. Although the *normal* oxygen cost of breathing at rest is less than 2% of resting oxygen consumption, up to 30% of total oxygen consumption may be used to move and aerate the lungs and chest wall during episodes of hyperventilation (Berne & Levy 1998). For patients who are habitually using more oxygen than usual to move air *at rest* (hyperventilating), the oxygen cost of breathing itself may limit their exercise capability.

A mechanical problem often coexists with this set of events. Chronic upper-chest breathers hyperinflate with exercise and reach the bony limits of their chest wall rapidly, and misinterpret the feeling of constriction as breathlessness/suffocation, or misattribute symptoms to

more sinister causes. (Chest wall pain due to overstretching of intercostal structures, the sequel to habitual upper-chest breathing, is a prime example of the patient thinking of heart pathology rather than musculoskeletal injury.) See Chapter 6 for consideration of musculoskeletal protocols, based on osteopathic methodology but with strong similarities to modern manipulative physiotherapy approaches.

Fear of effort becomes established, often triggered by unpleasant symptoms of breathlessness and fatigue. The latter may be central fatigue, with generalized feelings of low energy/unwellness, mediated in part by a shift of the acid-base balance (pH) toward alkalosis (Grossman & Wientjes 1989). Protection of pH is maintained by excretion of alkalis such as bicarbonate via the kidneys. Potassium and phosphates are also depleted (Magarian 1984), which causes muscle fatigue.

Lactic acid build-up in the skeletal muscles from compromised metabolic efficiency leads to aching and stiffness. Breathlessness in reaction to unbuffered acids reaching the central circulation triggers further hyperventilation (Lewis 1954).

Peripheral fatigue, where the venous system fails adequately to clear the accumulated waste products of metabolism from muscles during exercise, adds to the misery. The 'vicious circle' is complete. These patients then have the secondary problem of loss of condition (Fig. 7.11).

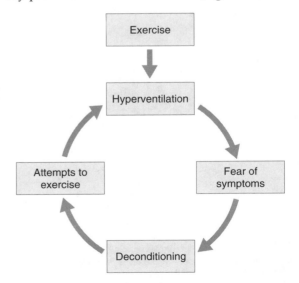

Figure 7.11 Deconditioning cycle.

Physical fitness is described in Altug and Miller's *Teacher's Guide for Fitness for Living* as 'the body's ability to meet the normal demands of everyday life – work and recreation – with ease and with enough margin to adequately cope with emergencies.' Patients who have been struggling with disordered breathing patterns and physiological sequelae often admit to falling far below this ideal. Some patients have fallen so far below they experience symptoms usually associated with heavy exercise while doing quite light activities.

⚠ **CAUTION:** The level of exercise a patient may undertake requires careful judgment with consideration as to age, nutritional status, exhaustion levels, and sleep patterns (see also p. 197).

A useful rule of thumb is to actively discourage fatigued patients from aerobic exercise until normal breathing and improved sleep patterns (adequate rest and restoration of homeostasis) are reestablished.

An excellent way of introducing discussion on effort and exercise is to view the 'human performance curve' and use it as a map (Nixon 1986, p. 132). Patients can pinpoint where they see themselves on the curve and this can be referred back to at regular intervals to check progress and provide an outcome measure (Fig. 7.12).

Fitness recommendations have changed emphasis from an exercise training/fitness to a physical activity/health model which uniquely incorporates *moderate* intensity and *intermittent* physical activity (Philips 1996). This is a more attractive prospect for most people – especially the drastically unfit, or those in sedentary jobs. Accumulated exercise times *gradually* increase towards a total of 30 minutes brisk activity a day, 6–7 days a week, which can be broken into 10-minute segments. Activity may be varied.

As little as 2 minutes three times a day may be a suitable starting point for the very unfit, or those suffering exhaustion, once normal breathing has become familiar.

Box 7.10 makes some recommendations on nutrition and exercise, and Box 7.11 outlines the role of the diaphragm in postural control.

Establishing an exercise program

A supervised session covering breathing with activity begins with a review of expected changes to breathing during exercise:

- Increases in respiration rates and tidal volumes in tandem with increased oxygen consumption (normal)
- Loss of the rest phase at the end of exhalation (normal)
- Upper-chest involvement during effort (normal)

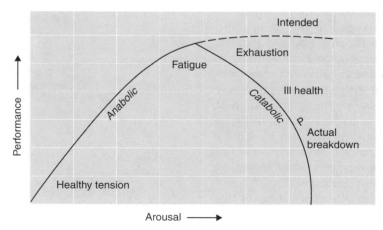

Figure 7.12 The human function curve. Performance relates to coping ability and efficiency. Arousal relates to effort and, at the higher levels, to struggle. P represents the 'catastrophic cliff edge' of instability where little further arousal is required to precipitate a breakdown. (Dr Peter Nixon.)

Box 7.10 Nutrition

- Good nutrition is an important aspect of fitness; many patients admit that their diet as well as their fitness levels is equally less than adequate.
- Fluctuating blood glucose levels may trigger symptoms in patients with high carbohydrate diets which produce rapid rises followed by sharp falls to fasting levels – or below (Timmons & Ley 1994).
- Patients are recommended to eat a breakfast which includes protein and to avoid going without food for more than 3 hours (Hough 1996).
- This fits in with a mid-morning and afternoon protein snack as well as the usual three meals a day.
- This is particularly relevant to patients who experience panic attacks or seizures which have been shown to be more likely to strike when blood glucose levels are low (Timmons & Ley 1994).
- Referral to a nutritionist may be warranted.

Box 7.11 The role of the diaphragm

- The role of the diaphragm and its non-respiratory contribution to postural control is of importance.
- Electromyographic (EMG) recordings of diaphragm activity show it is modulated concurrently for both respiration and postural control (Hodges et al 1997).
- Spinal stability may be compromised in patients with poor diaphragm action, or coexisting respiratory disorders.
- A 'warrant of fitness' to exercise should include low back and pelvic stability checks in patients complaining of low back pain (Allison et al 1998). (See Ch. 6.)

- Switching from nose to mouth breathing at extremes of effort keeping in mind that the very unfit will reach those extremes rapidly (normal)
- Breathlessness is not harmful, merely a signal to slow down or stop, recover, check breathing before continuing (stop drop flop).

Walking or climbing stairs is an easy way to observe breathing rates/patterns and pulse rates in response to exercise (see also Box 7.12). Using an oximeter to check SpO_2 saturations:

- Demonstrates normal values to anxious or skeptical patients
- May signal undiagnosed cardiopulmonary disease if oxygen desaturation accompanies breathlessness in falls below normal minimum levels (95%) during exercise. Further investigations would be indicated.

Box 7.12 Breathing patterns

A useful breathing pattern to adopt when checking patients walking is to have them initially:

- Inhale to two steps, and
- Exhale to three steps

in order to reestablish natural breathing rhythmicity. Ratios may be adapted according to age, levels of fitness, intensity of activity, or severity of BPDs or other concurrent respiratory diseases (e.g. 1 step, breathe in, 2 steps breathe out; 2 in, 3 out; 3 in, 4 out; 4 in, 5 out).

This pattern is also effective with stair climbing, when patients commonly take a large breath in and stop breathing as they ascend.

Once confident about breathing with exercise, patients can self-manage with individualized graduated programs if required, or resume regular gym or sports activities. The advantages regular enjoyable exercise brings are:

- Aerobic benefits (cardiovascular efficiency)
- Improved digestion/bowel function
- Improved sleeping patterns/relaxation responses
- Release of opiopeptoids into the bloodstream (e.g. mood and sleep enhancer, serotonin).
- Improvement/maintenance of bone density (important to those on long-term courses of steroids and to postmenopausal women).

REST AND SLEEP

A common and debilitating symptom experienced by patients with breathing pattern disorders is erratic sleep patterns/vivid dreaming. Recovery and repair for optimum physical and mental health depends on restful sleep and relaxed rest. Being deprived of this causes a great deal of stress, anxiety, and exhaustion to already overloaded body systems. Sleep regulating centers (SRCs) in the brainstem process information from different parts of the body – joint, organ, and muscle receptors – as well as from higher cortical levels, to either:

- induce sleep (lowered levels of stimulation to the SRC)
- encourage wakefulness/alertness (high SRC stimulation).

A calm mind as well as a relaxed body are prerequisites to restorative sleep.

Sleep involves two entirely different cycles in which significant changes to the respiratory system occur:

1. *Slow wave or quiet sleep*. This is deep and restful, characterized by reductions in peripheral vascular tone, blood pressure and respiratory and metabolic rates. CO_2 levels increase as hypercapnic responses are attenuated. Some dreaming may occur but these dreams are seldom remembered. This is considered the physical restoration phase.

2. *Rapid eye movement (REM) sleep*. Approximately every 90 minutes slow wave sleep changes to REM sleep which lasts between 5 and 30 minutes. Also called paradoxical sleep, because the brain is quite active during this phase, this sleep is thought to be linked to mood and emotional adaptions. Slight increases in heart and metabolic rates and blood pressure, irregular breathing, and reduction in tidal volumes occur; despite reduced muscle tone, including muscles of the upper airways, intercostals and accessory muscles (which dissociate from diaphragmatic activity; Hough 1996), muscle twitching and rapid eye movements can be observed. Dreams during this cycle are often remembered, at least in part (Berne & Levy 1998).

REM sleep may be absent in those suffering extreme tiredness, but returns after adequate rest/sleep.

A vicious cycle is established

People with chronic breathing pattern disorders who have low-level or fluctuating CO_2 levels by day commonly report startled waking at night, with rapid breathing. Having managed to fall asleep, CO_2 levels start to rise (reduced minute volumes) to higher than accustomed daily levels (Bootzin & Perlis 1992). This stimulates the respiratory centers to increase respiratory drives in order to reduce CO_2 to habitual daytime levels. Vivid dreams or nightmares are often experienced at this time, along with a pounding heart. Sleep itself becomes feared (Box 7.13)

Box 7.13 Sleep disturbances

This cycle may not exist in isolation. A sleep history assessment will determine other common causes of sleep disturbance such as:

- physical problems (e.g. chronic pain)
- drugs (whether prescribed or recreational) which are CNS stimulants (e.g. bronchodilators, caffeine, amphetamines, nicotine)
- environmental factors (e.g. crowded conditions, noise, pollution)
- behavioral reasons (e.g. boredom, daytime sleeping)
- psychiatric problems (e.g. clinical or reactive depression)
- social problems (e.g. unemployment, relationship problems, grief)
- upset diurnal rhythms (e.g. shift work)
- snoring bed partner
- sleep disorders such as obstructive sleep apnea
- addictions (e.g. alcoholism, drug dependence including hypnotics)

Noting these and finding relevant specialist agencies to address the underlying problem, where necessary, must be the first priority before dealing with the coexisting insomnia.

Re-establishing normal sleep patterns

- Breathing retraining: restoring low-volume, low chest breathing patterns during waking hours helps reestablish higher CO_2 tolerance by the respiratory centers
- Prior to sleep, or when sleep is broken, breathing awareness with total body relaxation helps reduce hyperarousal and promotes sleep
- Discussion about sleep rituals/preparation
- Commitment to an individualized sleep plan for 2–6 weeks.

Sleep hygiene checklist

Discuss how and why to:

- Instigate calming pre-sleep rituals to reduce hyperarousal (relaxing music, warm bath, avoidance of mental stimulants e.g. TV news, late night videos/cinema/theatre, debates/arguments)
- Reduce/stop dietary stimulants, e.g. replace coffee, chocolate, strong tea with decaffeinated, herbal teas or warm milk (see Ch. 3)

- Check soft drinks and over-the-counter (OTC) pain medication labels for caffeine levels
- Do not exceed 300 milligram recommended daily limit (the equivalent of three cups of coffee)
- Ban daytime naps (disturbs diurnal/circadian rhythms)
- Avoid late evening spicy or heavy meals
- Restrict late evening alcohol consumption (reduces upper airway muscle tone, triggering snoring/poor sleep architecture)
- Avoid late exercise/gym sessions (stimulating)
- Reduce stress levels (good and bad) in the bedroom – ban telephones, TV, Playstation, talk-back radio, reading, eating and drinking, or writing in bed – to reinforce bed as a place to sleep
- Making love is an exception. Deep post-orgasmic relaxation, however, only lasts 4–5 minutes: if sleep is not reached in that time, it is of no added benefit. Anxieties about sex may require specialist help.
- Keep evening fluid intake to a minimum to avoid bladder frequency.

These simple considerations, if adhered to, help restore restful and replenishing sleep.

Sleep retraining

Drug therapies may be required in some circumstances, such as:

- Severe chronic disabling insomnia causing extreme distress
- Transient sleep problems associated with shift-work or jet-lag
- Sleep disturbance related to emotional upheaval or serious illness.

One example (of many) behavioral modification guidelines is given below:

Non-pharmacological behavioral sleep retraining plan (based on Bootzin & Perlis 1992)

For the duration of retraining (2–6 weeks), the patient must designate a regular time to go to bed and a regular time to get up in the morning.

These times are not to be deviated from. The goal is to relearn the association of bed with sleep.

Going to sleep (e.g. 10 p.m.)

1. Once in bed, spend 2 minutes lying supine, practice slow, low-volume, abdominal nose breathing. Check tension areas. Stretch/relax.
2. Turn to usual sleeping position, e.g. left side-lying. Check the time.
3. If not asleep within 15 minutes, get out of bed, leave the room. Listen to calming music, or try light reading.
4. When sleepy, return to bed and repeat the sequence until sleep occurs.
5. Repeat if sleep is subsequently broken.

If nightmares and rapid breathing/panic wake the patient, use:

- Rescue breathing techniques to slow respirations and heart
- Relaxed breathing in supine (or prone) for 2 minutes before assuming the normal sleep position and returning to sleep.

Waking (e.g. 6.30 a.m.)

1. Stretch/check tension areas. Spend 2 minutes supine, repeating slow, low-volume, nose breathing techniques.
2. Get up and stay out of bed until the appointed bedtime.

This program is hard work, but if followed diligently may get results within 2 weeks, with 6 weeks as the cut-off point if no improvement is gained. For intractable problems, further investigations from a sleep specialist may be required.

TOWARD INDEPENDENCE

CREATING AN INDIVIDUAL PROGRAM

Having completed the detective work, and covered, where necessary, the six areas listed above, putting together an acceptable program for the patient to follow is the next step.

A workbook to fill in is useful for the first 2 weeks, both to check compliance and to keep the patient focused (see Ch. 10; modifications can be made to suit individual needs).

While the assessment session requires a lot of talk and inquiry, following sessions would be more action-based, with breathing retraining, education, and relaxation taking up the majority of time. As progress is made (and recorded), other specific topics, as judged appropriate, may be covered.

Weekly physiotherapy sessions will be needed until patients have stabilized and feel more confident in self-management skills. Appointments may then be spaced out with half-hour check-ups or telephone/email communications only required.

Recording objective markers at 2-monthly intervals – such as re-doing the Nijmegen score, rechecking thoracic trigger point pain levels, sleep changes, days off work/school – provides positive feedback to patients as well as outcome measures for data collection.

REFERENCES

Allison G T, Kendle K, Roll S, Schupelius J, Scott Q, Panizza J 1998 The role of the diaphragm during abdominal hollowing exercises. Australian Journal of Physiotherapy 44(2)

Altug Z, Miller M The natural exercise presciption. Clinical Management 9(3)

American College of Rheumatology 1990 Criteria for the classification of fibromyalgia, arthritis and rheumatism. 33: 160–172

Baldry, P 1993 Acupuncture, trigger points and muscular pain. Churchill Livingstone, Edinburgh

Benson H 1975 The relaxation response. William Morrow, New York

Berne R M, Levy M N 1998 Physiology, 4th edn. Mosby, New York, pp 546, 580

Bootzin R, Perlis M 1992 Non pharmacological treatments of insomnia. Journal of Clinical Psychology 53(6) (suppl)

Bradley D 1998 Hyperventilation syndrome/breathing pattern disorders. Tandem Press, Auckland, NZ

Caine M P, McConnell A 1998 The inspiratory muscles can be trained differentially to increase strength and endurance using a pressure thesbold inspiratory muscle training device. European Respiratory Journal 12: 85S

Carroll P 1997 Pulse oximetry: at your fingertips. RN (Feb): 22–27

Chaitow L 1996 Muscle energy techniques. Churchill Livingstone, Edinburgh

Chaitow L 2000 Trigger points and myofascial pain index. http://www.healingpeople.com/ht/EN/articles/2000/2/4/378.tmpl

Chesson R 1998 Psychosocial aspects of measurement. Physiotherapy 84(9): 435–438

Clifton-Smith T 1999 Breathe to succeed. Penguin NZ, Auckland, p 160

Conway A 1994 Breathing and feeling: capnography and the individually meaningful stressor. Biofeedback and Self Regulation 19(2): 135–140

Damas-Mora J, Davies L, Taylor W, Jenner F A 1980 Menstrual respiratory changes and symptoms. British Journal of Psychiatry 136: 492–497

Durbin C G 1994 Monitoring gas exchange. Respiratory Care 39: 123–137

Freedman R R, Woodward S 1992 Behavioural treatment of menopausal hot flushes: evaluation by ambulatory monitoring. American Journal of Obstetrics and Gynecology 167: 436–439

Gardner W N 1996 The pathophysiology of hyperventilation disorders. Chest 109: 516–534

Gilbert C 1999 Breathing and the cardiovascular system. Journal of Bodywork and Movement Therapies 3(4): 215–224

Glyn C J, Lloyd J W, Folkhard S 1981 Ventilatory response to intractable pain. Pain 11(2): 201–211

Grossman P, Wientjes C 1989 Respiratory disorders: asthma and hyperventilation syndrome. In: Turpin G (ed) Handbook of clinical psychophysiology. Wiley, New York, pp 519–554

Hanning C D, Alexander-Williams J M 1995 Pulse oximetry: a practical view. British Medical Journal 311: 367–311

Hodges P W, Butler J E, McKenzie D, Gandavia S C 1997 Contraction of the diaphragm during postural adjustments. Journal of Physiology 505: 239–248

Hough A 1992 Physiotherapy for survivors of torture. Physiotherapy 78(5): 323–328

Hough A 1996 Physiotherapy in respiratory care? Stanley Thornes, London

Howell J B L 1990 Behavioural breathlessness. Thorax 45: 287–292

Innocenti D M 1998 Hyperventilation. In: Pryor J, Webber B (eds) Physiotherapy for respiratory and cardiac problems. Churchill Livingstone, Edinburgh, pp 449–461

Jensen M P, Karoly P, Braver S 1986 The measurement of clinical pain intensity: a comparison of six methods. Pain 27: 117–126

Kabat Zin J 1995 Where ever you go there you are. Hyperion, New York

Kumar P, Clark M 1998 Clinical medicine, 4th edn. W B Saunders, Edinburgh, p 826

Lewis B I 1954 Chronic hyperventilation syndrome. JAMA 151: 1204–1208

Lisboa C 1997 Inspiratory muscle training in chronic airflow limitation: effect on exercise performance. Eur Resp J. 10: 1266–1274

Lum L C 1975 Hyperventilation: the tip and the iceberg. Journal of Psychosomatic Research 19: 375–383

Lum L C 1985 Psychogenic breathlessness and hyperventilation. Update 12 July, pp 99–111

McConnell A 1998 Inspiratory muscle training improves lung function and reduces exertional dyspnoea in mild/moderate asthmatics. Proceeding of the Medical Research Society. Clinical Science 95: 4P

Magarian G J 1982 Hyperventilation syndromes: infrequently recognised common expressions of anxiety and stress. Medicine 62: 219–236

Mitchell L 1988 Simple relaxation. John Murray, London

Nixon P G F 1986 Exhaustion: cardiac rehabilitation's starting point. Physiotherapy 72(5): 129–139

Nixon P G F, Freeman L J 1988 The 'think test': a further technique to elicit hyperventilation. Journal of the Royal Society of Medicine 81: 277–279

Novy M J, Edwards M J 1967 Respiratory problems in pregnancy. American Journal of Obstetrics and Gynecology (Dec 1): 1024–1045

Phillips W T 1996 Life style activity: current recommendations. Patient Management (Nov)

Pitman A 1996 Physiotherapy for hyperventilation video. Physiotherapy for Hyperventilation Group, c/o Anne Pitman, Physiotherapy Department. The London Clinic, 20 Devonshire Place, London, UK

Schleifer L M, Ley R 1994 End tidal CO_2 as an index of psychophysiological activity during VDU data entry work, and relaxation. Ergonomics 37(245): 261–266

Selye H 1956 The stress of life. McGraw Hill, New York

Timmons B H, Ley R 1994 Behavioural and psychological approaches to breathing disorders. Plenum, London

Tweeddale P M, Rowbottham I, McHardy G J R 1993 Breathing retraining: effect on anxiety and depression scores in behavioural breathlessness. Journal of Pyschosomatic Research 38(1): 11–21

Van Dixhoorn J, van Duivenvoorden H J 1985 Efficacy of Nijmegen questionnaire in recognition of the hyperventilation syndrome. Journal of Psychosomatic Research 29: 199–206

Vansteenkiste J, Rochette F, Demedts M 1991 Diagnostic tests of hyperventilation syndrome. European Respiratory Journal 4: 393–399

Weiner P 1992 Inspiratory muscle training combined with general exercise reconditioning in patients with COPD. Chest 102: 1351–1356

Weiner P 1995 Inspiratory muscle training during treatment with corticosteroids in humans. Chest 107: 1041–1044

Weiner P, Azgad Y, Ganan R 1992 Inspiratory muscle training in patients with bronchial asthma. Chest 102: 1357–1361

West J B 1995 Respiratory physiology, 4th edn. Williams and Wilkins, Philadelphia

West J B 2000 Respiratory physiology: the essentials. Lippincott, Williams and Wilkins, Philadelphia

Zigmond A S, Snaith R P 1983 The Hospital Anxiety and Depression Scale. Acta Psychiatrica Scandinavica 67: 361–370

8

Self-regulation of breathing

Christopher Gilbert (notes on relaxation response: Dinah Bradley)

INFLUENCING THE BREATHING, AND TEACHING SELF-REGULATION

This chapter focuses on interventions with a psychological component, including emotional factors, the breaking of habits, details and implications of self-regulation, psychotherapeutic techniques, and aspects of dealing with panic. As long as the mind and the intent are engaged, learning to breathe differently is a psychological process. This is especially true when disorders of the breathing pattern are based in disordered thinking and feeling. Changing such patterns is a bigger order than bringing about steadier breathing, and is not always necessary. Proceeding as if the breathing is simply excessive and trying to make it slower and less deep may be all that is needed. Because of the bidirectional relationship of body and mind, strictly physical or behavioral changes generally also have an impact on the emotional state. Theoretically, one person can come for improvement in the breathing pattern and end up feeling more psychologically stable, while another comes in for psychotherapy and ends up having more stable breathing.

A person with respiratory symptoms must choose how to interpret those symptoms, and this often determines what kind of practitioner to consult. With a combination of symptoms such as shortness of breath, chest tightness, light-headedness, and anxiety, most people would go first to a general practitioner. But if the tests come out negative, some may next consult a nutritionist, some an acupuncturist, some a chiropractor, some a psychotherapist, and some a physical therapist or osteopath. Thus the person is already displaying a biased belief about the source of the symptoms. Each of these disciplines (and others besides) has a valid approach to breathing problems, and each discipline will probably offer some relief through its particular approach to an identical set of symptoms – especially if the beliefs of the practitioner match the beliefs of the patient. This suggests that curative factors affect a multifactorial system which can be influenced from many directions.

Trying to guide or retrain someone's breathing usually involves teaching brief interventions which simulate natural relaxed breathing. With repeated practice and self-correction, the conscious intervention may become less conscious, perhaps habitual. Several books describe methods for retraining breathing along these lines, and they reflect careful observation and practice (Bradley 1998, Clifton-Smith 1999). This chapter offers a few general guidelines, with attention to the psychology of controlling the breath.

When the topic is 'learning to breathe better,' the teaching/learning situation as usually set up presents a quandary: the patient is informed of an erroneous breathing pattern and is offered help in learning to correct it. This exchange takes place during rational verbal interaction. But the breathing problem emerges from a system that is far from the rational verbal realm. Changing one's breathing is not the same as improving one's tennis serve or ski technique; breathing is a continuous process and fully automatic in the sense that it does not require conscious supervision. Also, since breathing is so essential to life, there are multiple controls and safeguards to ensure its operation. Teaching someone to interfere in this process is presumptuous. We can commandeer the breathing mechanism temporarily with full attention, but as soon as the mind wanders elsewhere, automatic mechanisms return.

Yet progress is quite possible. The interaction between voluntary and involuntary can be addressed with respect for the deep, protective systems which are trying to ensure adequate air exchange in spite of conflicting messages from various areas of the brain. The problems which create the need for breathing retraining may derive from emotional sources or from injuries, poor posture, or habits acquired through compensation for some other factor, as detailed in preceding chapters. Assuming there is no current structural or medical impediment to restoring normal breathing, the challenge is to allow the body to breathe on its own, in line with the metabolic needs of the moment. To change a chronic breathing pattern it is necessary to make the conscious intervention less conscious, more habitual.

If a chronic emotional state is contributing to the breathing problem, how could one change breathing in a long-term way? It would seem that both would have to be changed together. Yet if we consider that the mind is affected by the breathing as well as the reverse, the separation becomes artificial. The question posed emerges from assumptions about a mind–body dichotomy. We can talk about interaction, mutual influence, reciprocity, and synchrony until the distinction starts to seem like an artifact of language and ultimately pointless. Our English language preserves the mind/body distinction, but biological reality predates language.

Many breathing pattern problems can be seen as a too-tight coupling between the emotional life and breathing. This close interaction conflicts with regulation of breathing for strictly physical purposes, in the same way that eating can be influenced by psychological factors and begins to serve emotional needs. Voluntary regulation of the breath may also be opposed by emotional factors, sometimes serving as a brake on free abdominal expansion. The works of Wilhelm Reich and Alexander Lowen address this issue thoroughly (Gilbert 1999a).

In the case of hyperventilation, it is important to either interject a pause or create a slower exhale so that the volume of air flow per unit time is reduced. Patients often worry that they will be expected to monitor and control their breathing all the time. This is not practical or even possible. The degree of voluntary control over breathing is often below normal, and the trainer/therapist should not assume much native skill in the beginning.

When asked to pause at the end of an exhale, for example, many people simply cannot. They will partially comply, but will draw a slight amount of air in, either knowingly or unknowingly. When asked to exhale slowly, there may be little reversals, 'sneak breaths' on the way out. And if asked to not sigh so much (a very common problem in chronic hyperventilation), often the reverse happens instead: more sighing, as if thinking of the possibility stimulates more of it.

PAUSING THE BREATH

Breath-holding, voluntary apnea, is a simple place to begin. The breath can be stopped with the throat open so that air can still move easily in and out, or with the throat closed. Closing the throat is accomplished by pressing the back of the tongue against the soft palate so as to seal the air passage. This blocks all air movement, and can be achieved by preparing to pronounce a 'K' sound.

Stopping the breath is within everyone's repertoire. It is of course necessary when swimming underwater, and it is also part of the 'freezing' reflex. Vocalization requires interruption of the breathing cycle. We can also exhale forcefully, as when spitting or blowing out a flame. These are all manipulations of the breath for a specific purpose. But to meddle with the mechanism in the abstract is different in principle, and often feels threatening to those who most need it.

Interrupting the movement of air may bring out latent fears. Those very anxious about access to air at all times may ostensibly comply, but will still pull a little extra air in when asked to pause. This can be detected either with a strain gauge around the upper body or by close observation, or even a mirror held beneath the nostrils to collect the condensed moisture. The person may be unaware of this action. Breath-holding time is an indicator of a tendency to hyperventilate, if seen as excessive air hunger or as a fear of build-up of CO_2 – the so-called 'suffocation alarm' (see Klein 1993 for a discussion of this). Some patients cannot exceed 10 seconds of breath-holding at first; 30 seconds is reasonable; and 45 should be within reach. Using a pulse oximeter can display to the patient reassuring evidence that the O_2 saturation does not drop very much during breath-holding.

Interjecting a pause is the wedge, or 'foot in the door' of conscious control of breathing. It is useful to practice pausing with the throat both open and closed, to feel the difference. Once that is mastered, the next step would be a pause at the end of the exhale. This is a different act than a post-inhale pause and is usually harder and less familiar. Pausing without closing the throat is preferable, though there is no barrier to 'sneak breaths' this way. The object is to allow a complete exhale to 'happen', simply by releasing all breathing muscles and letting the movement subside, then resting just a moment before the next inhale.

In learning to pause the breath, it may seem just as logical to pause after the inhale as after the exhale. If the goal is to simply stop the loss of CO_2 in an urgent situation, then any method for accomplishing that is better than nothing. But there a few reasons why a post-exhale pause is better:

1. Pausing after the inhale, holding the lungs filled, creates tension and strain in the muscles of inhalation
2. Pausing after the inhale creates temporary hyperinflation, which works against relaxation and proper emptying of the lungs
3. Pausing after the exhale is more natural. The breathing system reduces volume by slowing the frequency, reducing the depth, and lengthening the post-exhalation pause. A post-inhale pause does not seem to occur naturally except when accompanying a state of suspense.

A count by the therapist is useful at first, at one count per second or less: '1–2–3 (in) 4–5–6 – (out) 7 (pause).' Then add one or two more counts to the pause segment. Then instead of counting each number, say in the same rhythm: 'in … out … pause …' Timing is not critical here; the depth will adjust to accommodate various ratios. It helps to focus attention on the sinking down of the chest, the deflating of the abdomen, the release of used air, and the quietness that ensues when all motion stops.

For individuals with anxiety about breathing, learning to do this means being desensitized.

Their uneasiness is being confronted by asking them to do what they usually avoid. Learning to tolerate a brief pause develops tolerance of CO_2 build-up, which may be important. Simply working with the breath in this way can provoke major fear if the person has had attacks of hyperventilation-linked panic. So it is important to go slowly, but also to convey that voluntary breathing control is worth learning because of the effects of relaxation. One must assume that an optimal breathing pattern is available underneath, if only the conscious mind can be induced to get out of the way.

SELF-MASTERY

When we ask a patient to breathe in a certain way we are encouraging self-mastery of a system which may have been a source of great fear and worry. Many patients are initially uneasy about following any directions to alter their breathing; such directions may initiate gasps or sighs, or else an apparent refusal to tamper with a biological process which they perceive as threatening. It would be the same in principle if a person were asked to drive a car for the first time, or better yet, to ride a horse, because a horse has a mind of its own and can move by itself. Trying to halt an episode of panicky hyperventilation may feel like trying to stop a runaway horse.

This alienation from a natural body function amounts to a withdrawal of responsibility, leaving the breathing process to be driven by emotional states. This alone constitutes a strong rationale for 'breathing exercises' – what is being exercised is voluntary control, with the intent of modifying or reversing influences from emotional centers.

Learning to interrupt out-of-control breathing is important, and so establishing some kind of entry point for conscious control is essential. This requires extending the conscious mind into a new, and sometimes frightening, realm. The breathing system may be the aspect of the body holding the most menace, by being associated with symptoms representing an uncontrollable aspect of the self. Breathing for some individuals is particularly linked to emotions; it may be a major route of emotional expression and represent something far more than simple air exchange. If so, requesting conscious regulation of this process is close to requesting conscious regulation of anger, grief, or feelings of abandonment – a much larger order. So it is not therapeutic to be frustrated with patients who balk at regulating the breath or have special difficulty with the task.

ACUTE HYPERVENTILATION

If a person is visibly hyperventilating, and it can be determined that the state is not due to organic factors but is generated and maintained by anxiety, this is not a medical emergency, only an emotional emergency. This is a condition frequently encountered in emergency medical departments, especially when chest discomfort is involved. A minor tranquilizer will terminate such episodes within a few minutes, but leaves the person with the conclusion that the solution to subsequent attacks lies in another pill.

The state of panicky hyperventilation can also be considered a state of heightened suggestibility. Brief hyperventilation is often used as the final 'push' to enter a hypnotic state, and many hypnotists routinely ask for deep breathing to facilitate entering a trance (Baykushev 1969). Cerebral hypoxia compromises orientation and perception of reality, and cognitive powers will usually be diminished. The emotional distress adds further to the need and willingness to be helped, and so anyone with a suggestion of authority or special knowledge is in a good position to do so.

Direct instruction works well here. For example: 'I can see you're very nervous and you're breathing pretty heavily. Would you like me to help you? You need to get control of your breathing, because it's a big part of the problem. Do you feel you're not getting enough air?' (*consider response*) 'You're getting plenty of air. You're breathing enough for three people! But the way you're breathing prevents your body from absorbing it. If you breathe more slowly, you'll start to absorb more oxygen. Let me help you. Watch my hand. Breathe with my hand.'

Then begin pacing the person's breathing with your hand, rising for inhale, falling for exhale, like a conductor, following the existing rhythm at first and then starting to lead it: in other words, *following, pacing, and leading*.

Following the person's breathing in the beginning imposes no requirement to change anything, but provides an external reflection of the breathing pattern. As the person's attention is fixated on the moving hand, the internally-directed drive is somewhat interrupted.

When there are signs of response to the hand slowing down slightly, change the magnitude of the movements, suggesting less volume as well as a slower rate. Questioning 'Do you feel a little better yet?' sets up the expectation that improvement is bound to happen. If the person is breathing through the mouth, suggest closing the mouth. If that is resisted, then suggest and demonstrate pursed-lips breathing to slow the exhale. Normally this procedure will bring about the desired results within 5 minutes, with perhaps an aftermath of the patient being shaken, with chest discomfort, but breathing and thinking normally again.

Fear of fear

A common idea when treating anxiety disorders is 'fear of fear.' With a simple phobia the object of fear is specific: dogs, deep water, heights, sharp objects. The alarm state rises up when close to the feared object or situation, and subsides upon withdrawal. It is rarely clear how much of the fear of the object itself (and the projected consequences) and how much is fear of the high-arousal state of fear itself.

In panic disorder, and usually in hyperventilation associated with anxiety, the fear becomes centered on the fear reaction itself. There may be avoidance of objects or situations which set off panic, but the essence of the panic is a fear of collapse, death, unconsciousness, insanity, or some similar catastrophe involving loss of control. In other words, it is fear of the fear state. Explaining this to a patient is sometimes helpful, and can initiate insight that can interrupt the cycle. But it usually takes more than explanation.

For this reason, tampering with a person's breathing, when breathing has been the object of fear, feels like unlocking the cage of a lion which once attacked. By the process of generalization (see Ch. 5), anything associated with the traumatic experience becomes a potential warning sign, and initiates avoidance.

'False equilibrium' and adaptation to imbalance

If the breathing pattern of hyperventilation is fairly fixed in the patient, it will feel familiar or even normal, regardless of the symptoms generated. This is partly due to the body's adaptation to the lower CO_2 levels, which includes reduction of bicarbonate buffer. The result is that achieving 'normal' breathing briefly will be opposed by the adaptation, which expects abnormal breathing to continue. Reduced breathing will raise CO_2 and may initiate a feeling of not getting enough air. If so, the patient may have become used to hyper-inflation, so that reduced volume and a full, relaxed exhale do not feel right. If mouth breathing has become a habit, the extra resistance of nose breathing will feel odd at first.

This adaptation to an imbalanced situation can be explained to the patient, depending on the level of comprehension, with the prediction that the patient's physiology will adjust in time to an improved, lower level of breathing. Presenting printed norms showing where CO_2 and oxygen saturation should be, can be convincing enough to motivate acceptance and home practice.

ASSESSMENT

There are several ways to evaluate breathing pattern disorders, particularly hyperventilation, and none reigns supreme. Arterial blood gas analysis is the medical approach for evaluating hyperventilation, but can only detect the state at the moment of the test. Behavioral observations and symptom checklists may seem less precise, but measure things over a longer time period. Chapter 2 carries details on assessment from the physiotherapist's perspective.

The following tools have in common an attempt to bring some objectivity to subjective impressions. They are described along with suggestions primarily for their use in clinical situations.

Anxiety Sensitivity Index

The Anxiety Sensitivity Index (ASI) measures the amount of concern about various symptoms of anxiety. The actual items of the ASI (see Ch. 5, p. 120) are a fair representation of the special fear state typical of most individuals with panic disorder. A large subset of this group has hyperventilation as a factor, whether as a source of the panic or a complicating consequence of the panic (Hegel & Ferguson 1997).

The ASI responses fall into four major categories, according to a factor analysis (Cox et al 1995):

1. Fear of cardiorespiratory distress and gastrointestinal symptoms
2. Fear of cognitive/psychological symptoms
3. Fear of symptoms visible to others (social fear)
4. Fear of fainting and trembling.

These are quite diverse factors, but all can lead to full-blown panic if the patient has no way to counteract excesses in these fears. Prior sensitivities to any of these issues would probably be magnified during an episode of hyperventilation, when the natural consequences of hypocapnia shift the body and mind toward instability or malfunction regarding:

- Disturbed cardiac and gastro-intestinal activity
- Dyspnea or unusual air hunger
- Racing, erratic, anxiety-tinged thinking, including possible dissociation and feelings of unreality
- Faintness, light-headedness, muscle twitches and tremors, weakness.

The fear of being afflicted in public, losing control and feeling helpless or humiliated, adds an extra layer of social fear that easily adds to the sense of danger and urgency, which is usually fed back into the psychophysiological storm going on, to further destabilize the system. It is the therapist's job to block this feedback and try to halt the generation of symptoms to begin with.

Variations from person to person in how these factors are manifested may be determined by each person's physiology: for instance, if a particular person's neurological system is more susceptible to P_{CO_2} drop, causing light-headedness, then that may become the person's major panic symptom. Personal history may be a deciding factor; for instance, a prior heart attack, an incident of severe pneumonia, or history of vomiting would make the person more sensitive to those symptoms as warning signs that a dreaded experience is recurring. Selective apprehension about particular symptoms is a third factor: if a relative died of a heart attack or brain tumor, for example, then any disturbance in those systems will be more salient than usual.

Once this test is given and scored, however, one has only a number. Clinical effectiveness requires more than that. Use of the ASI encourages differentiation of a monolithic 'attack' into its components, which then can lead to inquiry about personal history, the experiences of close friends and relatives, and beliefs about the meaning of the symptoms. With this information in hand it is easier to begin correcting what seems to be a latent phobia, or an unopposed phobic potential – a susceptibility which becomes activated by evidence of the symptom appearing.

When presented with this sort of analysis, some patients will begin to understand that their reaction to, and interpretation of, the symptoms is an integral part of the episode. There has been some debate as to whether the hyperventilation-based panic attack is primary, giving rise to anxiety, or whether the anxiety is primary, set off by perhaps unconscious associations or emotional factors such as suppressed anger. After the onset of an attack, this debate becomes academic, because the two factors of interpretation and physiological disturbance become so intertwined that intervention becomes the main priority.

So when assessing a patient who has signs of acute or chronic hyperventilation, adding the ASI to the evaluation takes only a few minutes and provides additional data *about the person who has the problem*, as opposed to data about the problem itself (objective data such as respiration rate, CO_2 readings, reported symptoms, etc.). Knowing that the person scores especially high, compared to the ASI norms, suggests a subjective factor at work which amplifies the apparent symptom picture. Discovering this, one might switch the therapeutic focus from reducing symptoms to examining what the person assumes about the meaning of the symptoms.

Nijmegen questionnaire

Most of hyperventilation's 'signs and symptoms' as listed in the Nijmegen questionnaire and similar scales are not specific for hyperventilation, and often occur during periods of anxiety regardless of whether CO_2 is depleted (Han et al 1998, Wientjes & Grossman 1994). Items of the scale are to be found in Chapter 7 along with discussion of its use. Some researchers have concluded that reporting of symptoms is influenced by psychological factors as well as by actual CO_2 levels. So there is much room for uncertainty in distinguishing between hyperventilation and an 'anxiety state.' The fact that a patient reports dyspnea, cardiac symptoms, or even peripheral tingling cannot be considered objective in the same way that an instrument reading is; the tendency to notice something and to report it is itself a powerful variable, and appears to be as much psychological as physiological.

The Nijmegen questionnaire has shown itself to correlate well with other objective signs of hyperventilation: 80% of high scores reported that their symptoms matched the sensations felt after a provocation test (van Dixhoorn and Duivenvoorden 1985). It is useful as a screening test and is certainly safer and simpler than the provocation test. Repeated administration of its 16 items can show improvement during a course of treatment, and provides a good foundation for discussion of symptoms.

Recently, Moscariello et al (1999) added to the validation of this questionnaire by provoking hyperventilation through maximal exercise on a cycle ergometer. Subjects were patients referred to a pulmonary center with 'suspected hyperventilation syndrome.' Failure of the $PaCO_2$ to return to baseline within 10 minutes after exercise stopped was considered slow recovery. A certain cut-off point was used on the Nijmegen questionnaire to designate the 'hyperventilating' group. In 88% of the subjects there was agreement in classification between the two tests, supporting the notion that either test can predict results of the other, and that they measure the same characteristics.

The variance in self-reporting because of psychological characteristics is not limited to respiratory complaints. It also applies to irritable bowel syndrome, for example; research has determined that the tendency to experience and report bowel pain, bloating, and abdominal cramping function correlates with psychological indicators of anxiety and depression as much as with objective laboratory findings. These variables also tend to correlate with a tendency to consult medical practitioners. An extensive sampling of individuals who had never complained to a doctor of irritable bowel symptoms revealed that such symptoms were relatively common, but did not bother them or at least did not motivate doctor visits. The psychological coping in these people was apparently more effective (Whitehead et al 1988).

When relating such conclusions to respiratory symptoms, it is important to consider the psychological and cultural context within which an individual is functioning. There may be something helpful which a practitioner can do with words and emotional communication that cannot be done by manipulation or breathing training alone. Even the structural and postural changes which give rise to some breathing problems may in some instances be physical expressions of chronic feeling states. If so, correcting them at the 'distal' point of expression may be of limited value and symptom-focused, analogous to an allopathic medicine approach.

Hyperventilation provocation test

This test is often used to rapidly determine whether a person's symptom complaints can be reproduced by hyperventilating, on demand. The regimen is usually rather extreme, such as one deep breath per second for 3 minutes. This is sufficient to create paresthesias and light-headedness in nearly anyone. One minute of vigorous breathing may be sufficient (see Timmons 1994, p. 283, on this issue). The rationale is that a similar hypocapnic state develops more gradually from a less extreme form of hyperventilation, and reproducing it quickly by vigorous hyperventilation is a matter of time economy. The physician or therapist often has a paper bag ready to help, in theory, to terminate the state by rebreathing air with a higher concentration of CO_2 (but see Ch. 9 for a discussion of this).

⚠ **CAUTION:** Provocation of symptoms of hyperventilation carries some risk (see Ch. 2), and if there is any reason to suspect a compromised cardiovascular system, an increased risk of stroke, or possibility of seizure, asking someone to hyperventilate may not be wise because of the stress on the brain, heart, and blood vessels. Vigorous hyperventilation does stress the cardiovascular system, can initiate anginal pain in those who are susceptible, and could reduce cardiac blood supply enough to stop the heart. The mechanism of action is partly smooth-muscle vasoconstriction; coronary blood vessels are not immune to this effect, which operates also on the bronchi, esophagus and gastrointestinal tract, and cerebral blood vessels.

The nervous system is also affected by low CO_2 and the resulting alkalosis, and nerve conduction within the heart can be disrupted (Nixon 1989, 1993a, b). A large Japanese study compared patients with angina to control subjects. After hyperventilating for 6 minutes, 62% of the angina subjects developed clear signs of ischemic electrocardiographic changes indicating coronary spasm, and none of the control group did. This study implied that hyperventilation is a specific and reliable test for diagnosing coronary artery spasm (Nakao et al 1997) and is quite potent for disrupting the heart function in susceptible individuals.

In the practice of neurology, using hyperventilation to provoke latent defects in a physiological system has long been employed to detect the abnormal spikes and discharges which indicate seizure susceptibility. The cerebral circulation is stressed by hyperventilation during EEG monitoring; the rapid development of hypoxia increases the chance of seizure activity. So if the person has a history of seizure activity, it should be clear why provoking hyperventilation for testing purposes is not recommended.

Most people hyperventilate now and then in the course of normal activities. This probably does not equal what is requested during a hyperventilation 'challenge' during which a capnometer may be used to confirm that sufficient hypocapnia occurs – usually 20 mmHg or below. Complying with such a procedure removes any natural restraints the person may have, which may be protecting against seizure or anginal pain.

Therefore, before considering the hyperventilation provocation test it is prudent, as a minimal precaution, to check for susceptibility to seizures, lung disease, which compromises breathing, and heart trouble or chest pains which could be angina. 'If in doubt, leave it out' – or substitute the hyperventilation provocation *suggestion* test. To do this, simply describe a proposed test in which the patient would be asked to breathe fast and deep for a short time to see what happens. If the response is apprehension, refusal, or obvious discomfort (often accompanied by hyperventilation!) this suggests that the patient probably knows already that symptoms might be provoked, in which case demonstration of this fact would be superfluous, as well as insensitive.

There are positive and negative aspects to provoking hyperventilation as a diagnostic aid. When familiar symptoms are made to appear and then recede by a simple breathing manipulation, some patients will be surprised and intrigued, and this will begin a process of considering the symptoms as potentially controllable, rather than implacable and mysterious, appearing without warning or reason. But since natural breathing increases are rarely as drastic as during a provocation test, the transfer of insight to real life can be difficult. The maneuver of 'proving' to the patient something about the source of the symptoms may take away some of the fear, but not necessarily, because reducing the magnitude of breathing during an episode of hyperventilation still takes training and practice.

In spite of the risk, the provocation test is routinely performed by researchers in the field, sometimes with emergency resuscitation equipment available and sometimes not. The advantage of having a patient deliberately hyperventilate is that it can be reversed by controlled breathing, and this can prove to be a powerful demonstration.

There is a greater complication, however, inherent in the HVPT as usually practiced: it implies that the symptoms are entirely due to CO_2 depletion. Several factors work against this conclusion, related to the power of context and the difference between the testing situation and real life: the occurrence of strong emotion in natural situations, the lack of safety and support, and the lack of clear triggers for the sensations. Provocation of hyperventilation in the office or hospital setting does not reproduce the usual context in which the symptoms occur. Therefore, symptoms provoked in this way may not match what is experienced naturally, leading to false conclusions.

Modified provocation

A two-step educational maneuver can be very effective in recruiting the patient's interest and cooperation, especially if the hyperventilation involves panic attacks. (This is not suitable for cases where even mild hyperventilation could be dangerous.)

The first step would be explaining in detail the physiological route by which excessive breathing can create such symptoms. The second step would be requesting a very brief bout of hyperventilation to demonstrate that the symptoms can be created and eliminated by restoring normal breathing.

This 'provocation of the symptoms' can be quite gentle, consisting of perhaps five deep open-mouthed breaths in 15 seconds, emphasizing complete exhalations to maximize CO_2 clearance. Reassurance should be provided beforehand that any sensations which appear can be quickly reversed by terminating the hyperventilation. A capnometer if available will furnish some objective data, but the patient's sensations are valuable data also.

From this brief provocation, the beginning or 'edge' of the panic symptoms commonly appears quickly in many patients: slight light-headedness or faintness, peripheral or lip tingling, chest tightness, or general uneasiness. Since these changes were predicted and their reversal promised, panic is less likely to occur.

The reversal consists of returning to slow, normal breathing, mouth closed, pausing briefly at the end of each exhale if possible. Usually within 2–3 minutes the patient feels normal again. This symptom reversal, together with explanation and discussion, offers clear evidence to the patient that the symptoms (and the fear) are potentially controllable.

Delayed recovery

One marker of a tendency to hyperventilate is delayed recovery of Pa_{CO_2} following a hyperventilation provocation test. This was originally studied in detail by Hardonk & Beumer (1979). These researchers standardized the hyperventilation phase to one deep breath per second for 3 minutes, after which the subjects were asked to stop and resume normal breathing. The researchers used this procedure to compare a control group with patients already diagnosed by other means as having hyperventilation syndrome. There was a large variation in the time elapsed before baseline level was achieved, sometimes as long as 15 minutes. After studying differences between the two groups, they determined that the best-discriminating criterion was a ratio of 1.5 or larger between percent CO_2 at rest (before the test) and percent CO_2 at 3 minutes. For example, if the baseline reading was 40 torr and the post-hyperventilation level 3 minutes into the recovery was 25, this would yield a ratio of 1.6 and therefore would qualify as hyperventilation. A reading of 32 would yield a ratio of 1.25 and would fall below the diagnostic criterion (Fig. 8.1).

The reason for this phenomenon is unknown; Folgering (1988) describes it as 'irradiation' of cortical activity to the brainstem in resemblance to a 'flywheel' effect. In other words, an after-discharge persists even though the individual intended to resume normal breathing. Another factor related to this is the finding that hyperventilators tend to judge their breathing normal again, following a provocation test, even though

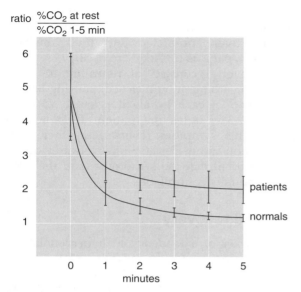

Figure 8.1 The relationship between the ratio %CO_2 at rest and %CO_2 after 1 through 5 minutes recovery from 3 minutes of hyperventilation. Vertical lines are standard deviations. Normals returned more quickly to their resting values than patients (chronic hyperventilators). A ratio of 1 signifies complete recovery. (From Hardouk & Beumer 1979.)

it has still not recovered (King et al 1990). This may mean that their set point for 'normal' was altered because of habituation to a chronic hypocapnic state.

This 'delayed recovery' test distinguishes individuals who complain of chronic symptoms typical of hyperventilation, and so if they actually are hyperventilating, they probably do so a lot of the time. However, this test might not pick out the individual who hyperventilates occasionally in response to a particular emotional state (this is the category defined by Conway et al (1988) and also referred to by Gardner (1996).) Individuals who occasionally lapse into this state are less likely to have the prolonged recovery time from hyperventilation. This may mean that they are less dominated by a feeling state which overstimulates breathing.

'Think test'

Peter Nixon, a London cardiologist, pointed out the inadequacies of the simple HVPT, observing that episodes of hyperventilation are often triggered by moments of strong emotion. His technique requires more active involvement by the practitioner, but is more likely to recreate the conditions under which the symptoms have appeared.

His procedure (detailed in Nixon & Freeman 1988) starts with a HVPT duplicating the standard protocol of 60 breaths per minute for 3 minutes, with the P_{aCO_2} required to fall below 19 mmHg. (His 57 subjects all had cardiovascular symptoms of various sorts.)

During the 3-minute recovery period, P_{CO_2} was monitored for return to baseline according to the Hardonk & Beumer criterion. Then subjects were asked to 'close their eyes and recreate in their minds a time and place where they had experienced their typical symptoms: they were invited to think back and remember all the feelings and sensations which were present at the time' (p. 277). Also, topics that had seemed emotionally significant during the initial history taking were brought up again, and the patients were asked to recall those feelings and sensations. The criterion for this phase was a fall of more than 10 mmHg maintained for 1 minute or more.

Using this more personal experience-based testing, the researchers found many positive responses in subjects who would not have been labeled 'hyperventilators' according to the delayed recovery test. 60% actually met the second criterion, and only seven would have been identified by the previous provocation test. (One subject, incidentally, had a grand mal seizure during this phase; he was not a known epileptic.)

This result fits with the observations cited in Chapter 5, of Conway and colleagues, including that hyperventilation often occurs occasionally in certain people in response to strong emotion, but that they do not hyperventilate routinely. This group also is less likely to display the delayed recovery from hyperventilation; that trait is more likely in those who could be termed chronic hyperventilators, and perhaps are doing it out of habit or else some fairly steady emotional state.

It should not be necessary to put patients through the first provocation procedure in order to test them with the second. Nixon & Freeman speculate that the prior hyperventilation sensitized the subjects, reducing cerebral blood flow in comparison with flow to lower brain centers such as the amygdala, which are more involved in emotionality. However, clinical work is not research; the goals are different. Discussing situations and events which were associated with an 'attack' is likely to disrupt the breathing pattern somewhat, and with either capnometry monitoring or close observation, this disruption can be focused upon as an opportunity for self-knowledge and self-regulation.

BREATHING TRAINING

Biofeedback

The following descriptions use end-tidal CO_2 feedback, using a capnometer, to illustrate some strategies for teaching breathing control. The principles, though, are general, and some can be adapted to other kinds of biofeedback.

Monitoring and display of end-tidal CO_2 can be valuable for reversing the behavior of hyperventilating, whether it is an occasional event or a chronic condition. The basic instrument samples exhaled air by either a mask, nasal cannula, or a thin tube at the nostril. Most commonly, the instrument's display panel shows the breath-by-breath measurement as digits, either mmHg (torr) or as percentage of the exhaled air. There is often a CO_2 waveform display also. End-tidal CO_2 correlates well with arterial CO_2 (in the absence of lung disease or heavy exercise) and so serves to indicate the degree of blood saturation with CO_2.

The monitoring set-up can be used for clinician information only, for spot displays to the patient, or for continuous biofeedback. Interpreting the data correctly requires a bit of explaining, but once it is clear in the patient's mind what is desirable in the CO_2 trace, a good learning situation is established.

There are several things that can be done clinically with a capnometer. It can:

- Check on adequacy of breathing (presence of hyperventilation) at any moment

- Observe the slope of recovery after a provocation test
- Demonstrate the effects of emotional recall
- Show the effect of various manipulations: slow breathing, rapid breathing, breath-holding, sighing, and brief exercise
- Provide feedback on attempts to relax and slow the breathing
- Assess the variability ('steadiness') of the breathing pattern during various conditions.

1. Checking for presence of hyperventilation

Provided the capnometer is switched on and warmed up, a single reading of end-tidal CO_2 ($PetCO_2$) can be obtained in a matter of seconds, barely more than the time it takes to exhale into the sampling line. This reading does not necessarily imply anything beyond that moment. The normal range is 35–45 mmHg; by convention, 30 mmHg is a rough dividing point for signifying hyperventilation below that point. $PaCO_2$ fluctuates continuously and is more labile in some people than others. A single deep breath can push the next breath's CO_2 content temporarily below 30 torr, while suspending breathing for 30 seconds may result in the next breath reading close to 50.

Blood gas measurements in the medical setting are usually done via arterial puncture. This is a less trivial procedure than venipuncture, so since repeat measurements are not routine, the single value of $PaCO_2$ is taken to represent a steady state. Like end-tidal measurements, this represents one moment only, but more information is available with a blood gas measurement. The values of oxygen saturation plus the partial pressure of oxygen and bicarbonate help to clarify the meaning of the $PaCO_2$ reading.

With capnometry, a series of end-tidal readings is easily obtained and begins to outline the pattern of breathing. Since both the depth of inhalation and the rate of breathing combine to determine total air flow, it is difficult to decide by observation alone whether an individual is actually hyperventilating. The florid cases are obvious: heaving chest and rapid breathing. But with a more subtle deviation from normal, sampling the exhalations for a minute or two adds objective information which would permit the conclusion that the person is truly hyperventilating. It may be a habitual style, it may be because of what was just discussed, or it may be expressing anxiety about the measurement process. But the information is a beginning. If certain symptoms are being reported (light-headedness, chest discomfort, confusion, etc.) and the $PetCO_2$ is low as well, then making this explanation can be very helpful.

2. Rate of recovery of CO_2 after hyperventilation provocation

The procedure of provoking hyperventilation in order to observe speed and completeness of recovery requires a capnometer, since the test was developed around end-tidal CO_2 measurements. Following Hardonk & Beumer's standard procedure of 3 minutes of deep breathing, one per second, still allows variability in respiratory variables, but the timing of the breaths and requiring a certain degree of drop in measured CO_2 at least provide some standardization. Some researchers use 20 torr as a criterion for adequate hyperventilation. In clinical use one looks for 'indications' and 'apparent tendencies' rather than arbitrary pass–fail cut-off points, and determining hyperventilation on the basis of one test is unwise in any case.

With those reservations, using this procedure to observe the rate of recovery can be very useful both for the clinician and for the patient. The addition of O_2 saturation monitoring via pulse oximeter adds even more information. The rate of recovery after the patient is asked to 'resume normal breathing' is assumed to depend primarily on minute volume rather than some constitutional physiological variable.

Patients may be unaware of brief periods of apnea, most often at the end of an exhale. Such interruptions of breathing rhythm are normal to some extent, since breathing is driven by CO_2 level, and if CO_2 stays low the pattern may alternate between continued hyperventilation and loss of respiratory drive. This area has not been much studied, but O_2 saturation can drop because of cessation of breathing. This is what happens when some swimmers prepare for an underwater dive by intentionally hyperventilating; by depleting their blood CO_2 they are removing the marker that serves as a signal for 'air hunger.' Thus the swimmer can remain underwater a little longer before the urge to breathe becomes overpowering. It feels as if there is more oxygen available, but in truth the warning mechanism has been disabled, making blackout a more imminent danger.

Demonstrating to patients how long it takes to return to normal, baseline CO_2 levels with a capnometer can underscore the point that their breathing has persistent physiological consequences. If oximetry monitoring shows a drop in O_2 saturation in the process of recovering normal breathing, that is useful information also. Breath-holding is relatively easier after hyperventilation (as in the underwater swimming example), but while it may return CO_2 levels to normal more quickly, it is also depriving the body of continuous oxygen supply. The instability and oscillation between the two extremes may be characteristic of those who chronically hyperventilate.

In any case, patients should be led to understand that an experience of strong negative emotion can be prolonged partly through breathing not returning to normal; this makes them more susceptible to recurrence of the disturbing feeling. Thus an argument, for example, might go on longer than necessary because the state of outrage or insult is reverberating with excessive breathing. A state of fright might persist also, defined partly by mental phenomena and partly by continued low CO_2.

The above illustrates the principle of psycho-physiological reverberation between the two aspects of a person, a curious interaction between mind and body. Such resonance provides an opportunity to intervene from two different directions: change the thinking–feeling state and the breathing will change. Change the breathing and the thinking–feeling state will change.

3. Demonstrating the effects of emotional recall

The work of Conway (see Ch. 5) as well as Dudley (1969) and others has demonstrated the extreme 'thinness' of the interface between emotions and breathing in certain people. If the respiratory system is acting out each emotional state that runs through the mind, and is forever preparing for some new imaginary threat, then physiological stability will be significantly compromised. Using the capnometer (or any other kind of breathing monitor) helps to magnify and sharpen patients' awareness of their breathing responses to various emotional states (Fig. 8.2). This information is of course useful to the therapist also, not only to confirm that the breathing reacts strongly to induced emotion, but also to show more precisely which topics and emotions affect the breathing. But until this information is understood by the patient it is not of much practical use. The capnometer can be used like any other psychophysiological monitoring instrument, in the manner of a polygraph examination, except that the goal is to detect strong emotional responses without the motive of detecting deception (see Case study 8.1).

Most often connections such as the ones in the case study are not so clear or retrievable, but it is usually enough to ask the patient to describe a recent instance of hyperventilating while being monitored with the capnometer. Normally this request elicits a detailed image from which the patient retrieves details, but in the process the whole response begins to start up again. The capnometer will show a drop in CO_2, and often the

breathing change is obvious: mouth and chest breathing at an irregular rate. The point is made, then, that thinking about the symptoms can actually recreate the symptoms. Distraction from this experience of recall (or simply giving instructions to breathe normally) will restore normal breathing and thus a rise in CO_2. Seeing such evidence of mental manipulation usually impresses the patient with how self-generated the symptoms actually are. With an adequate sense of self-power, or efficacy, this fact can be translated into more active control.

4. Show the effect of various breathing manipulations

Most of the inappropriate breathing changes which create problems happen naturally without conscious intent, unless one ascribes intent to less ostensibly conscious parts of the person. An individual does not usually decide to suspend breathing in order to think more clearly in an emergency; breathing just stops. In this sense breathing is fully automatic in the way that stomach contractions are. Yet the abundant nerve connections from the cortex to the breathing centers permit us to direct our breathing very thoroughly. The most basic neural control centers in the pons and medulla receive inputs from chemoreceptors for fine-tuning of breathing variables, but they also receive input from the limbic

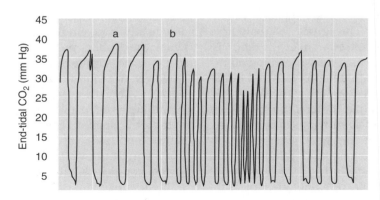

Figure 8.2 Capnogram showing drop in 36-year-old male patient's end tidal CO_2 while relaxing (a) and (b) starting to think (with frustration) about a missed job promotion. Trace duration was 90 seconds. Each wave represents a breath: peaks are end-points of exhalations.

Case study 8.1

A 32-year-old woman with panic attacks and hyperventilation was being monitored by a capnometer while discussing the origin of a recent panic attack. She was asked to recount, with eyes closed, the various aspects of the context where the attack occurred, remembering and imagining 'being there.' She had intended to visit a friend's house, but on the way began to feel chest tightness, dyspnea, and light-headedness. She began to worry about being able to control the car and as she continued driving toward the friend's house, this worry escalated into panic over the possibility of crashing. She stopped the car, tried to calm her breathing and rapid heartbeat, and finally felt able to drive back home.

Recalling and describing this whole episode dropped her CO_2 about 20%, especially as she described pulling the car over and becoming convinced that she could not drive safely. She could not state what set off the incident, but assumed it came 'out of the blue' or else was connected somehow with driving. She denied any uneasiness about the woman she was visiting, or the neighborhood, or the car itself. She speculated that her panicky breathing might be connected with the chest tightness the last time she had panicked.

To pursue the question of what triggered her attack, I asked her to visualize each stage of the trip and briefly mention the associations she had to these images. The capnometer was recording, and intervals of silence permitted adequate samples of her breathing.

As she spoke more about driving toward the woman's house, her breathing became faster and the CO_2 level dropped from 39 to 28–30 in about a minute. As I mentioned this to her, she confirmed that she was now feeling some chest tightness and rapid heartbeat again. Suddenly she remembered that her friend sometimes took care of a relative's dog, chaining it in the back yard. This had major psychological meaning for her because she had once walked into someone else's back yard and was attacked by a dog. This connection became clear to her for the first time; it was as if her 'warning system' was operating beneath her awareness. The mere possibility of the friend keeping a dog that day had set off anticipatory hyperventilation, and her attention went to the resulting symptoms instead of to the real cause.

Understanding this was a revelation to her and led to greater understanding of the concept of 'triggers' activating her alarms. Without this understanding, teaching her to control her breathing in order to approach her friend's house might not have been successful, because it would be opposed by the 'hidden alarm' being activated.

structures (emotional input) from the reticular formation when the person is awake (general arousal, alertness), and from the cerebral cortex via corticospinal neurons for full voluntary control. It is this last pathway that can be practiced, or 'exercised' in order to strengthen its dominance over breathing patterns.

If the end-tidal CO_2 is initially low (<35 torr), slow breathing may be requested directly, and the capnometer will most likely reflect a rise in CO_2 toward normal. This gives the patient a sense of potential control, but a likely question is: 'Will I have to be thinking of my breathing all the time?' The next step is to demonstrate that thinking of other things, creating other mental states, is sufficient to normalize the breathing without focusing on it directly. Removing or minimizing the feedback helps in this goal. Eyes closed is better, to promote imagery and remove visual distraction. Speaking softly to the patient about the seashore, mountains, or some other pleasant and relaxing experience will usually induce a calm state which reduces breathing volume temporarily, with a corresponding rise in CO_2. The implication of this for the patient should be clear. Assigning home practice, perhaps with a prepared audio tape in the therapist's voice, or listening to peaceful music, can provide structure for the necessary rehabilitation practice.

Rapid breathing

The full hyperventilation provocation test is stressful to some people more than others, physiologically and emotionally. Of course, that is what the testing process is trying to discover. There is no strong reason in the clinical setting, however, to request a drastic change in breathing such as a breath every second for 3 minutes, or breathing as deep and fast as possible until major symptoms appear. The test is difficult to standardize unless a capnometer is available. If the goal is not to test a body of subjects under consistent conditions but to work with one person in a therapeutic manner, then the individual patient 'becomes the experiment.' A more moderate and exploratory procedure is more appropriate in such cases.

A request to breathe slightly faster and/or deeper is usually adequate, and more acceptable to the patient. While monitoring by capnometer, the breathing is mildly accelerated to see what will happen, both psychologically and objectively. The capnometer should confirm a lowering of $PaCO_2$ and the patient may or may not feel the beginning of symptoms. At that point it is fine to back off by slowing the breathing, and observe whether the $PaCO_2$ rises and whether there is a diminution of any symptoms.

Apart from demonstrating a possible relationship between breathing volume and the twin variables of sensations and $PaCO_2$, this gentle acceleration provides practice in subtle sensing and adjusting of the breathing. It is easy to breathe fast and deep, and it is easy to hold the breath, but these are ends of a continuum rather than a dichotomy. Infinite points of adjustment are more useful for matching metabolic need, but the patient may have to practice to discover this. The 'discovery' may occur at unconscious levels, in the same manner as motor skills learning, and since the goal is to return the breathing system to automatic and minimize conscious or emotional interference, the normalizing of breathing may really be returning breathing regulation to more automatic functions.

Breath-holding

Many researchers have observed the reduced tolerance for breath-holding in hyperventilators and commented on it as indicating a higher sensitivity to CO_2 build-up. This may be because of a lower level of bicarbonate buffer, which might normally oppose the higher acidity though not the actual CO_2 rise. It is easy enough to test this capacity by requesting a breath-hold without hyperventilating beforehand. One would think that if hyperventilating before underwater swimming, for example, increases the breath-holding time by depleting CO_2 (see Ch. 2) then a chronic hyperventilator would have a head start here, but it seems to work in the opposite way.

Breath-holding times of 10–15 seconds are common when individuals fitting the hyperventilation profile are tested, which is below the normal, usually estimated as 30 seconds. This cannot be too meaningful a test, however, without controlling the style of the delivering the instructions. Presumably the build-up of the urge to breathe will be opposed by the will to please the experimenter, to appear normal, to achieve a high score in something, or some other motivation which may increase the tolerance of an uneasy sensation.

Apart from using breath-holding time as a possible diagnostic aid, there are two other uses:

1. When using a capnometer, breath-holding provides a good demonstration of how PCO_2 and breathing interact. Holding after a moderate inhale for as long as possible, the patient will see CO_2 trace reading zero, and when the breath is finally released, the trace will rise higher than it was before. A person who had a hard time rising above 35 torr might see 40 or 45 for a few breaths, as the accumulated CO_2 is released. This can be pointed out as a fast way to alleviate symptoms of hyperventilation and possibly terminate a panic attack, although not the best way; interrupting the natural breathing cycle induces a rebound air hunger for the next few breaths. It can be offered as a quick alternative to the 'paper bag' remedy. The point can be made that if breath-holding raises $PaCO_2$ quickly by restricting air exchange, the slow, limited breathing will raise $PaCO_2$ also, though more slowly.

2. Using breath-holding as training to tolerate air hunger is valuable and easily practiced. This amounts to suggesting voluntary apnea for brief periods. Resisting the urge to breathe, postponing the next breath, may be in the same category as resisting an urge to smoke, drink, or eat. The idea of going on an 'air diet' (Figure 8.3) clarifies the goal. It should be explained that the rising urge to breathe is caused by CO_2 build-up and not a drop in oxygen; the latter does not contribute to breathing drive until the oxygen content falls much lower. This is why hyperventilating before swimming underwater prolongs tolerance for submersion. At first, most people will hold the breath after inhaling, with throat stoppage (back of tongue against soft palate) but one should work toward a pause after an exhale, with no throat stoppage. This simulates the

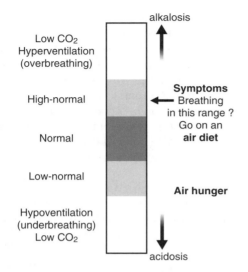

Figure 8.3 Chronic hyperventilation in principle resembles overeating: perhaps to avoid feeling out of air, some people overbreathe, depleting their systems of carbon dioxide and provoking symptoms associated with alkalosis. (Reproduced with kind permission from Gilbert 1998.)

natural breathing pattern of one count in, one count out, and one count rest. (See Buteyko notes in Ch. 9.)

Exercise

To demonstrate that more CO_2 is generated when muscles are working, suggesting light exercise on-the-spot is useful. Not every patient can be talked into deep knee bends with a capnometer sampling tube taped to their upper lip, but when they try it, it is memorable. A few squats will push the CO_2 up 10–15%. The rise is not immediate, but within 30 seconds should be apparent. This is not an exercise or endurance test, but is meant to educate the patient as to alternative ways to raise CO_2 during a hyperventilation episode. Most people during panic feel a strong urge to move around, possibly to escape where they are, and this urge for activity is strong. So cooperating with this urge generates the extra CO_2 that the body 'expects' and the discrepancy between breathing volume and breathing demand should lessen. It also provides the impression of a remedy, which is psychologically important, placebo-style.

Many other clinical techniques are available in Fried (1993). From his long experience with capnometry and with hyperventilation, he describes the use of music, imagery, biofeedback, EEG monitoring, and other approaches combined with a capnometer to normalize breathing pattern problems.

Other biofeedback

Most practitioners will not have access to a capnometer, but may wish to use some method of displaying breathing information to the patient to aid in learning to control breathing. What follows is a summary of useful ways to do this:

Strain gauges

Sensors consist of expandable tubes, belts, or bellows placed either around the abdomen (1-channel) or around the abdomen and chest (2-channel). The feedback display may consist of a chart recorder, a biofeedback screen, or other display. With two channels, the relative movements of each breathing region may be displayed for comparison. The patient can see instantly the effect of chest or abdominal expansion. The feedback is vivid and comprehensible. It is helpful for practicing abdominal breathing, for detecting paradoxical breathing, for enhancing awareness of breathing, and for helping transfer this awareness to inner sensing.

The drawbacks: attaching the sensors can be intrusive, since it requires fastening the expansion gauges around the thorax and abdomen (over the clothing). The gauges can slip down and change the measurements. Also, the gauges are hard to calibrate to objective volume quantities, and they are best used as a relative measure of volume and direction of movement (in–out) for comparison within the subject.

Surface electromyography (EMG)

Adhesive electrodes can be placed over many muscles involved in breathing. The display may be by a meter or LED light bar gauge, or on a stand-alone battery-operated instrument, via chart recorder, or via computerized processing and analysis. This last is a part of most modern biofeedback setups, and provides a display and recording of the raw signal, the processed, rectified signal (single line), a bar graph display for different locations simultaneously, various graphic transformations such as circles, random color arrays, and games in which the body functions as the game controller. Thresholds may be set for goals of relaxing. Sound can be provided for biofeedback, and toggled on or off depending on threshold settings. The most common general strategy is to inhibit use of accessory breathing muscles during inhalation.

Muscle sites

1. Trapezius Either one or both sides may be monitored at once. Electrodes are placed over the upper trapezius, with the ground elsewhere. The display shows a rising and falling trace proportional to the magnitude of muscle contraction. The greater the movement, the more the trapezius is participating in the inhalation. When the signal is minimized, upward shoulder movement is inhibited and air is directed lower down in the body. The patient can attempt to breathe exclusively with the lower abdominal muscles and inhibit trapezius movement altogether. Though probably not natural, attempting to achieve this builds control and the ability to inhibit shoulder breathing.

2. Scalenes Located midway between trapezius and sternocleidomastoid (SCM) muscles on the side of the neck, these muscles attach variously to the clavicle and 1 and 2 ribs to elevate them, thus increasing the volume of the upper chest. They are less easily isolated and monitored than the trapezius, but it is worthwhile learning to inhibit their contractions for normal breathing. This delegates more of the work of inhalation to the lower costal and diaphragmatic muscles (Figs. 8.4 and 8.5).

3. Sternocleidomastoid This muscle mainly turns the head to the side, but it also aids in lifting the clavicles and expanding the chest. If the scalenes are active in quiet breathing, then the SCM will probably be also. It can be hard to isolate with the electrodes since it moves laterally under the skin, so the patient's head must be held still and facing straight ahead (see Ch. 6 for more discussion of these muscles).

Temperature feedback

A biofeedback thermometer with fast response and small thermistor can be used to monitor and display the difference in temperature between inhaled and exhaled air. The tip of the wire thermistor is taped onto the upper lip in the airstream outside the nostril without touching the skin. Depending on ambient temperature the difference between inhaled and exhaled air is usually between 2 and 10°F, sufficient to mark the breathing cycle. Though insensitive to location of breathing (chest vs. abdomen) it does verify nasal as opposed to mouth breathing. This display is very sensitive to speed of exhale during exhale, and is useful for reinforcing slower exhalation. Audio feedback can enhance the experience.

All of these biofeedback modes can be helpful as temporary learning aids. People with 'bad breathing' habits often seem relatively unaware of proprioceptive sensations; this may be a subtle perceptual or sensory deficit or a habituation to 'error signals' that arise from habitual chest breathing, mouth breathing, or excessive speed. The biofeedback information helps to direct conscious attention to the relevant sensations. The goal is to sensitize the patient to how suboptimal breathing feels compared with optimal breathing. Other methods such as hand-on-abdomen, the practitioner's hands on shoulders, breathing into a candle flame, lying prone on the floor (for feedback from whatever area is expanding most), and mirror feedback can all help to extend conscious control to the breathing realm.

Sighing

Frequent sighing is frequently mentioned by researchers and clinicians alike as a sign of the chronic hyperventilator. It contributes to breathing instability and has been interpreted variously as responses to surges of emotion, an expression

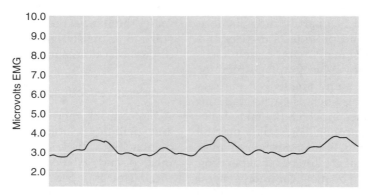

Figure 8.4 EMG tracing of scalene muscle (side of neck) during normal breathing (three breaths) with abdominal expansion and shoulders relaxed.

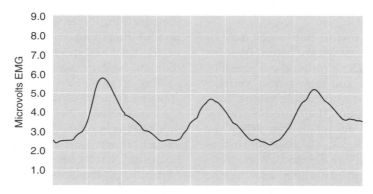

Figure 8.5 EMG tracing of scalene muscle (three breaths) with abdominal movement restricted; accessory muscles recruited.

of dyspnea, hypersensitivity to rising CO_2 levels, and an attempt to loosen tight breathing muscles. A recent study (Wilhelm et al 2001) looked at this variable in more detail by monitoring breathing volumes, timing, and end-tidal CO_2 in panic disorder patients and others. Compared to controls, sighing was more frequent in those with panic disorder, sighs were deeper, and return to baseline was slower. The authors concluded that the lower baseline CO_2 present in those with panic disorder was not explainable by minute volume in general, but by frequency and depth of sighing, plus slower recovery. The sighs did not occur following a rise in CO_2 and they did not appear to be attempts to correct for pauses in breathing.

This suggests that training steadiness of breathing and suppression of sighing is import-

ant for reducing hyperventilation. The explanations of individuals vary as to why they sigh so often, and they may be rationalizations for a behavior that occurs spontaneously for unknown reasons. Teaching tolerance of whatever feeling precedes sighing is sometimes successful, given sufficient self-observation. Also, teaching to limit the size of the sigh may work, plus keeping the mouth closed during a sigh. A quick swallow can terminate a sigh.

The relaxation response

The relaxation response is a term coined nearly 30 years ago by Mirian Klipper and the then associate professor of medicine at Harvard Medical School, Herbert Benson MD. It was used to describe the conscious initiation in the body of a protective mechanism to counter the effects of anxiety and the 'fright, fight or flight' reaction to stress (Benson & Klipper 1988). First described by Dr Walter B. Cannon, a professor of physiology at Harvard Medical School at the turn of last century, the 'fight-or-flight' response was seen as an 'emergency reaction' where increases in blood pressure, heart rate, breathing and increased body metabolism were recorded. Benson believed that the more this reaction was activated the more likely high blood pressure was to develop, especially if the responses it was designed to provide – fighting or fleeing – were continually repressed.

Benson, who was also director of the hypertension section of Boston's Beth Israel Hospital, was curious to find the cause of 'essential hypertension' (of unknown cause) which affected a very high percentage of his patients. Often put down to 'stress' he determined to find out more about the then inadequately studied subject. An ill-defined and overused word, stress has come to mean different things in different areas of health care. But whatever its origin – emotional, environmental, occupational, or physiological – learning how to switch off the signs and symptoms of stress by evoking this response has been exhaustively researched and documented as well as put into a practical guide for patient use by Benson and his colleagues.

Taking centuries-old Eastern meditation techniques and the claims that physiological functions could be altered by practicing these methods was the basis of the Harvard group's exploration. Prior to this, it was generally accepted in orthodox medicine that control over the automatic functions of the body was beyond conscious control. But the Harvard studies revealed what practitioners of Eastern yogic and meditational techniques had understood empirically for many centuries – that mechanisms in the unconscious autonomic nervous system could be altered by both mental and physical relaxation techniques to slow heart, breathing, and metabolic rates and reduce both mental and physical tension. Acknowledging the age-old universality of the techniques examined, the group came up

with a term and method acceptable to most skeptical Western stress sufferers.

The four basic elements for the effective practice of the relaxation response are:

1. A quiet environment to help reduce external stimuli
2. An object to dwell on, which can be either a word or sound to repeat, or something to gaze at such as a flower or symbol
3. A passive attitude by letting all thoughts and distractions float away (this appears to be the most important factor in eliciting the response)
4. A comfortable position in sitting to prevent falling asleep.

(These four elements put together while lying down help promote sleep.)

The recommended practice, developed at Harvard's Thorndike Memorial Laboratory, is to schedule two sessions daily of between 10 and 20 minutes. Sitting comfortably, the patient relaxes the muscles from the feet up, and then focuses on breathing in and out through the nose and silently saying the word 'one' at the end of each exhalation. A simple technique to use, without attachment to any cult or philosophy, the relaxation response is an acceptable method to teach patients who fear ancient or 'godless' practices or who cannot afford to pay to attend other types of courses.

Clinical tips

In practice, this technique is best taught once abdominal nose breathing patterns have been restored. Some patients may have already felt the relaxed pause at the end of exhalation, and the new sensation of 'letting the in-breath start itself,' and appreciate its calming qualities.

The majority of patients, when asked if they practice any form of relaxation, usually answer in the negative or exclaim they never have enough time to 'sit round doing nothing.' Reinforcing the need to take 'time out' can be made more acceptable if the patient perceives they are doing something (even if it is 'doing nothing').

As mentioned above, patients with strong religious affiliations may balk at any technique which smacks of a philosophy other than their own. Packaging it as all-in-one method which includes:

- continued breathing retraining
- 'time out'
- relaxation

makes it acceptable to most. Accepting that many people have to work long hours in stressful jobs and find it hard to practice such commonly taught methods as transcendental meditation (TM), which requires 20-minute sessions twice a day, teaching 'mini relaxes' to practice throughout the day becomes an equally acceptable way of turning on the relaxation response and reducing hyperarousal levels. (This compares with the more recent exercise prescriptions stating several short sessions of exercise daily are as effective as the more prolonged sessions previously required.)

Patients can learn to switch on their relaxation response while reclining by tuning in to light abdominal nose breathing, concentrating on the exhale and the silently repeated word 'one' (or whatever they choose to focus on).

Taking blood pressure readings before and after a relaxation session in patients who have hypertension may be helpful, although often the very sight of a sphygmomanometer cuff is enough to instantly raise the patient's blood pressure ('white coat fever').

A session discussing and practicing this technique in the sitting position for further daily practice equips the patient with physical coping skills to deal with stressors wherever they occur in daily life.

Cognitive therapy

An important step in this process is helping the patient to deal with the rapid, fairly automatic assumptions being made about the meaning of the symptoms. Rapid heartbeat, for instance, could represent impending heart attack. With that interpretation dominating, it is no wonder that a panic attack ensues. Mild dyspnea resulting perhaps from a tensed diaphragm muscle could be interpreted as impending suffocation, light-headedness as about to lose consciousness, tingling fingers as an approaching stroke, and so on.

Helping the patient to reinterpret these 'symptoms' as mere sensations which result from the hyperventilation coupled with a cognitive proneness to catastrophizing, provides a very new angle on things.

The concept of automatic thoughts has been developed by the cognitive therapy school (Salkovskis 1988) and holds that such thoughts emerge from underlying assumptions about what things mean. The deepest level of belief might be 'I am at particular risk from heart attack because there is heart disease in my family.' Given that belief, the individual will be predisposed to react to benign chest sensations, heart palpitations, or tachycardia as a confirmation of these deeply held beliefs. The automaticity of this process means that the matter is not necessarily referred to the conscious mind for decision; it has already been decided. The conscious mind becomes occupied instead with the next step, such as deciding where the closest hospital is. This anxiety will feed back into the physiological system which is producing the symptom, sustaining the state or provoking it to even greater levels of alarm.

One should question the patient about the assumed meaning of symptoms related to hyperventilation. Teaching control of breathing without explanation may not be sufficient, even though the chest or neurological symptoms abate, if the patient covertly decides that a heart attack has been averted. Intervening at a higher cognitive level – challenging the assumption that the sensations signal approaching disaster – can interrupt a disruptive and very persistent vicious cycle. Clark (1986) and Salkovskis et al (1996) represent this clinical approach, and find that breathing retraining can often be bypassed when the implicit meaning of the hyperventilation symptoms is uncovered, challenged, and changed.

Cognitive therapy takes account of thinking errors, but tends to stay at the conscious level of mental life. Emotional interference with breathing can be quite complex; the state of confusion and disorientation resulting from hyperventilation can be rewarding or punishing. The act of hyperventilating can create depression, agoraphobia, and fear of death; the symptoms may lead to misdiagnosis of schizophrenia, hysteria, conduct disorders, and hypochondria. It can aggravate pre-existing psychiatric disorders. Fensterheim (1994) reviews these matters and stresses the prevalence of fear of death in people who hyperventilate. This can include a general feeling of doom or imminent death, the fear of death or loss of a significant person, and fear of fatal medical illness.

Non-cardiac chest pain

When chest pain or tightness occur, it is usually attributed at first to problems in the heart, especially if there is a family history or other risk factors. If cardiac examination shows no heart problems, other explanations will be considered: asthma, muscle tension, esophageal disorders, or arthritis of the rib–sternal joints. The pain may be labeled 'angina pectoris' if associated with physical exertion. If the chest symptoms coincide with emotional stress, however, diagnosis becomes

more complicated because stress is associated with a style of breathing which can generate pain or tightness in the chest. Although the discomfort occurs in the heart region, it is not necessarily related to the heart. Unpleasant sensations can arise from intercostal and other breathing muscles due to prolonged upper chest breathing, with or without hyperventilation.

Restriction of abdominal breathing forces the chest and shoulder muscles to do the work of breathing. This may come about from tight clothing, a habit of bracing the abdominal muscles, or from simply inhibiting abdominal expansion for reasons of personal appearance. Friedman (1945) did the definitive experiment in this area by tight strapping of the abdomen and lower ribs of normal volunteers. Chest pain developed within a day or two, and the trouble was exacerbated during exercise. Also, patients already suffering from chest pain (called in those days 'neurocirculatory asthenia') had their chests strapped to

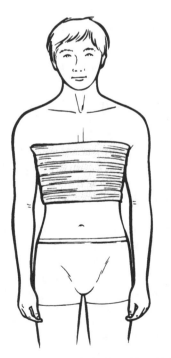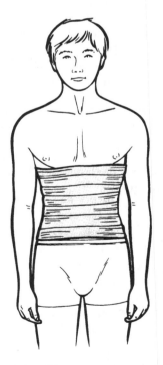

Figure 8.6 Non-cardiac pain related to faulty breathing. Habitual thoracic breathing can create angina-like chest pain from overuse of accessory breathing muscles. Such pain was abolished within 2 days by tight strapping of the upper chest to prevent expansion, and could be created in normal subjects by tight strapping of the abdomen and lower ribs. (Reproduced with kind permission from Gilbert 1999b.)

prevent the exaggerated thoracic breathing which Friedman considered was causing the pain. Forced to adopt more abdominal breathing, these patients lost their pain within 2 days, but it reappeared when the strapping was removed and their habitual breathing returned (Fig. 8.6).

This is not to suggest that incorrect breathing does not affect the heart; Nixon (1989, 1993a, 1994) has reviewed and documented the effect of chronic hyperventilation on the heart itself. He has focused on the physiological consequences of a continuing personal struggle to close the gap between existing performance and what seems required. He calls this the 'effort syndrome,' which stimulates hyperventilation via preparation for effort. This worsens the situation by unbalancing the autonomic nervous system toward the sympathetic end, triggering tachycardia, rise in blood pressure, and ultimately exhaustion as more effort is expended for less and less return. Homeostatic priorities are sacrificed. Hyperventilation over time disrupts the balance of potassium, magnesium, phosphorus and calcium which play intricate interlinked roles in maintaining proper cardiac function. Ultimately, the loss of alkaline buffer (see Ch. 3) and increase of lactic acid production reduces tolerance for exercise. This is apparent in the lower threshold for anaerobic muscle metabolism during standard exercise testing, indicating metabolic acidosis. Details can be found in Nixon (1994) and in Von Schéele & Van Schéele (1999).

A large number of cases of non-cardiac chest pain are eventually diagnosed as 'functional' and are most likely attributable to chronic hyperventilation (Bass & Wade 1984). Cardiovascular symptoms are reported by nearly all panic patients. An intervention study (De Guire et al 1992) attempted to reduce symptoms in patients who reported chest pain, palpitations, shortness of breath, arrhythmias, tachycardia, and paresthesias. Breathing retraining, the main intervention, consisted of teaching slower, more abdominal breathing. Some patients also received more involved explanations and training with respiratory strain gauges and CO_2 feedback. Significant improvement occurred in 6 weeks, and included reduced respiratory rate, increased end-tidal CO_2, and reduction in symptoms. Reduced breathing rate and the subject's belief that they were maintaining paced abdominal breathing were the strongest predictors of success. Exposure to the strain gauges and CO_2 feedback did not enhance the results.

At follow-up 3 years later, the improvements had held, with an average 10% rise in CO_2 levels and a drop from 16 to 10 breaths per minute, and corresponding drop in symptom occurrence. Potts and colleagues (1999) obtained similar success with 60 patients having chest pain but normal coronary arteries. Belief in their efficacy contributed to symptomatic improvement in this study also; those who still attributed their chest pain to heart disease had poorer outcomes.

The conclusion from these studies seems to be that teaching improved breathing to people having non-cardiac chest symptoms is quite feasible in a matter of weeks, and can bring substantial relief. Expectation and belief in one's ability to control breathing are involved, though this may interact with success in learning the breathing techniques.

Respiratory sinus arrhythmia (RSA)

This term refers to the cyclic rise and fall of the heart rate in rhythm with breathing. Laymen tend to consider a steady, unvarying heartbeat a good sign, perhaps because skipped beats, palpitations, extra beats, and a racing heart all seem to involve deviations from clock-like steadiness. The truth is actually the opposite: a heartbeat that is steady like a metronome is not generally a sign of health, and if chronic, usually indicates high stress and/or cardiac damage.

In a relaxed, healthy person, the heart rate normally rises part way through each inhalation, and then drops with the exhalation. The range of variation in beats per minute can range from fewer than 5 to more than 30, but averages between 8 and 14. RSA is often used as an index of general vagal tone since there is a waxing and waning of parasympathetic influence with each breath when the autonomic nervous system is properly balanced. Deeper breathing amplifies the variability; atropine, a parasympathetic inhibitor, will abolish RSA, as will anxiety and other influences which tip the balance toward sympathetic dominance.

Much basic physiological research is being done now in this area, and a certain amount of clinical research as well. The general assumption is that learning to increase the RSA can promote a healthier balance between sympathetic and parasympathetic dominance. Chronic disorders which involve autonomic imbalance, such as asthma, do seem to respond to the slow steady breathing involved in RSA training. Current research often uses the term 'resonant frequency biofeedback training,' which refers to using heart rate feedback for seeking a resonance between the breathing rhythm and the Traub-Hering-Mayer wave, which is tied to blood pressure regulation. The ideal breathing rate should be determined for each individual, but in most people a rate around six breaths per minute, or one complete breath every 10 seconds, establishes the resonance. That frequency is often mentioned as optimal by yoga practitioners and others who work with breathing relaxation.

Lehrer et al (1997) trained a number of asthmatics to increase RSA amplitude via RSA biofeedback, and compared their outcomes to others who learned an enhanced abdominal breathing technique by other means. Respiratory impedance (a measure of bronchoconstriction) was reduced in the RSA-trained group only. This provided confirmation for results reported from the Center for Medical Rehabilitation for Children in St Petersburg, Russia, where RSA biofeedback has been used for several years to treat thousands of children with bronchial asthma (Smetankin 1997) with a claimed 70% rate of success. Another study (Lehrer et al 2000) found improvements in spirometic measures in asthmatic children trained with RSA biofeedback.

The theory behind why RSA training should work has to do with exercising baroreceptor reflexes which regulate blood pressure. This is hypothesized to strengthen homeostatic activity, and this in turn helps modulate and limit stress-induced perturbations which may affect the entire autonomic nervous system. By this means, 'parasympathetic rebound' following stress-induced sympathetic arousal would be inhibited. This rebound phenomenon is thought to be a factor in asthma. Sympathetic dominance provokes bronchodilation (thus, adrenaline as an emergency treatment for asthma attacks) but when the body strives to recover its balance the rebound can go too far toward parasympathetic dominance, which is associated with bronchoconstriction.

Monitoring this variable can involve very elaborate electrocardiographic equipment, but any device which can display heart rate and updates rapidly can give rough biofeedback. Simply palpating the pulse will give an indication of whether the heartbeat rises and falls with the breathing. More details on this technique and other cardiovascular aspects of breathing can be found in Gilbert (1999b).

Van Dixhoorn

In the area of cardiac rehabilitation, one of the largest studies of cardiac rehabilitation including breathing based relaxation was done in The Netherlands by Jan van Dixhoorn (van Dixhoorn et al 1989, van Dixhoorn & Duivenvoorden 1989). In this study 156 survivors of recent heart attacks were randomly divided into two groups. All patients participated in standard aerobic conditioning exercises, but members in one group received an additional 6 hours of individual instruction in a simple relaxation technique which centered on breathing. This was a short-term intervention, a matter of weeks, but follow-up data were collected for several years afterward.

The main conclusions relevant here were that incidence of subsequent heart trouble was lower in the relaxation-plus-exercise compared with the exercise-only group. The breathing-based relaxation procedure provided a clear advantage over aerobic training alone. Breathing rate at follow-up was reduced, and respiratory sinus arrhythmia was stronger in the relaxation group, indicating lowered sympathetic tone. The average heart rate of relaxation-trained patients was lower, as was the incidence of ST-segment depression (meaning less evidence of myocardial ischemia). The changes in breathing persisted at a 2-year follow-up. Serious cardiac incidents occurred in 37% of the exercise group, compared to 17% in the relaxation group. A 5-year follow-up analysis showed that hospitalizations for cardiac problems were still lower in the relaxation group, and that the cost of the extra relaxation training intervention had been more than offset by the reduction of medical costs. All this resulted from 6 hours of instruction.

Method used The way that the author Jan van Dixhoorn taught relaxation via breathing is unique (Box 8.1). The essence of the technique consisted of comparing one's state (physical, mental, emotional) before and after the relaxation procedure, and noting the difference. Improved body awareness, rather than performance of a particular physical routine, was considered central to the entire intervention, and the desired respiratory change was coupled to passive awareness and self-observation. Breathing-based relaxation was integrated into daily routines by practicing in a variety of positions and situations.

Box 8.1 Van Dixhoorn's breathing techniques used in cardiac rehabilitation

- Deemphasize the idea of 'exercises' and 'performance'
- Emphasize self-observation and self-awareness, with many brief interventions throughout the day
- Practice both 'active relaxation' (during movement) and 'passive relaxation'
- Separate the intervention into two components: relaxed breathing and self-observation
- Encourage awareness and involvement of entire body in breathing
- Use manual touch to facilitate awareness of abdominal expansion, muscular tension, and participation of the ribs and back
- Use EMG biofeedback from the forehead
- Encourage experimentation with breathing variables (depth, rate, location, ease, regularity)
- Patient's hand placed on abdomen, with the direction: 'The hand notices what the body does'
- Directing attention to subtle body changes during exhale vs. inhale, such as the distance between sternum and pubic bone, magnitude of lumbar and cervical curves

---

Van Dixhoorn's recommended rest breaks were defined as exercises in self-awareness rather than 'relaxation' which his population of cardiac patients would have considered synonymous with being lazy or 'falling behind.' Van Dixhoorn's intervention neatly sidestepped this conflict by assigning a 'before and after' cognitive comparison. To do this requires entering an objective state that disrupts ongoing emotional states which contribute to stress.

In the six individual training sessions van Dixhoorn and his colleagues used several methods to initiate a self-awareness which was considered the key to restoring homeostatic balance (van Dixhoorn & Duivenvoorden 1989). In his words: 'The patient learned to elicit and observe a "shift" in the respiratory pattern, such that inspiration expanded both the lower abdomen and the costal margin, and expiration was moderated and slow' (van Dixhoorn et al 1990). Pursed-lips breathing to make the air movement audible increased breathing awareness further.

Van Dixhoorn went beyond encouraging diaphragmatic movement to improving the coordination of diaphragm action with other respiratory muscles in the abdomen, back, and chest. Efficient breathing actually involves movement of the whole trunk, the pelvis, spine, and sternum. He noted, for instance, that the top of the pelvis rotates subtly forward during inhalation, that the lumbar curve increases while the cervical curve decreases, and that the distance between the symphysis pubis and the sternum increases. Individualized instruction sometimes included manual touch to focus attention and to provide tactile feedback. For instance, he would place his hands on the abdomen or lower back and instruct the patient to 'breathe into my hands.' This gentle and personal instruction downplayed prescribing the 'proper' proper way to breathe. He encouraged patients instead to experiment with depth, rate, location, and timing, and then observe any differences in feeling state.

REFERENCES

Bass C, Wade C 1984 Chest pain with normal coronary arteries: a comparative study of psychiatric and social morbidity. Psychological Medicine 14: 51–61

Baykushev S 1969 Hyperventilation as an accelerated hypnotic induction technique. International Journal of Clinical and Experimental Hypnosis 17(1): 20–24

Benson H, Klipper M Z 1988 The relaxation response. Collins, London

Bradley D 1998 Hyperventilation syndrome, 3rd edn. Tandem Press, North Shore City, NZ. Hunter House, San Francisco, 2001.

Clark D M 1986 A cognitive approach to panic. Behaviour Research and Therapy 24: 461–470

Clifton-Smith T 1999 Breathe to succeed. Penguin Books, Auckland, NZ

Conway A V, Freeman L J, Nixon P G F 1988 Hypnotic examination of trigger factors in the hyperventilation syndrome. American Journal of Clinical Hypnosis 30: 296–304

Cox B J, Parker J D A, Swinson R P 1995 An examination of levels of agoraphobic anxiety in panic disorder. Behaviour Research and Therapy 33: 57–62

DeGuire S, Gevirtz R, Kawahara Y, Maguire W 1992 Hyperventilation syndrome and the assessment of treatment for functional cardiac symptoms. American Journal of Cardiology 70: 673–677

Dudley D L 1969 Psychophysiology of respiration in health and disease. Appleton-Century-Crofts, New York

Fensterheim H 1994 Hyperventilation and psychopathology: a clinical perspective. In: Timmons B H, Ley R (eds) Behavioral and psychological approaches to breathing disorders. Plenum, New York

Folgering H 1988 Diagnostic criteria for the hyperventilation syndrome. Respiratory Psychophysiology 50: 133–140

Fried R 1993 The psychology and physiology of breathing. Plenum, New York

Friedman M 1945 Studies concerning the aetiology and pathogenesis of neurocirculatory asthenia: IV. The respiratory manifestations of neurocirculatory asthenia. American Heart Journal 30: 557–566

Gardner W N 1996 The pathophysiology of hyperventilation disorders. Chest 109: 516–534

Gilbert C 1998 Hyperventilation and the body. Journal of Bodywork and Movement Therapies 2(3): 190

Gilbert C 1999a Breathing: the legacy of Wilhelm Reich. Journal of Bodywork and Movement Therapies 3(2): 97–106

Gilbert C 1999b Breathing and the cardiovascular system. Journal of Bodywork and Movement Therapies 3(4): 215–224

Han J N, Stegen K, Schepers R, Van den Bergh O, Van de Woestijne K P 1998 Subjective symptoms and breathing pattern at rest and following hyperventilation in anxiety and somatoform disorders. Journal of Psychosomatic Research 45(6): 519–532

Hardonk H J, Beumer H M 1979 Hyperventilation syndrome. In: Vinken P J, Bruyn G W (eds) Handbook of Clinical Neurology 38: 1 Amsterdam

Hegel M T, Ferguson R J 1997 Psychophysiological assessment of respiratory function in panic disorder:

evidence for a hyperventilation subtype. Psychosomatic Medicine 59: 224–230

King J C, Rosen S, Nixon P G F 1990 Failure of perception of hypocapnia: physiological and clinical implications. Journal of the Royal Society of Medicine 83: 765–767

Klein D F 1993 False suffocation alarms, spontaneous panics, and related conditions: an integrative hypothesis. Archives of General Psychiatry 50: 306–317

Lehrer P, Carr R E, Smetankine A et al 1997 Respiratory sinus arrhythmia versus neck/trapezius EMG and incentive inspirometry biofeedback for asthma: a pilot study. Applied Psychophysiology and Biofeedback 22(2): 95–109

Lehrer P, Smetankin A, Potapova T 2000 Respiratory sinus arrhythmia biofeedback therapy for asthma: a report of 20 unmedicated pediatric cases using the Smetankin method. Applied Psychophysiology and Biofeedback 25(3): 193–200

Moscariello A, Molle J P, Wattiez A, Dejonghe M, Thiriaux J, Gillard C 1999 The hyperventilation syndrome (HVS): diagnostic tests. Chest 116, 3358

Nakao K, Ohgushi M, Yoshimura M et al 1997 Hyperventilation as a specific test for diagnosis of coronary artery spasm. American Journal of Cardiology 80(5): 545–549

Nixon P G F 1989 Hyperventilation and cardiac symptoms. Internal Medicine 10(12): 67–84

Nixon P G F 1993a The grey area of effort syndrome and hyperventilation: from Thomas Lewis to today. Journal of the Royal College of Physicians 27: 37–383

Nixon P G F 1993b The broken heart – counteraction by SABRES. Journal of the Royal Society of Medicine 86: 468–471

Nixon P G F 1994 Effort syndrome: hyperventilation and reduction of anaerobic threshold. Biofeedback and Self-Regulation 19: 155–169

Nixon P G F, Freeman L J 1988 The 'think test': a further technique to elicit hyperventilation. Journal of the Royal Society of Medicine 81: 277–279

Potts S G, Lewin R, Fox K A, Johnstone E C 1999 Group psychological treatment for chest pain with normal coronary arteries. Quarterly Journal of Medicine 92: 81–86

Salkovskis P M 1988 Phenomenology, assessment, and the cognitive model of panic. In: Rachman S, Maser J D (eds) Panic: psychological perspectives. Erlbaum, Hillsdale, NJ

Salkovskis P M, Clark D M, Gelder M G 1996 Cognitive-behavior links in the persistence of panic. Behaviour Research and Therapy 34(5/6): 453–458

Smetankin A 1997 Biofeedback developments in Russia: progress in the biofeedback treatment of childhood asthma. Biofeedback Newsmagazine 25: 8–11, 17

Timmons B H 1994 Breathing-related issues in therapy. In: Timmons B H, Ley R (eds) Behavioral and psychological approaches to breathing disorders. Plenum, New York

van Dixhoorn J, Duivenvoorden H J 1985 Efficacy of Nijmegen questionnaire in recognition of the hyperventilation syndrome. Journal of Psychosomatic Research 29: 199–206

van Dixhoorn J, Duivenvoorden H J 1989 Breathing awareness as a relaxation method in cardiac rehabilitation. In: Stress and tension control – III. Plenum, New York, pp 19–36 van Dixhoorn J, Duivenvoorden H J, Stall J A, Pool J 1989 Physical training and relaxation therapy in cardiac rehabilitation assessed through a composite criterion for training outcome. American Heart Journal 118(3): 545–552

van Dixhoorn J, Duivenvoorden J A, Pool J 1990 Success and failure of exercise training after myocardial infarction: is the outcome predictable? Journal of American College of Cardiology 15: 974–982

von Schéele B H C, von Schéele I A M 1999 The measurement of respiratory and metabolic parameters of patients and controls before and after incremental exercise on bicycle: supporting the effort syndrome hypothesis? Applied Psychophysiology and Biofeedback 24(3): 167–177

Whitehead W E, Bosmajian L, Zonderman A B, Costa P T, Schuster M M 1988 Symptoms of psychologic distress associated with irritable bowel syndrome: comparison of community and medical clinic samples. Gastroenterology 95(3): 709–714

Wilhelm F H, Trabert W, Roth W T 2001 Characteristics of sighing in panic disorder. Biological Psychiatry 49(7): April 1, 606–614

Wientjes C J E, Grossman P 1994 Over-reactivity of the psyche or of the soma? Interindividual associations between psychosomatic symptoms, anxiety, heart rate and end-tidal partial carbon dioxide pressure. Psychosomatic Medicine 56: 533–540

9

Other breathing issues

Leon Chaitow, Dinah Bradley &
Christopher Gilbert

INTRODUCTION

In this chapter we have compiled information on a variety of methods and modalities which seem to have no natural home in any of the preceding chapters, but which we thought it important to include. The discussion in this chapter of a particular topic does not necessarily signify that the authors advocate its application. Specifically, there are reservations among the authors relative to the Buteyko system, as well as to aspects of the somewhat bizarre intranasal bodywork approach.

Because methods are being used clinically by some health care professionals (including perspectives deriving from Traditional Chinese Medicine, yoga and Buteyko methods, among others), we felt it important to provide at least a thumbnail impression of the methodology and underlying concepts, and where necessary, a word of caution.

Other topics covered include the apparently light-hearted look at hyperventilating chickens, which despite the humor inherent in the topic offers important lessons relative to the biochemistry of the process, and the use of carbonated water.

This chapter therefore contains topics which do not fit comfortably elsewhere in the text but which it was felt were deserving of inclusion in order to offer balance to the text as a whole. They are listed below, in the order in which they appear in the chapter:

1. Air travel and hyperventilation
2. The Buteyko method
3. Exercise induced hyperventilation

4. Chickens who breathe too much
5. Intranasal manipulation
6. Musicians (woodwind and brass)
7. Nasal strips
8. Paper bag therapy
9. Sleep apneas
10. Stage fright
11. Traditional Chinese Medicine and respiratory dysfunction
12. Yoga and breathing (including alternate nostril breathing)

AIR TRAVEL AND HYPERVENTILATION

Chronic hyperventilators are put at extra risk on long haul flights where aircraft may reach 35 000 or 37 000 feet above sea level for up to 10–12 hours. Cabins are pressurized to prevent altitude hypoxia and ensure the comfort of the traveler. Older aircraft (Boeing 737s for example) relied entirely on fresh air flowing through all the aircraft's sections. However, more fuel-efficient methods have been devised in recent years which recycle used air mixed with fresh air in varying proportions, reducing at times the levels of available oxygen.

A British charity, the Oxford-based Aviation Health Institute (AHI), is one of many authorities who have shown concern at the declining quality of cabin air since the oil crisis in the late 1970s. Disturbed at the number of flight attendants with recurring health problems such as influenza-like eye, nose, and throat complaints, dizziness, and headaches, they were also concerned with reported breathing and fainting episodes among small children and passengers over 50 years of age.

Angina attacks have been reported in normal subjects, triggered by hyperventilation during long flights in response to lower available circulating oxygen (O_2). Respiration rates increase to maintain adequate O_2 levels and carbon dioxide (CO_2) is flushed out of the lungs at too great a rate. Preceded by chest pains, pins and needles, dry throat, or nausea, coronary artery spasming may have dire consequences for people with pre-existing coronary heart disease (CHD). Flight attendants may offer paper bags to rebreathe CO_2

(see p. 233). Anginine (nitroglycerine) tablets, if given early enough, are more effective as they relax and dilate the coronary arteries. Passengers who have CHD should be encouraged to keep their medication at hand and to use it immediately symptoms occur and notify the flight attendant.

In the case of both normal and at-risk passengers, low oxygen levels make an increased respiratory rate a normal response. However, those with existing chronic hyperventilation problems would experience discomfort or even angina faster that non-hyperventilators because of their already lowered CO_2 levels.

Hyperventilation is a classic manifestation of 'fear of flying' and those suffering this (even on shorter flights) may experience signs and symptoms of hypocapnia. Recent reports published on so-called 'economy class syndrome', where potentially life-threatening deep vein thromboses/pulmonary emboli may occur from clots arising from pooling of blood in feet and legs and cramped conditions, have further increased travelers' anxieties. People most susceptible to this are those who drink too much alcohol or use sleeping pills, or are overweight. Fear of flying courses help and should cover these issues. They base much of their training and conditioning on maintaining breathing control as well as cognitive skills to manage fear.

THE BUTEYKO METHOD

A breathing retraining approach devised by Dr Konstantin Buteyko in Russia in the 1960s is now being taught in many Western countries, particularly in the UK, USA, Australia, and New Zealand.

The main objective of Buteyko training appears to be to increase the individual's tolerance for CO_2, using a series of simple, self-applied exercises. The key features include (Buteyko Alternative Approach Manual 1996):

- Encouraging shallow breathing (hypoventilation) so that the individual becomes accustomed to a sense of slight 'lack of air.'
- Use of a 'control pause' as an exercise, in which normal exhalation is held until a

'distinct sensation' of 'slight lack of air' is experienced, at which time breathing recommences, *without loss of control of the shallow rhythm* (i.e. the control pause is not followed by a deep breath).

- The control pause is practiced a number of times daily to encourage an increase in CO_2 tolerance.
- 'First aid' use of a 'maximum pause' is suggested, in which the exhaled breath is held until moderate discomfort is experienced, at which time breathing recommences, *without loss of control of the shallow rhythm* (i.e. the maximum pause is not followed by a deep breath). The maximum pause is used to relieve the symptoms of hyperventilation (similar to rebreathing CO_2 from a paper bag).

⚠ **CAUTION:** Buteyko instructors suggest that caution should be used regarding use of the maximum pause in the case of patients with cardiovascular or kidney disease, hypertension, epilepsy, or diabetes.

- Nasal breathing, including encouraging the use of mouth taping at night to prevent mouth breathing. A 25 mm-wide, paper-based surgical tape is suggested for this purpose. Contraindications include anyone who has just taken sleeping tablets or consumed alcohol or is feeling nauseous (and presumably anyone who is wary of having the mouth taped).

Buteyko teaching encourages other factors such as improved posture, relaxation, regular physical exercise, and reduction in stimulants such as caffeine. Buteyko (1991) explains the background to his method as follows:

Thirty-seven years have passed since the time I found the cause of several of the most widespread diseases which belong to so called 'civilised diseases' (bronchial, cardiovascular, allergic etc). These diseases have one common cause – alveolar hyperventilation or deep breathing. It had occurred to me: reduction in depth of breathing or normalisation of breathing may treat such diseases. An experimental study proved the validity of this presumption; more so it was based on the laws of physiology, biochem-

istry, biology and other disciplines … The essence of the method is a decrease in the depth of breathing by will power and by relaxation of breathing muscles until one achieves a slight feeling of lack of air. All mentally healthy adults and children from the age of three can use the method.

Such claims have not surprisingly attracted concern and more recently, attempts at scientific validation. Only one major study, which admits to flaws in its methodology, has appeared in a mainstream peer-reviewed journal to date.

Research

Evidence of efficacy of the method was sought in a prospective, blinded, randomized study comparing the effect of the Buteyko breathing technique (BBT) with control classes in 39 subjects with asthma (Bowler et al 1998).

Intervention trial participants underwent training simultaneously in two separate groups. Teaching occurred over 7 days, with each session lasting for 60–90 minutes.

Buteyko training for the treatment group consisted of the teaching of a series of exercises in which subjects reduced the depth and frequency of respiration. Breath-holding exercises measured the impact of this training and gauged progress. Participants were encouraged to practice these exercises several times a day.

In the control group, subjects were given general asthma education and relaxation techniques, and were taught abdominal breathing exercises which did not involve hypoventilation.

The main outcome measures used were medication use, morning peak expiratory flow (PEF), forced expiratory volume in one second (FEV_1), end-tidal (ET) CO_2, resting minute volume (MV), and quality of life (QOL) score, measured at 3 months. The results showed:

- There was no change in daily PEF or FEV_1 noted in either group.
- At 3 months, the BBT group had a median reduction in daily $beta_2$-agonist dose of 904 µg (range, 29 µg to 3129 µg), whereas the control group had a median reduction of 57 µg (range, – 2343 µg to 1143 µg) ($P = 0.002$).

- The daily inhaled steroid dose fell 49% (range, – 100% to 150%) for the BBT group and 0 (range, –82% to +100%) for the control group ($P = 0.06$).
- A trend toward greater improvement in quality of life score was noted for BBT subjects ($P = 0.09$).
- Initial minute volume (MV) was high and similar in both groups, but by 3 months, MV was lower in the BBT group than in the control group ($P = 0.004$).
- End tidal CO_2 was low in both groups and did not change with treatment.

The researchers concluded that those practicing BBT reduced hyperventilation and their use of beta$_2$-agonists. A trend toward reduced inhaled steroid use and better quality of life was observed in these patients without objective changes in measures of airway caliber.

Comment

Buteyko is one among many other modalities which may help reduce medication usage and/or relieve or prevent hyperventilation-induced asthma – including exercise/improved cardiopulmonary fitness, inspiratory muscle training (IMT), breathing reeducation, asthma education, relaxation, and environmental control. The Buteyko method may suit those with mild to moderate asthma who display anxiety over their diagnosis and drug regimen, and who also carry out all other environmental, dietary, and fitness recommendations.

Parents whose children have been trained in the BBT method must be vigilant in monitoring symptoms if inhaled steroid medications are reduced. They should be encouraged to let their family doctor know what they are doing. Some doctors are extremely wary of the method, especially those who have had to attend children with severe asthma attacks who had cut out their preventor (inhaled steroid) medication. Children have been known to reduce their medications to please their anxious parents. If symptoms worsen and bronchoconstriction and airway inflammation increases, hypoventilating (BBT) allows CO_2 levels

to rise above normal, while O_2 levels drop (hypoxia), ushering in a severe attack. But most family doctors, if they are kept informed will support a parent's right to choose any alternative therapies provided the child is not put at risk.

EXERCISE-INDUCED HYPERVENTILATION

While asthma is clearly the most common cause of exercise-induced dyspnea it is not the only cause of breathlessness during exercise. People who exercise regularly and have been tested at their gyms or sports clubs and pronounced fit may complain of breathlessness disproportionate to their fitness levels (Howell 1990). An excessive ventilatory response to exercise may bring on chest discomfort which is commonly perceived as dyspnea. These symptoms are thought to be triggered by hyperventilation-induced hypocapnia and, because they do not respond to inhaled beta agonists, indicate an absence of bronchospasm.

Clinicians assessing exercise-fit HVS/BPD patients frequently find a musculoskeletal element to their dysfunction. A common finding is entrenched upper-chest breathing patterns, often accompanied by chronic mouth breathing. Perhaps due to upper body overtraining, these patients tend to hyperinflate their chests at rest and hyperventilate rapidly on starting exercise. The associated dyspnea limits their activity. Breathing retraining with abdominal/diaphragmatic strengthening has been shown to be effective. Studies done on inspiratory muscle training with pressure threshold devices (Caine & McConnell 1998) showed improvements in both strength and endurance and improvement in athletic performance.

A study by Chambers and colleagues (1988) showed decreased end-tidal CO_2 in some exercise-induced dyspnea patients diagnosed with functional cardiovascular syndromes. (These syndromes encompass psychological, cardiovascular, and respiratory symptoms in varying proportions with non-cardiac chest pain as a primary symptom.) While these patients exhibited no overt signs of classic HVS, chest pains could be reproduced by inducing hypocapnia with voluntary hyperventilation. The authors speculated that such patients might have an abnormality of respiratory control during exercise.

Among more recent research, a study on children and adolescents by Hammo & Weinberger (1999) revealed that some children who were initially diagnosed as having asthma were in fact hyperventilating when they exercised. The physiological changes in airflow and gas exchange that ocurred during standardized treadmill exercise were examined in patients previously diagnosed with exercise-induced asthma, whose histories were atypical, or where conventional treatments, including an inhaled beta agonist, did not alleviate symptoms.

Thirty-two patients aged between 8 and 18 during a 1-year period fitted these criteria and underwent exercise testing. Seventeen of the children tested had no shortness of breath as previously experienced, and had normal respiratory function. Shortness of breath was reproduced in the other 15 children, with only four of those exhibiting findings consistent with asthma, including coughing, wheezing, and decreases in FEV_1 of more than 15%. The remaining 11 children experienced chest tightness and dyspnea with no wheeze or cough, and no changes in their lung function measurements. However, this group had significantly lower carbon dioxide levels than those measured in the other children, suggesting these children were hyperventilating in response to effort.

Hammo & Weinberger state:

mechanisms of normal respiratory control during exercise remain a controversial subject. The rapid increase in ventilation documented to occur at the start of exercise suggests a neurogenic stimulus, although undefined humoral factors cannot be excluded as influencing control of ventilation during sustained exercise. The decreased end tidal CO_2 during exercise in our patients could therefore potentially result from insensitivity of afferent receptors to a lowered PCO_2, or efferent neural factors of central origin overdriving ventilation. Whether of central origin or due to a receptor abnormality, the 11 children and adolescents we identified with chest tightness associated with exercise-induced hypocapnia, and the adult patients with similar symptoms undergoing cardiac stress testing described by Chambers

et al (1988) appear to represent an abnormality of ventilatory homeostasis during exercise.

They also note:

CO_2 levels normally decrease somewhat during heavy exercise when the anaerobic threshold is exceeded and a degree of respiratory alkalosis begins to compensate for the metabolic lactic acidosis that occurs at sustained high exercise levels. The decreased end-tidal CO_2 in our patients therefore does not by itself distinguish between inappropriate and compensatory hyperventilation. The similarity of symptoms described by Bass et al (1991) among adults with chest discomfort during exercise supports the hypothesis that primary hyperventilation contributed to the symptoms associated with the end-tidal CO_2 in our patients.

Their research showed that many children and adolescents with chest discomfort or pain may be misdiagnosed and treated as having exercise-induced asthma when they in fact are hyperventilating. Their findings also examine parallels in the adult population where chest discomfort is more likely to be diagnosed as cardiac in origin, and both groups require careful investigation as to the true causes of their complaints.

Box 9.1 examines the case of the hyperventilating chickens.

INTRANASAL MANIPULATION

Intranasal work is a method which is sometimes employed during the 10-session series of structural integration processing developed by Dr Ida Rolf (Rolf 1976). Other schools such as those training neuromuscular therapists are now copying or developing on this work, according to Rolfer Tom Myers (2001). Myers writes:

Dr Rolf died in 1979, and the history of how intranasal work came to be included in the Rolfing series is not clear. Dr Rolf herself acknowledged yoga and osteopathy as the two main taproots for her work. Yoga, as she practiced it earlier in her life, included 'kriyas' or cleansing practices, one of which reportedly involved passing a cloth through the nasal passages. More likely the source of the nasal work was seminars that Ida Rolf took with William Sutherland DO, the founder of cranial osteopathy.

Myers suggests that employing intranasal technique should ideally involve prior preparation of the client's connective tissues, and that the technique may be contraindicated in cases of current

---

Box 9.1 Chickens that breathe too much

This book focuses on breathing pattern disorders in humans, but the following account illustrates the biochemical principles presented in Chapter 3, manifested in another species under particular conditions. Agricultural researchers studied chickens confined in commercial egg-laying facilities (Odom et al 1985). During the hot summer months the eggshells become thinner, leading to increased breakage and decreased profits for the owners. This outcome was finally traced to the chickens panting to cool themselves. Under these conditions the blood chemistry shifts to alkaline, carbonate content drops, calcium is lost, and eggshells become fragile.

Chicken farmers have tried many solutions over the years, including adding powdered cement to the chicken feed in order to harden the shells. Once hyperventilation was suggested as a contributing cause, installing costly air-conditioning for the chickens seemed the only answer. But the researchers cited above tried replacing the plain drinking water with carbonated water. A controlled experiment ensued, with 400 hens on carbonated water and another 400 on plain water. This strategy produced a very significant difference in eggshell breakage, and it was calculated that the money saved by egg producers would more than offset the extra cost of providing carbonated water.

Calcium carbonate is a major ingredient of bones and also of eggshells; it was being drawn out of the body because of the hyperventilating. Drinking carbonated liquid (dissolved CO_2 is what makes water 'carbonated') replaced the missing ingredient in the diet of the overheated chickens (CO_2 is carried in the blood primarily as carbonic acid), and egg production rose. This is the reverse of what some endurance runners do by ingesting bicarbonate of soda to increase blood alkalinity (see Ch. 3) to counteract build-up of lactic acid. In the case of the hyperventilating chickens, acidity is needed to restore pH balance, and adding carbonated water neatly balances the losses caused by hyperventilation.

Though unresearched so far, it would follow that human hyperventilators might seek out carbonated beverages in an unconscious effort to rebalance their pH. This author (CG) encountered two clinical cases in which the patients reported, after questioning, a sharp increase in consumption of carbonated beverages around the time they experienced emotional traumas which initiated chronic hyperventilation. One woman had been puzzled over her new craving for 1–2 liters per day of plain soda water.

Animals in general shift their food preferences and priorities depending on nutritional status; this may extend to compensating for respiratory alkalosis.

---

acute sinus or other pharyngeal infection, recent facial trauma, the use of anticoagulant drugs, or hemophilia, or patients on the extreme end of psychophysiological sensitivity, as well as anyone habitually using ('snorting') cocaine.

⚠ Neither the intranasal nor the nasal specific ('balloon' method) described briefly in this text should be attempted without a thorough training in their usage, as well as a full understanding of the risks involved and a signed informed consent form from the patient. There also exist legal proscriptions forbidding the entry to body orifices by therapists, with or without patient permission, in many states of the USA and elsewhere. *Reporting of the methods in this text should absolutely not be seen as a recommendation for their use.*

The structural integration method

Myers (2001) reports:

In structural integration [i.e. Rolfing] practice, intranasal work is done with the little finger, gloved and lubricated, with great sensitivity and concentra-tion, with ultimate slowness and client communica-tion, and only after the entire rest of the body has been prepared for this work by detailed myofascial processing. The direct purpose in introducing a finger into the nose is to widen, open, and loosen the soft-tissues surrounding the nasal cavity.

Myers states:

Once into the vestibule, the finger encounters the 'gate' around the nasal passage, formed by the maxillary bones laterally and interiorly, and the nasal septum medially. When the vestibular gate has 'melted' open (forcing is neither called for nor advisable), the fingertip emerges into the wider chamber of the nasal cavity. In the deeper part of the nasal passage, the vomer bone, rather than the carti-laginous nasal septum, forms the medial wall, and the palatine bone forms the floor behind the maxilla. Superior to this are the nasal conchae as well as the nasal and lacrimal bones. None of these bones are touched directly. It is the contention of structural integration, and the rationale for this part of its technique library, that the tendency is for these turbinates to migrate medially, thus reducing such contact and rendering the inner passages, between the turbinates and the septum, less open. This compels more reliance on the outermost passage, between the first turbinate and the maxilla, though this passage may also be reduced in the general narrowing of the facial structure. Thus the idea in the intra-nasal work is to move the turbinates laterally away from the septum. The turbinates are located not only one above the other but one behind the other, so that they would be encountered sequentially by the practitioner's finger.

Additional foci of the method include evaluation of the position of the turbinates, 'the doors to the facial sinuses.' The efficacy reported (anecdotally) of enhanced sinus drainage by means of intranasal work is a principal justification for its application. Myers also reports that he has:

found many deviated septa to be responsive to treatment, with the results of increased opening being very gratefully received by clients. The cartilage, we must admit, occasionally crackles disconcertingly when directed toward the midline, but we have had no reports of post-session pain or disturbance related to these sounds. Intraosseous strain within the vomer caused by cranial torque or shear forces can also be eased by sustained attention in this direction.

Habitual use of cocaine and other recreational drugs, which can break down the cartilage of the septum, is a contraindication for this type of manipulation, especially in immature or elderly individuals.

The balloon method (nasal specific technique)

A method involving the inflation of small balloons (finger cots) within the nose was developed in the 1930s as a means of altering intranasal deviations or obstructions.

This method employs a minimum of two finger cots (one inside the other), which are inserted into the nasal cavity with the outer one lubricated. The first is secured to the nipple on the bulb of a blood pressure cuff, which is used to inflate them. The inflated cots follow the path of least resistance posteriorly into the nasopharynx. Dr Douglas Lewis, past head of the department of physical medicine at Bastyr University in Seattle, Washington, USA, describes the effect as equivalent to 'a high-velocity, low amplitude thrust' commonly employed in osteopathic or chiropractic manipulation. Lewis has used this

method for a variety of problems, including sinusitis, as well as opening the nasal passages for breathing. This treatment is 'not pleasant at the moment of inflation,' according to Lewis, but due to its efficacy, patients frequently request, however reluctantly, for him to repeat it (reported in Myers 2001).

According to Folweiler & Lynch (1995):

It is common for the patient to hear 'cracking' or 'popping' sounds within the skull during the technique. Occasionally, they can be perceived by the practitioner. Tenderness following the treatment along the median palatine suture and other facial sutures is common, persisting for a few days after treatment. Epistaxis (nose bleed) can occur, but is not commonly long in duration nor large in volume.

The 'balloon' treatment is primarily employed for chronic sinusitis and other nasal complaints. 'The nasal specific technique, when used in conjunction with other therapies, may be useful in treating chronic sinus inflammation and pain,' speculate Folweiler & Lynch. They go on to hypothesize as to the mechanism of such relief:

Numerous theories could be used to explain the benefits of the nasal specific technique for chronic sinusitis. One such explanation may be the direct elimination of mucus from the nasal passages by the force of the inflated cot, thus reducing pressure and pain and allowing increased sinus and nasal drainage. It is also possible that pressure against the thin, slightly pliable bones surrounding the sinuses allows equalization of pressure in the sinus to that of the atmosphere. It is also possible that a neural reflex exists by which the nasal specific technique causes mucus thinning and/or altered discharge. Manually compressing edematous tissues may result in a vascular response that leads to normalization of function.

MUSICIANS (WOODWIND AND BRASS)

Brandfonbrener (2000) has summarized many of the influences relative to breathing dysfunction and the playing of musical instruments: 'All blown instruments have multiple risk factors for medical problems involving the respiratory and musculoskeletal systems. However, both musically and medically one must distinguish between the woodwinds and brass.' The risks relative to the playing of woodwinds relate to the extremes of breathing requirements and not just to the volume of air required to achieve the pressures necessary. The least stressful efforts relate to the flute, while the greatest force is required when playing double reeds, oboe, and bassoon. Here the problem relates to maintaining the volume of contained air while slowly releasing this at very high pressure. Air flow requirements for the clarinet are between those for flute and oboe.

The pressures and contortions necessary for playing woodwinds, involving the *embouchure* – the complex made up of the mechanical mouthpiece and the biophysiological stomatognathic (mouth) structures – are capable of affecting 'the facial muscles, bones, skin, mucous membranes, nerve, tongue and teeth.'

With brass instruments, the most serious negative influences relate to the structures which constitute the biophysiological components of the *embouchure*. The effects will be determined by individual characteristics as well as the type of mouthpiece chosen and the style of playing.

Breathing-related medical problems relating to woodwind and brass players

- *Pneumothorax*: Brandfonbrener reports that his clinical experience suggests that people with a predisposition who play wind or brass instruments are at increased risk of pneumothorax.
- *Hypopharyngeal dilatation*: there are anecdotal reports of hypopharyngeal dilatation in trumpet players.
- *Asthma*: Brandfonbrener states that he has 'treated a number of musicians, especially low brass players, in whom playing the instrument appeared responsible for the onset of an exercise-induced asthma equivalent. In all cases, patients were benefited by the use of an inhaled bronchodilator prior to playing.'

NASAL STRIPS

Nasal strips (such as Breathe Right™) are an over-the-counter commercial product designed to give temporary relief to people with nasal congestion or nasal septal deviations. The strips resemble a band-aid which adheres to either side of the nostrils. A built-in plastic spring encourages the strip to flatten and so spreads the nostrils, increasing nasal airflow.

Nasal strips have received publicity in the popular media as being of benefit to performing athletes by enhancing nasal airflow, particularly in sports where participants are required to wear mouth guards. This claim has come under scrutiny from sports scientists who have rejected any suggestion of improvement in oxygen uptake by athletes, but have acknowledged they may be helpful to athletes suffering nasal congestion.

Invented by an allergy sufferer in 1987, nasal strips were cleared by the US Food & Drug Agency as a medical device to improve nose breathing. Nasal strips were subsequently cleared to be marketed for the reduction or elimination of snoring. While of no help to snorers with obstructive, restrictive, or central sleep apneas, many noisy mouth breathers who were unable to nose breathe because of allergy or sinus problems have claimed benefit – as have their sleeping partners.

People who have experienced increased nasal resistance due to cartilage degradation, a natural aging process (Edelstein 1996), have found nasal strips beneficial during sleep. At the other end of the spectrum, children with allergies or chronic sinus problems can use them safely to help reinforce nose breathing patterns.

⚠ Warning. Some individuals may be allergic to the adhesive on the strips.

PAPER BAG THERAPY

To terminate an episode of acute hyperventilation, many handbooks, articles, and texts recommend breathing into a paper bag, with the rationale that exhaled CO_2 will be conserved and reabsorbed. Since hyperventilation is known to be associated with a deficit of CO_2, this explanation seemed quite valid, and so experimental research was apparently not done until the late 1980s. A simple attribution of panic symptoms to low CO_2 was being challenged by findings that many people could hyperventilate for as long as an hour without ill effects, dropping their CO_2 to half of normal. Subjects who were already prone to panic in response to lactate or breathing high levels of CO_2 were likely to panic with hyperventilation also. Thus a possibility emerged that something other than actual blood CO_2 level could be responsible for panic, as well as other symptoms of hyperventilation.

This popular remedy was finally tested (van den Hout et al 1987) with two experiments. In the first, 12 normal volunteers hyperventilated for 2 minutes and then followed one of two procedures: either breathing into a paper bag for 3 more minutes or attempting to resume normal breathing unaided. In both cases end-tidal $Paco_2$ was monitored continuously, and subjects were asked to report when any physical symptoms had disappeared. (Each subject participated in both conditions, randomized as to order.) Symptoms were reported gone in an average 67 seconds when subjects were rebreathing, and in 96 seconds when not rebreathing. There was large variance, but the difference was significant.

The CO_2 recovered more quickly in the rebreathing group, climbing significantly higher than in the non-rebreathing condition. This recovery was limited to the duration of paper bag breathing; when it was removed, the CO_2 quickly dropped to the non-rebreathing level.

The data up to this point seem to confirm the supposition that restoring CO_2 by the paper bag technique helps hyperventilators recover faster from their symptoms. A significant point in the experimental procedure, however, was that all subjects were told at the beginning that the bag rebreathing should make symptoms go away. Thus this expectation was operating whatever condition a subject started with. Given a different research goal, this pre-test information would be considered sloppy experimental procedure, biasing the subjects toward believing that the rebreathing would be effective rather than letting them discover it for themselves. But the experiments were being carried out in a department of medical psychology, and the focus of the research was on a psychological variable.

Belief and expectation

The second experiment was very different; a new group of subjects was given the same explanation about how rebreathing CO_2 was effective for terminating any sensations and symptoms of hyperventilation. The paper bag apparatus was exchanged for a mouthpiece and a system of tubes and valves which could be opened or closed surreptitiously. Subjects were told that they would be rebreathing their exhaled CO_2 in two separate trials because the experiment was about test–retest reliability. This was a deception; the procedure of the first experiment was repeated exactly (one trial with rebreathing exhaled CO_2 and one trial without).

The CO_2 recovery pattern duplicated the results of the first experiment: faster restoration with rebreathing CO_2 than without. Disappearance of symptoms, however, took the same amount of time in each condition, averaging around 60 seconds. This time, presence or absence of rebreathing had no apparent effect on disappearance of symptoms. The experimenters concluded that the significant factor was not change in CO_2, but expectation and belief that rebreathing CO_2 would terminate the hyperventilation-related sensations.

Medical risk

Another study not involving deception was done by Michael Callaham (1989, 1997). After describing several cases of deaths associated with using a paper bag to terminate what seemed to be hyperventilation, the author describes not only the CO_2 recovery with rebreathing into a paper bag, but also the drastic drop in Pao_2. Air in a paper bag rapidly becomes depleted of oxygen when breathed and rebreathed. (The bags used were 2.25 liters, larger than a standard lunch bag.) Normal values of arterial Pao_2 are 80–100 mmHg, with 100 being more desirable. There was considerable variation among the subjects in oxygen loss, but the mean maximal drop was 26 mmHg. In a person with normal oxygenation, a drop of that magnitude would still be in the low-normal range where hemoglobin saturation is high enough to prevent significant hypoxia. However, if oxygenation is compromised due to pulmonary disease or cardiac insuffiency, the starting level of oxygen will be lower, and the bag rebreathing would plunge the person's PaO_2 into the range where cardiac arrhythmia and unconsciousness are likely.

⚠ Thus there is danger in using the paper bag rebreathing method when an individual's oxygen saturation and oxygenation status are not known. The technique causes rapid deprivation of oxygen, while raising the CO_2 only moderately. Callaham describes several cases in which death followed the paper bag maneuver, recommended in the erroneous belief that symptoms were due to anxiety-based hyperventilation. One death resulted from a pulmonary embolism, another from myocardial infarction, and another from emphysema. Sometimes the paper bag recommendation is given by phone, where no auxiliary tests are possible. Emergency personnel may assume that symptoms of peripheral tingling, breathlessness, weakness, and chest tightness represent hyperventilation and advise the paper bag remedy. However, these sensations can also represent dire emergencies which are worsened by reducing one's oxygenation.

These medical risks should be measured against the apparent illusory nature of the paper bag remedy for panic symptoms. It is probably most dangerous when the subject's medical history is not known, but new conditions can appear at any time. Callaham suggests that since the reassuring presence and advice of a health professional is the most important treatment for acute hyperventilation, having the person breathe into cupped hands combines the same placebo effect with greater safety, since it does not limit oxygen or elevate CO_2 at all.

These tests were done with subjects holding the paper bag tightly sealed against the face. Even small gaps and leaks moderate the effect on O_2 and CO_2. Many clinicians who recommend the paper bag technique, realizing the rapid loss of oxygen that occurs, advise that a gap be left between the bag and the face. Holding the bag loosely allows a flow of fresh air, which reduces the danger. Still,

Callaham concludes: 'Bag rebreathing may alleviate the anxiety, but increases the risk of hypoxemia and its complications. [It] is a potentially very risky procedure in a small subgroup of patients, and should never be instituted unless myocardial ischemia can be ruled out and the patient's oxygenation is known by measurement of arterial blood gases or through pulse oximetry' (p. 628).

SLEEP APNEAS

Sleep apnea is defined as cessation of breathing for at least 10 seconds during sleep. This may happen up to 300–400 times per night, and is often accompanied by thunderous snoring. Soft tissues in the upper airways relax during rapid eye movement (REM) sleep to levels below those experienced during waking hours. As the airway becomes blocked, huge increases in upper airways resistances occur. The inspiratory muscles respond by contracting more forcefully, causing increased negative intrathoracic pressures to try and unblock the airways. Breathing stops, carbon dioxide levels rise, while oxygen levels drop. (Oxygen saturations may drop as low as 75%): 'This is analogous to breathing through a wet soda straw. As you pull air through the straw it actually closes more tightly' (Downey & Perkin 2000, p. 408). As a consequence, the patient rouses to a lighter sleep level or may wake briefly, muscle tone returns to the upper airways and normal breathing is reestablished – until the next deep sleep phase.

Sufferers typically wake unrefreshed, with headaches due to hypercapnia and hypoxia, and are prone to daytime sleepiness and poor concentration, with sometimes disastrous results (e.g. falling asleep at the wheel).

Women suffer this disorder less than men, possibly because of the protective action of progesterone, which acts as a respiratory drive, and less tendency to fat deposition round the neck area. Of those with sleep apnea, 10% have chronic obstructive airways disease (COAD), sometimes referred to as the 'overlap syndrome.' The condition is made worse by smoking and high alcohol intake (Hough 1996, p. 83).

Obstructive sleep apnea (OSA) is the commonest form of apnea and is usually associated with obesity. Patients of normal body weight who have abnormal craniofacial configurations may also be at risk from, for instance, a small or recessed chin, with narrowed upper airway spaces. The adverse consequences of OSA are listed in Box 9.2 and the common clinical features are listed in Box 9.3.

Restrictive sleep apneas may occur in people who have preexisting musculoskeletal breathing impairment. Disorders such as diaphragmatic paralysis, ankylosing spondylitis, or severe scoliosis or kyphoscoliosis reduce respiratory reserves and so, during the normal inhibition of accessory muscles during REM sleep, breathing stops.

Central sleep apneas with the loss of normal respiratory drive and rhythmicity are caused by abnormalities in the central nervous system's breathing control centers. With the absence of behavioral control of breathing during sleep, it is thought both hypoxic and hypercapnic responses are depressed. Patients with central sleep apnea seldom complain of daytime sleepiness, but commonly report experiencing insomnia. Pure central sleep apnea is rare. Often patients have components of both central and obstructive disturbances.

Sleep disordered breathing. Infants and children may suffer sleep disordered breathing from, for instance, chronic nasal obstruction, enlarged tonsils and/or adenoids, obesity, or craniofacial anomalies. As with adults, snoring is the defining symptom of OSA in the young. If untreated, OSA in children can have adverse effects on their schooling in particular and behavior in general.

Sudden infant death syndrome (SIDS) is the leading cause of death in infants under the age of 1 year. *Apparent life threatening events* (ALTEs) is the term used for skin colour and muscle tone changes where the baby appears to be dying. The exact relationship between SIDS and ALTEs is not known, but there is a suggestion that OAS may be a risk factor in both. The worldwide Back to Sleep campaign's recommendation to put infants down to sleep supine has substantially reduced SIDS by 15–20% (American Academy of Pediatrics 1996).

Assessment of sleep-related breathing problems

Pulse oximetry is often required as a precursor to further laboratory studies. An oximeter with a paper strip recorder is used to monitor oxygen saturations overnight, while the patient sleeps. This can be done at home, using a portable oximeter. A pattern of sharp drops in SpO2 levels, followed by sharp increases, is indicative of sleep related breathing problems. These are further investigated by a polysomnograph (PSG), performed in a laboratory setting. This requires an overnight stay in a sleep study unit, attached to various electrodes which monitor chest, abdominal, and eye movements during sleep, a chin electromyograph to detect muscle tension changes, and an electroencephalograph to monitor brain wave pattern variations. Diagnosis is made from the findings.

Treatment and management of OSA

The first steps in treatment are behavioral. First by weight loss, cessation of smoking, alcohol consumption and use of sedatives or hypnotics, and

---

Box 9.2 Obstructive sleep apnea: adverse consequences (From Scanlan et al 1999 with permission)

Cardiopulmonary
Nocturnal dysrhythmias
Diurnal hypertension
Pulmonary hypertension
Right or left ventricular failure
Myocardial infarction
Stroke

Neurobehavioral
Excessive daytime sleepiness
Diminished quality of life
Adverse personality change
Motor vehicle accidents

Box 9.3 OSA: Common clinical features (From Scanlan et al 1999 with permission)

Male
Age over 40 years
Upper body obesity (neck > 16.5 inches)
Habitual snoring
Complaint of fatigue or daytime sleepiness
Diurnal hypertension

avoidance of sleeping in supine. The 'tennis ball technique' where a ball is stitched into the back of the patient's nightwear at shoulder-blade level sometimes helps. Discussion about the risk factors of untreated OSA is important and may help with motivation and compliance (see Box 9.2 above). Patients from all groups must create their own tactics to prevent falling asleep while driving.

Continuous positive airway pressure (CPAP) therapy is at present the front-line medical therapy in the treatment of OSA. Pressure via a nasal mask pneumatically splints open the upper airways, preventing collapse and allowing normalized sleep patterns. Reversal of OSA related problems such as impotence, pulmonary hypertension and right heart failure, daytime sleepiness and lethargy are some of the benefits of CPAP. It may act as a catalyst to weight loss, which in turn could lead to discontinuation of CPAP (Bradley 1993).

Surgical interventions include removal of the uvula and part of the soft palate (uvulopalatopharyngoplasty or UPPP) by laser-assisted surgery. It has a success rate of less than 50% in eliminating OSA but may alleviate snoring. It is not currently being recommended as treatment for OSA (Egan 1999, p. 565).

OSA patients are sometimes referred for breathing retraining as they may have developed secondary hyperventilation problems due to fatigue. Restoration of nose/diaphragm breathing by day to prevent the added distressing signs and symptoms of HVS/BPDs is an important part of patient education/behavioral training.

STAGE FRIGHT

Arcier (2000) looks at the phenomenon of stage fright, but fails to highlight hyperventilation as a likely part of the etiology, although 'rapid breathing' is listed as one among many symptoms. Others include: 'quickening and pounding of the heart beat, dry mouth … shaking, fast breathing, sweat, a lump in the throat, digestive trouble, stomachache, muscular tension and concentration loss.' Arcier reports that a study involving over 2000 professional musicians from four orchestras showed that 24% considered stage fright a health problem, with 16% considering it to be a 'serious health problem':

- Of the 2000 musicians, 19% of females, and 14% of males reported stage fright
- The most prevalent age group reporting stage fright was between 35 and 45 years of age
- Wind instrument players were the group most involved (22% of those reporting stage fright).

The specific connection between stage fright and hyperventilation was examined by Suzanne Widmer and colleagues (Widmer et al 1997). Though no breathing or blood samples were obtained, the Nijmegen questionnaire was given to 141 musicians, along with an assessment of their general anxiety (Spielberger State-Trait Anxiety Inventory) and a measure of their experienced performance anxiety. The Nijmegen questionnaire is the most accepted symptom-list measure of hyperventilation, and it was correlated 0.71 with a combined score from the two anxiety measures.

For further analysis the authors divided subjects into three levels based on reported anxiety. The amount of hyperventilation-related symptoms more than doubled for performance-related situations from the lowest to the highest anxiety level. This makes it likely that the anxiety experienced had at least a component of hyperventilation; many of the Nijmegen questionnaire's items can be explained by cerebral hypoxia and reduced CO_2. Females were much more common than males in the high-anxiety group; when the Nijmegen/anxiety correlations were done separately based on gender, they were 0.78 for women and 0.52 for men. Overall, around 30% of all musicians reported reaching crucial levels of hyperventilation during performances.

The authors encouraged consideration of the hyperventilation factor within the wider context of performance anxiety, which might include general trait anxiety, perfectionism, and other personality factors, inadequate preparation and technique, and memories of previous episodes of performance anxiety. The fact that musical performers are using their bodies in very precise ways makes stability of the physiological substrate very important. Muscle control, nervous system integrity, perceptual accuracy, memory, and cognition can all be affected by lowered $P\text{CO}_2$ and shifts in the acid-base balance.

TRADITIONAL CHINESE MEDICINE AND RESPIRATORY DYSFUNCTION

Disorders of breathing rhythm are treated in Traditional Chinese Medicine (TCM) by a combination of herbal medicine, manual therapy, and acupuncture. In order fully to understand the language of TCM, acceptance is required of the use of what may appear at times to be 'quaint' – and sometimes meaningless – terms are used. However, these terms have very real meanings within the TCM model, and can often be translated into expressions which equate with Western physiology. For example, in discussing dyspnea, the terms 'heart Qi, blood Yin (or Yang) deficiencies' may be translated as a 'congestive heart condition' in Western terminology. Similarly the extreme shortness of breath noted in pneumonia might be described in TCM as 'Internal deficiency, attributable to Lung Qi and Yin deficiency' while the phrase 'the lungs descending function' may refer to coughing (Ryan & Shattuck 1994).

Herbal approaches

TCM includes a wide range of herbal medications, commonly used in complex formulations involving combinations of a dozen or more substances. Chinese herbal compounds usually include a principal herb, combined with another single herb which strongly assists the principal herb or which has a secondary function. These two are assisted in their function by a number of other herbs which act synergistically with the first two or which modify their actions. Finally other 'messenger' herbs are added to the formulation to ensure appropriate delivery and use of the compound.

⚠ It is worth cautioning that some of the herbs commonly used in TCM have been found to have high (plant) steroid levels or to contain plant alkaloids which are considered potentially dangerous either on their own or in combination with prescribed medications (Werbach & Murray

1996). For example Ma Huang is a frequent ingredient of TCM herbal combinations, especially those targeting treatment of the common cold, asthma, hay fever, bronchitis, edema, arthritis, fever, hypotension, and hives. It is also used in 'weight loss' formulations. This formulation contains *Ephedra sinica*, which is banned from over the counter sale in the UK and the USA.

The meaning of 'Qi'

The word 'Qi' which is usually translated into English as 'vital energy' actually has a wider meaning in TCM: 'TCM asserts that the body is possessed of Qi, which is at once its energy, life force, and material substance. Qi regulates bodily function and simultaneously *is* the body's activity as well as the material structures associated with it.' Early translations of the word Qi include: 'that which fills the body', 'that which means life,' 'breath,' 'vapours,' and 'wind' (Ryan & Shattuck 1994).

The meaning of 'Lung'

Where breathing is concerned it may be useful to compare the meaning of the word 'Lung' in TCM with the meaning of the word, as understood in Western anatomy/physiology, in order to see what there is in common:

The Chinese Lung and the Western lung share some similarity. They both relate to the intake of air and include some of the same physical structures. But the Chinese concept takes the physical organ as only one component of a larger functional group which includes the processes of extracting Qi from the environment in the form of air, circulating Qi along with fluids, and [offering] overall body protection. The Lung, then, is involved with fluid metabolism and transportation in the Chinese concept. It moves fluids down to the Kidney and around the body, especially the skin and pores. The relationship to the skin includes the body hair and sweat glands, and the secretion of sweat. Finally the Lung is related to protection from 'External Invasion' [seen in TCM to include both infection and climatic influences] … and is associated with the emotion of sadness or grieving. (Ryan & Shattuck 1994)

Although there is no direct reference to the exchange of gases in TCM's understanding of

Lung function, it is not difficult to see the similarities between Western thinking and TCM's concepts as to what the lung (Lung) does, ranging from a defensive role in immune function to pumping actions as it 'moves fluids around the body,' as well as in a relationship between breathing and emotions.

Assessment

In assessing the background to breathing (and other) disorders, TCM practitioners evaluate the status of the patient using a variety of differentiating approaches, including the patient's obvious presenting signs and symptoms, as well as tongue diagnosis (in which the color and state of the tongue is noted in order to evaluate the patient's current pathophysiological status, for example using descriptors for the appearance of the tongue such as 'pale,' 'fat,' 'moist,' 'dry,' 'yellow,' etc., etc.); and pulse diagnosis which involves palpating three different positions of the wrist pulse, each taken at three depths (in which what is palpated is described using words such as 'wiry,' 'rapid,' 'empty,' 'thin,' 'superficial,' 'thready,' 'bounding,' or any of a host of other words, each considered to have a particular significance in terms of energy balance relative to particular organs and functions).

Acupuncture points relative to respiratory dysfunction

Several points which are regularly used in acupuncture (and acupressure) relate directly to symptoms which are linked to altered breathing function. For example:

- *Lung 1* which is found in the first intercostal space, slightly lateral to the mamillary line. According to Austin (1974), this point is used to treat dyspnea, and as a general point for 'pulmonary affections.' Mann (1963) supports use of Lung 1 for dyspnea as well as for 'fullness of chest, oppression, pneumonia and pleurisy.'
- *Lung 10* (on the palmar surface of the hand just below the head of the first metacarpal) is used to treat anxiety as well as dyspnea.

- For rhinitis/sinusitis GB (Gall bladder) 20, 14, and Yintang (special point midway between eyebrows) (R. Newman Turner DO BAc, personal communication, 2001).
- Also for rhinitis/sinusitis Li (Large intestine) 20 and Li 19, points on the lateral external crease of the nasal alae and Li 4 (HoKu) on the dorsum of the hand in the interosseous muscle between the thumb and index finger (Chari 1988).

These points are also useful acupressure points.

Chinese bodywork (Tui-na)

Tui-na forms that branch of TCM which has as its Western equivalent physical/orthopedic medicine. McCarthy (1998) states, 'Tuina is, in the main, a physical therapy but it also uses traditional Chinese "bioenergetic" principles in its application.' The objectives of Tui-na as practiced in the West are (McCarthy 1998):

- The promotion of Qi movement in the channels
- Mobilization of joints to improve articulation
- Optimization of fluid flow (blood and lymph) through the microcirculatory system
- Release of muscle cramp or spasm to help reintegrate structure
- Tonification of muscular tissue in prolapse to recover function.

The techniques used have some similarities as well as considerable differences compared with Western manual approaches, and include soft tissue rolling, rubbing, tapping, 'sweeping,' grasping, chopping and 'scrubbing' methods (Figs 9.1–9.3). Tui-na joint mobilization closely resembles osteopathic methodology.

Example of TCM bodywork application to breathing related disorder

Chengnan (1993) describes the application of Chinese bodywork in a case of syncope. The TCM etiology in the case of fainting is described (in part) as follows: 'Harassment and covering of *Clear Apertures* by adverse uprising of *Vital*

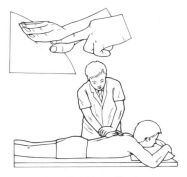

Rou Fa (Kneading)

Figure 9.1 Vibration and kneading with palm on trapezius, superior and inferior aspect of serratus posterior, erector spinae and lumbo-sacral areas. (Reproduced with kind permission from McCarthy 1998.)

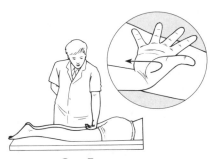

Gun Fa
(Rolling technique)

Figure 9.2 Rolling technique to trapezius, mid-thoracic, lumbar, gluteal and posterior aspect of the lower limb areas. (Reproduced with kind permission from McCarthy 1998.)

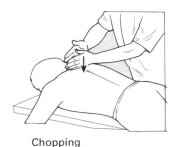

Chopping

Figure 9.3 Light chopping with both hands on trapezius and mid-thoracic areas. (Reproduced with kind permission from McCarthy 1998.)

Energy due to indignation of fright; failure of *Clear Yang* to ascend due to the sinking of *Spleen-Stomach* energy; obstruction of *Clear Apertures* by the rushing up of *Blood* during violent anger; collapse of *Vital Energy* from loss of blood; *Dampness-Phlegm* cover *Clear Apertures* ...' As in the discussion (above) as to the 'meaning' of Lung, in TCM, it is clear that the words used (spleen, stomach, blood, etc.) have different meanings in the context of the TCM model.

Chengnan discusses the signs, symptoms, and therapeutic principles before describing Tui-na approaches to syncope when it is due to 'excess of vital energy'. 'First aid – open passes and dredge apertures. After resuscitation, push the chest with the thenar mound, relieve the chest with dotting [tapping] and vibrating, push and wipe to divide the ribs, scratch the back, rectify limbs and fingers.'

Clarification

The fact that only acupuncture, manual, and herbal methods have been discussed in this segment should not be taken to suggest that these are the only methods used in TCM which also incorporates dietary therapy, tai chi and Qigong (which incorporates exercise, relaxation, breath and balance training, as well as 'energy' work).

YOGA THERAPY AND BREATHING

Yoga therapy represents the merging of traditional yoga practices and modern medical methods (Monro 1997). Yoga therapy employs a graded set of asanas (postures) and pranayama practices (breathing exercises). The effects are claimed to include:

- relaxation, strengthening and balancing of muscles
- mobilization of joints
- improvements of posture
- reflex influences
- improvement in breathing function, calming of the nervous system, promotion of homeostatic influences on digestive, cardiovascular, endocrine and other systems.

Research evidence to validate the claims of either yoga therapy or traditional yoga methods is scanty; however, some verification exists:

• In a study by Nagarathna & Nagendra (1985), 106 individuals with asthma were divided into a treatment and control group, matched for age, sex, and severity of the condition. There were significantly greater improvements in the yoga group in weekly number of asthmatic attacks and in scores for drug usage as well as peak flow rates, which were still evident at 4-year follow-up.

• Cappo & Holmes (1984) used a pranayama breathing pattern (inhale quickly/exhale slowly) in their study, which compared the effects on arousal of that pattern with patterns of slow inhalation/rapid exhalation, as well as inhalation and exhalation at the same rate, and also with control groups (distraction control, and no treatment control). All three breathing pattern groups reduced their overall rate to six cycles per minute for a period of 5 minutes during the evaluations. The results showed that 'inhaling quickly and exhaling slowly [the pranayama pattern] was consistently effective for reducing physiological (skin resistance) and psychological (subjective cognitive arousal) during anticipation and confrontation periods.'

• This result is consistent with yoga teaching about the value of slow exhalation. Van Lysebeth (1971) points out: 'Every other point in the breathing cycle involves muscle tension; so absolute relaxation can occur only when the exhale is complete.' The point of equilibrium, the rest point between exhale and inhale, is a moment when the breathing apparatus is motionless. Cutting short the end of the exhale means that the exhale is incomplete and that the breathing muscles never quite relax between breaths. This may result in retention of more 'used' air than normal, and also can promote chronic hyperinflation and hypertonic neck and shoulder muscles.

• A study of patients with congestive heart failure attempted to produce improvements by teaching the yoga 'complete breath.' This is a 3-stage breath that fills, in sequence, the abdomen, lower chest and upper chest, then reverses the order with the exhale. Breathing this way produces a natural breathing rate of about six breaths per minute. The chronic heart conditions led to subnormal O_2 saturation, limited exercise tolerance, and dyspnea; these all improved significantly with continued practice of the yoga breathing, and sensations of dyspnea diminished. By improving the ventilation-perfusion ratios as well as alveolar ventilation, this style of breathing optimized breathing and made the most of available function. Respiratory efficiency improved and irregularity was reduced (instability in O_2 saturation was associated with instability in breathing frequency and amplitude). The 'spontaneous' breathing rate (the rate at which subjects breathed when they thought they were unobserved) dropped from 13 to less than 8 (Bernardi et al 1993).

The heart and lungs operate in many ways as a cardiorespiratory unit. Breathing and heart action are closely related, and their synchronization stabilizes the autonomic nervous system (see Ch. 8).

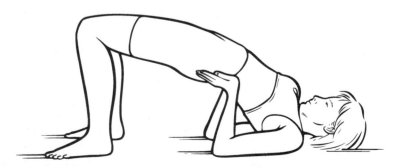

Figure 9.4 Bridge: promotes diaphragmatic breathing. (Reproduced with kind permission from Monro 1997.)

Yoga breathing emphasizes full use of the diaphragm in breathing (Fig. 9.4). The diaphragm is attached by fascia to the heart's pericardium in such a way that diaphragmatic movement provides a massaging action to the heart. Also, the vena cava, which carries freshly oxygenated blood from the lungs to the heart, passes through the diaphragm and is alternately squeezed and released during breathing. This action promotes a periodic acceleration of blood flow toward the heart. As Andrew Thomas (1993) states: 'The fully and correctly operating diaphragm is thus a second heart.'

Yogic alternate nostril breathing
(Box 9.4; Fig. 9.5)

In health one nostril is more dominant than the other at any given time in terms of the volume of

---

Box 9.4 Alternate-nostril breathing

1. In a sitting position, hold one hand at the nose so that each nostril can be closed by pressing on its side with the thumb or the ring finger. Fold the index and middle fingers down
2. Block the left nostril and breathe in through the right nostril
3. Block the right nostril and exhale through the left nostril
4. Keep the right nostril blocked and inhale through the left nostril
5. Block the left nostril and inhale through the right nostril
6. Repeat the sequence 15–20 times. Try to make the exhale last twice as long as the inhale

---

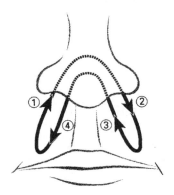

Figure 9.5 Alternate nostril breathing. The air stream is directed alternately through each nostril by gently occluding the opposite nostril. This is thought to harmonize the two hemispheres of the brain, creating a balance between sympathetic and parasympathetic dominance. (Reproduced with kind permission from Gilbert 1999.)

air flow. There is an alternation every $1\frac{1}{2}$ to 3 hours throughout the 24-hour cycle, with one nostril being more open than the other (Gilbert 1999). Evidence suggests that whichever nostril is more open, the opposite hemisphere of the brain is slightly more active, and in yoga this is utilized to enhance different activities related to particular hemispheric functions. These traditional yogic intuitions and observations have been confirmed by modern research in which EEG readings from the brain have been found to correlate with increased hemispheric activity with the currently dominant nostril (Rossi 1991, Shannahoff-Khalsa 1991, Block et al 1989). Some yoga breathing exercises alternate between the two nostrils, breath by breath, with the intent of regulating the balance between the two hemispheres. This is thought to promote proper alternation between sympathetic and parasympathetic nervous system functions.

REFERENCES

American Academy of Paediatrics 1996
American Pharmaceutical Association 1986 Handbook of nonprescription drugs, 8th edn. American Pharmaceutical Association, Washington DC, p 183
Arcier A-F 2000 Stage fright. In: Tubiana R, Amadio O (eds) Medical problems of the instrumentalist musician. Martin Dunitz, London
Austin M 1974 Acupuncture therapy. Turnstone Books, London

Bass C, Chambers J B, Gardner W N 1991 Hyperventilation provocation in patients with chest pain and a negative treadmill exercise test. Journal of Psychosomatic Research 35: 83–85.
Bernardi L, Spadacini G, Bellwon J, Hajric R, Roskamm H, Frey A W 1998 Effect of breathing rate on oxygen saturation and exercise performance in chronic heart failure. Lancet 351(9112): 1308(4)

Block E, Arnott D, Quigley B, Lynch W 1989 Unilateral nostril breathing influences literalized cognitive performance. Brain and Cognition 9(2): 181–190

Bowler S, Green A, Mitchell C 1998 Buteyko breathing techniques in asthma: a blinded randomised controlled trial. Medical Journal of Australia 169: 575–578

Bradley T D 1993 Unexpected presentations of sleep apnoea. British Medical Journal 306: 1260–1262

Brandfonbrener A 2000 Epidemiology and risk factors. In: Tubiana R, Amadio O (eds) Medical problems of the instrumentalist musician. Martin Dunitz, London

Buteyko K 1991 Buteyko Method: the experience of the implementation in medical practice. Titul, Odessa (in Russian)

Buteyko alternative approach manual 1996

Caine M P, McConnell A K 1998 The inspiratory muscles can be trained differentially to increase strength or endurance using a pressure threshold inspiratory muscle training device. European Respiratory Journal: abstract PO455

Callaham M 1989 Hypoxic hazards of traditional paper bag rebreathing in hyperventilating patients. Annals of Emergency Medicine 18(6)(June)

Callaham M 1997 Panic disorders, hyperventilation, and the dreaded brown paper bag (letter). Annals of Emergency Medicine 30 (6) (December): 838

Cappo B, Holmes D 1984 Utility of prolonged respiratory exhalation for reducing physiological and psychological arousal in non-threatening and threatening situations. Journal of Psychosomatic Research 28(4): 265–273

Chambers J B, Kiff P J, Gardner W N, Jackson G, Bass C 1988 Value of measuring end-tidal partial pressure of carbon dioxide as an adjunct to treadmill exercise testing. British Medical Journal 296: 1281–1285

Chari P 1988 Acupuncture therapy in allergic rhinitis. American Journal of Acupuncture 16 (2)

Chengnan Sun 1993 Chinese bodywork. Pacific View Press, Berkeley, CA

Downey R, Perkin R 2000 Assessment of sleep and breathing. In: Wilkins K S (ed) Clinical assessment in respiratory care, 4th edn. Mosby, St Louis

Edelstein D R 1996 Aging of the normal nose in adults. Laryngoscope 106 (September): 1–25

Egan D 1999 Fundamentals of respiratory care. Mosby, St Louis

Folweiler D, Lynch O 1995 Journal of Manipulative and Physiological Therapeutics 18: 38–42

Gilbert C 1999 Yoga and breathing. Journal of Bodywork and Movement Therapies 3(1): 44–54

Hammo-A, Weinberger-MM 1999 Exercise-induced hyperventilation: a pseudoasthma syndrome. Annals-of-Allergy-Asthma-and-Immunology 1999 Jun; 82(6): 574–8 (18 ref)

Hough A 1996 Physiotherapy in respiratory care. Stanley Thornes, Cheltenham

Howell J B 1990 Behavioural breathlessness. Thorax 45: 287–292

McCarthy M 1998 Fibromyalgia: a Chinese Medicine view. Journal of Bodywork and Movement Therapies 2(4): 203–207

Mann F 1963 The treatment of disease by acupuncture. Heinemann Medical, London

Monro R 1997 Yoga therapy. Journal of Bodywork and Movement Therapies 1(4): 215–218

Myers T 2001 Some thoughts on intra-nasal work. Journal of Bodywork and Movement Therapies 5(2)

Nagarathna R, Nagendra H 1985 Yoga for bronchial asthma – a controlled study. British Medical Journal 291: 172–174

Odom T W, Harrison P C, Darre M J 1985 The effects of drinking carbonated water on the egg shell quality of single comb white leghorn hens exposed to high environmental temperature. Poultry Science 64: 594–596

Rolf I 1976 Rolfing. Dennis Landman, San Francisco

Rossi E 1991 The twenty-minute break: using the new science of ultradian rhythms. Jeremy Tarcher, New York

Ryan M K, Shattuck A 1994 Treating AIDS with Chinese Medicine. Pacific View Press, Berkeley, CA

Shannahoff-Khalsa D 1991 Lateralised rhythms of the central and autonomic nervous system. International Journal of Psychophysiology 11(3): 222–251

Thomas A P 1993 Yoga and cardiovascular function. Journal of the International Association of Yoga Therapists 4: 39–41

Scanlan C L, Wilkins R L, Stoller J K 1999 Egans fundamentals of respiratory care. Mosby, St Louis

Tinkelman D 1977 Ephedrine therapy in asthmatic children. Journal of the American Medical Association 237: 553–557

van den Hout M A, Boek C, van der Molen G M, Jansen A, Griez E 1988 Rebreathing to cope with hyperventilation: experimental tests of the paper bag method. Journal of Behavioral Medicine 11 (3): 303–310

Van Lysebeth A 1971 Yoga self-taught. Harper and Row, New York, p 32

Werbach M, Murray M 1996 Botanical influences on illness. Third Line Press, Tarzana, California

Widmer S, Conway A, Cohen S, Davies P 1997 Hyperventilation: a correlate and predictor of debilitating performance anxiety in musicians. Medical Problems of Performing Artists 12(4): 97–106

10

Self-help approaches

Leon Chaitow, Dinah Bradley &
Christopher Gilbert

INTRODUCTION

In the end, the degree of effort an individual puts into his or her own rehabilitation towards more normal breathing patterns will determine the outcome. Breathing retraining has to be self-applied; it cannot be 'done' to the patient. If patient compliance is to be achieved, self-help strategies – whether involving lifestyle and dietary modification (if appropriate), relaxation, postural and breathing methods, or methods aimed at releasing tense tight muscles – need to be understandable, safe and easy to perform. The methods listed in this chapter conform to these needs. Some derive from well-researched methods (antiarousal breathing and autogenic training, for example) while others have proved themselves in practice to the satisfaction of one or more of the authors. Although there are many other methods, those presented in this chapter represent a selection that are commended; they may be reproduced free of copyright for individual patient use.

REDUCING SHOULDER MOVEMENT DURING BREATHING

Stand in front of a mirror and breathe, and notice whether your shoulders rise. If so, there is a strategy you can use to reduce this tendency.

Before starting one of the breathing exercises outlined in this chapter, sit in a chair with arms and place your elbows and forearms fully supported by the chair arms (Fig. 10.1). Slowly exhale through pursed lips, and then, as you inhale through your nose, push gently down onto the chair arms to 'lock' the shoulder muscles, preventing them from rising. As you exhale release the downward pressure. Repeat throughout the exercise.

As a substitute for the strategy described above, especially if there is no armchair available, sit with your hands interlocked, palms upward, on your lap.

As you inhale, lightly but firmly push the pads of your fingers against the backs of the hands, and release this pressure when you slowly exhale. This reduces the ability of the muscles above the shoulders to contract, and will lessen the tendency for the shoulders to rise.

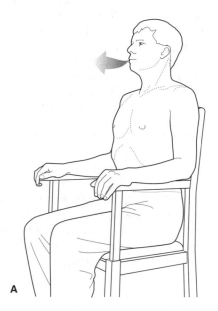
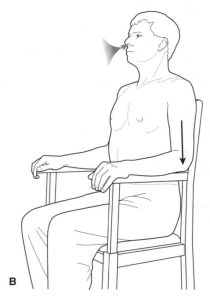
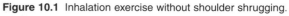

Figure 10.1 Inhalation exercise without shoulder shrugging.

ANTI-AROUSAL BREATHING EXERCISE

Place yourself in a comfortable (ideally seated/reclining) position, exhale FULLY through your partially open mouth, lips just barely separated. This outbreath should be slowly performed. Imagine that a candle flame is about 6 inches from your mouth and exhale (blowing a thin stream of air) in such a way as to not blow the candle out.

As you exhale, count silently to yourself to establish the length of the outbreath. An effective method for counting one second at a time is to say (silently) 'one hundred, two hundred, three hundred, etc.' Each count then lasts about one second.

When you have exhaled fully, *without causing any sense of strain* to yourself in any way, allow the inhalation which follows to be full, free, and uncontrolled. The complete exhalation which preceded the inhalation will have created a 'coiled spring' which you do not have to control in order to inhale. Once again, count to yourself to establish how long your inbreath lasts. The counting is necessary because the timing of the inhalation and exhalation phase of breathing is a major feature of this exercise.

Without pausing to hold the breath, exhale FULLY, through the mouth, blowing the air in a thin stream (again you should count to yourself at the same speed). Continue to repeat the inhalation and the exhalation for not less than 30 cycles of in and out.

The objective is that in time (some weeks of practicing this daily) you should, without strain, achieve an inhalation phase which lasts for 2–3 seconds while the exhalation phase lasts from 6–7 seconds. Most importantly, the exhalation should be slow and continuous. It is no use breathing the air out in 2 seconds and then simply waiting until the count reaches 6, 7, or 8 before inhaling again.

By the time you have completed 15 or so cycles, any sense of anxiety which you previously felt should be much reduced. Also, if pain is a problem this should also have lessened.

Apart from ALWAYS practicing this once or twice daily, it is useful to repeat the exercise for a few minutes (about five cycles of inhalation/exhalation takes a minute) every hour if you are anxious or whenever stress seems to be increasing. At the very least it should be practiced on waking, and before bedtime, and if at all possible before meals.

© Harcourt Publishers Ltd 2002   Chaitow L, Bradley D, Gilbert C *Multidisciplinary Approaches to Breathing Pattern Disorders*. Churchill Livingstone, Edinburgh

AUTOGENIC TRAINING RELAXATION

Relaxation exercises focus on the body and its responses to stress, trying to reverse these, while meditation tries to bring about a calming of the mind and through this a relaxation response.

Autogenic training (AT) is a form of exercise which combines the best of both relaxation and meditation. The modified AT exercise described below offers a way of achieving effective relaxation:

Exercise for effective relaxation

Every day, at least once, for 10 minutes at a time, do the following:

- Lie on the floor or bed in a comfortable position, small cushion under the head, knees bent if that makes the back feel easier, eyes closed.
- Practise the anti-arousal breathing exercise (or some other relaxing breathing exercise) for a few minutes before you start the AT exercise.
- Focus attention on your dominant (say right) hand/arm and silently say to yourself 'My right arm (or hand) feels heavy.'
- Try to sense the arm relaxed and heavy, its weight sinking into the surface it rests on. Feel its weight. Over a period of about a minute repeat the affirmation ('My arm/hand feels heavy') several times and try to stay focused on its weight and heaviness.
- You will almost certainly lose focus as your mind wanders from time to time. This is part of the training in the exercise – to stay focused, so don't be upset, just go back to the arm and its heaviness which you may or may not be able to sense.
- If it does feel heavy, stay with it and enjoy the sense of release – of letting go – that comes with it.
- Next, focus on your other hand/arm and you do exactly the same thing for about a minute.
- Move to the left leg and then the right leg, for about a minute each, with the same messages and focused attention on each.
- Go back to your right hand/arm and this time affirm a message which tells you that you

sense a greater degree of warmth there – 'My hand is feeling warm (or hot).'
- After a minute or so, go to the left hand/arm, then the left leg and then finally the right leg, each time with the 'warming' message and focused attention. If warmth is sensed, stay with it for a while and feel it spread. Enjoy it.
- Finally focus on your forehead and affirm that it feels cool and refreshed. Hold this cool and calm thought for a minute before completing the exercise. Finish by clenching your fists, bending your elbows and stretching out your arms. The exercise is complete.

By repeating the whole exercise at least once a day you will gradually find you can stay focused on each region and sensation.

Explanation

'Heaviness' represents what you feel when muscles relax and 'warmth' is what you feel when your circulation to an area is increased, while 'coolness' is the opposite, a reduction in circulation for a short while – usually followed by an increase due to the overall relaxation of the muscles.

Measurable changes occur in circulation and temperature in the regions being focused on during these training sessions. Success requires persistence – daily use for at least 6 weeks – before benefits are noticed, usually a sense of relaxation and better sleep.

How to use these skills for health enhancement by visualizing change

- If there is pain or discomfort related to muscle tension, AT training can be used to focus on the area and by getting that area to 'feel' heavy this will reduce tension.
- If there is pain related to poor circulation the 'warmth' instruction can be used to improve it.
- If there is inflammation related to pain this can be reduced by 'thinking' the area 'cool.'

The new skills gained by AT can be used to focus on any area – and most importantly helps to allow you to be able to stay focused – to intro-duce other images, 'seeing' in the mind's eye a stiff joint easing and moving, or a congested swollen area melting back to normality, or any other helpful change which would ease whatever health problem there might be.

⚠ AT trainers strongly urge that you avoid AT focus on vital functions, such as those relating to the heart, or to the breathing pattern in the case of anyone with a breathing disorder, unless a trained instructor is providing guidance and supervision.

Chaitow L, Bradley D, Gilbert C *Multidisciplinary Approaches to Breathing Pattern Disorders*. Churchill Livingstone, Edinburgh

COULD YOU BE HYPERVENTILATING AND NOT KNOW IT?

Most people, even many doctors, have the notion that hyperventilation is always obvious: heaving chest, open mouth, eyes wide with anxiety or excitement. Such a person, though standing still, can appear to be running a race, pushing way too much air through the system. This picture of 'acute' hyperventilation is often associated with panic, but sometimes it goes along with excitement, anger, or frustration. It is dramatic and recognizable, but it is not the only kind. When hyperventilation is more subtle and chronic, it is hard to detect. Hyperventilation (defined simply as breathing too much for the body's needs) can be nearly invisible, and may continue for hours or days. And it can cause plenty of problems (Fig. 10.2).

Blood tests or a chemical analysis of exhaled air, if done at the right time, can help make the diagnosis. Here some clues to raise your suspicion:

- Rapid, irregular breathing (over 16 breaths per minute)
- Primarily mouth breathing

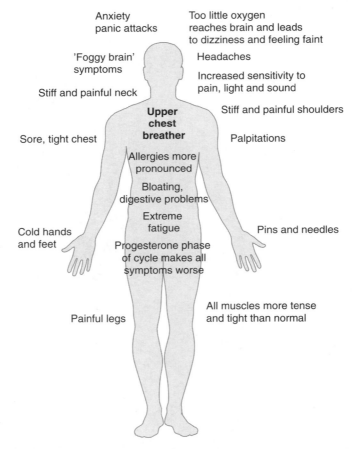

Figure 10.2 The symptoms which result from upper-chest breathing patterns (overbreathing as well as true hyperventilation) are caused by *too much carbon dioxide being breathed out* rather than too little oxygen being breathed in. This breathing pattern is often a habit we have learned from childhood. When we breathe out too much carbon dioxide, the blood becomes too alkaline, and all the symptoms listed in this picture can appear within a few seconds. The tightness in the chest, neck, and shoulder muscles produced by breathing like this, as well as the anxiety caused by the carbon dioxide imbalance, both make the breathing worse. To recover the tight muscles need to be released, and the patient needs to learn how to breathe in a better way.

- Breathing more in the upper chest than the abdomen
- Premature fatigue or exhaustion.

Try hyperventilating for just 12 breaths – fast and deep, both – and you will probably begin to feel dizzy (**do not do it if you have a heart condition**). You may feel your fingers and face tingle, your vision may dim or get spotty, and your whole body may feel different. Muscle weakness, rapid heart beat, sweating, disorientation, and dizziness are common. If brought on intentionally, the symptoms are easily reversed by holding your breath, breathing more slowly, or perhaps breathing into cupped hands.

Now imagine having some of those symptoms without knowing why. Subtle, chronic hyperventilation can result in effects such as those above, but they are hard to diagnose because they resemble many other diseases and conditions. A vague sense of anxiety, 'something not right' with the breathing, chronically cold hands, poor digestion, light-headedness, confusion, exhaustion … Lots of other medical problems can cause these symptoms, and doctors will look for them first before thinking of hyperventilation.

What is happening?

With both chronic and acute hyperventilation the problem is *not* too much oxygen. The bloodstream can only absorb so much of it, and the excess gets breathed right back out again, unchanged. The effects of hyperventilation come from breathing out too much carbon dioxide (CO_2). This gas is the byproduct of metabolism, especially muscle contraction, something like the smoke and ash of simply being alive. It is dumped from the tissues into the bloodstream and excreted by the lungs.

On its way to the lungs, however, CO_2 performs the essential function of maintaining the body's acid-base balance. It is carried in the blood mainly as carbonic acid. If you hold your breath, your blood, your entire body, really, starts to become more acidic. If you breathe more than your body needs, your body begins to turn alkaline. And that interferes with many

physiological functions: the diameter of blood vessels is reduced, for one thing, so it is harder for oxygen to be released into the tissues. The blood is saturated with oxygen from all that breathing but it is not being delivered as readily to the body. This explains the dizziness, tingling, muscle weakness, confusion, etc. – the brain and the nervous system are being short-changed of oxygen. Hyperventilation affects the heart also, causing it to beat faster; at the same time the coronary blood vessels are constricting.

Overbreathing is often developed during a time of unusual stress (Figs 10.3 and 10.4), and becomes a bad habit. It might also reflect chronic anxiety or anger, which stimulates the body to prepare to run or fight. If there is no

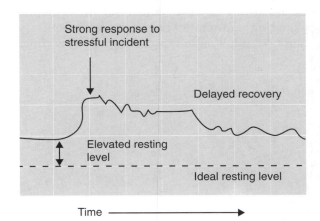

Figure 10.3 Excessive stress response. This general picture of an excessive stress response, with delayed recovery, can apply to any aspect of the body – muscles, breathing, blood pressure, intestines, heart rate – as well as to thoughts and feelings. Excessive stress is often caused by negative emotions which become chronic, run in the background, and begin to dominate a person's daily life in both body and mind.

Examples:

- Resentment, bitterness, hot-tempered, quick to anger
- Reflexive fear of social disapproval, disease, or loss of control
- Time urgency
- Performance pressure
- Guilt over not doing enough

Hypervigilance – perpetual watchfulness for whatever is maintaining the negative emotion – is often associated with these states. As the stress response is magnified and prolonged, it becomes harder and harder to feel calm.

Chaitow L, Bradley D, Gilbert C *Multidisciplinary Approaches to Breathing Pattern Disorders*. Churchill Livingstone, Edinburgh

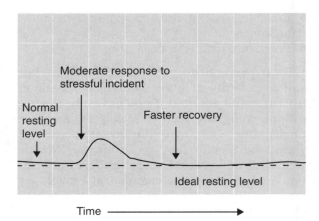

Figure 10.4 Normal stress response. An improved response to stress. This could refer to any function of the body as well as to thoughts and feelings. Note the three components: **1** lower resting level, or baseline; **2** more moderate response; **3** faster smoother recovery. This improvement could be created in a crude way by tranquilizers, or by practice of self-regulation. Biofeedback, hypnosis, progressive relaxation, and meditation are four common procedures for bringing about these changes.

good medical reason for the hyperventilation (and there are some) then reducing the volume of breathing is the cure. But this means changing automatic behavior, because it is hard to think about breathing all the time.

There are good books and audio tapes available for changing one's breathing pattern; for more personalized help, physical therapists and respiratory therapists are usually the ones to see.

 Chaitow L, Bradley D, Gilbert C *Multidisciplinary Approaches to Breathing Pattern Disorders*. Churchill Livingstone, Edinburgh

COMBINED RELAXATION EXERCISE

1. Pause

When you decide it is time to relax, first clear your mind of any thoughts, worries, and problems that do not require action for the next 5–10 minutes. Commit yourself to a time period devoted to reducing tension and restoring your overall balance. Adopt a comfortable position in a private place.

2. Breathing

Observe and begin to regulate your breathing. Check for tightness in your abdomen, shoulders, lower back, throat, and chest. Develop smooth abdominal breathing with a steady, slow rhythm. Breathe with your nose; relax more with each exhale.

3. Muscles

While maintaining this breathing rhythm, scan your body briefly for muscles that are tight or braced. Release these, and then systematically relax each area, letting go more and more. Imagine the joints loosening. Watch for feelings of heaviness and warmth in your arms and legs.

4. Circulation

While maintaining easy breathing and relaxed muscles, attempt to warm your hands from within. Imagine that your circulation is expanding to the most remote regions of your body. If you feel any pressure in your head, imagine the pressure draining downward.

5. Thinking

Look ahead to the next few hours and visualize yourself functioning in a more relaxed and balanced manner. If something is bothering you right now, consider whether you can let it go. Then breathe deeply and try to hold on to the feeling of relaxation as you resume your normal activities.

   Chaitow L, Bradley D, Gilbert C *Multidisciplinary Approaches to Breathing Pattern Disorders*. Churchill Livingstone, Edinburgh

BRUGGER'S RELIEF POSITION
(Fig. 10.5)

This position should be adopted for a few minutes, several times a day, especially if you have to spend much of the day seated, for example at a desk or computer.

- Sit very close ('perch') to the edge of your chair, arms hanging down at your side.
- Place your feet directly below your knees and then move them slightly more apart and turn them slightly outward.
- Roll your pelvis slightly forward to produce a very small degree of arching of your low back.
- Ease your sternum (breastbone) slightly forward and up.
- Turn your arms outward so that the palms face forward.
- Separate your fingers until your thumbs face slightly backward.
- Tuck your chin in gently.
- Maintain this posture while you practice four or five cycles of slow breathing to a pattern such as that outlined under the heading 'anti-arousal breathing' (above).
- Repeat this whenever you sense muscle tension during sitting, or if you feel the need for deeper breathing.
- This 'relief' posture ensures that the chest can be as free and open as possible and reverses many of the stresses caused by long periods of sitting.

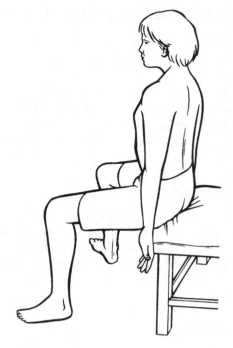

Figure 10.5 The Brugger relief position. (Reproduced with kind permission from C. Liebenson. Motivating pain patients to become more active. Journal of Bodywork and movement Therapies 3(3), July 1999, p. 149)

DIETARY STRATEGIES

Self-help strategies for allergies and food sensitivities

The identification of foods to which we are allergic or intolerant can be difficult. In some cases the culprit is obvious, and we therefore avoid the food, in other cases we may need to undertake detective work in order to identify the foods which are best avoided.

There are various strategies. The first to be described involves a process of exclusion and then challenge.

Exclusion

Make notes of the answers to the following questions:

1. List any foods or drinks that you know disagree with you, or which produce allergic reactions (skin blotches, palpitations, feelings of exhaustion, agitation, or other symptoms).

   NOTES

2. List any food or beverage that you eat or drink at least once a day.

   NOTES

3. List any foods or drink that if you were unable to obtain, would make you feel really deprived.

   NOTES

4. List any food that you sometimes have a definite craving for.

   NOTES

5. What sort of food or drink is it that you use for snacks? List these.

   NOTES

6. Are there foods which you have begun to eat (or drink) more of recently?

   NOTES

7. Read the following list of foods and underline twice any that you eat at least every day, and underline once those that you eat three or more times a week:
   Bread (and other wheat products); milk; potato; tomato; fish; cane sugar or its products; breakfast food; sausages or preserved meat; cheese; coffee; rice; pork; peanuts; corn or its products; margarine; beetroot or beet-sugar; tea; yogurt; soya products; beef; chicken; alcoholic drinks; cake; biscuits; oranges or other citrus fruits; eggs; chocolate; lamb; artificial sweeteners; soft drinks; pasta.

When it comes to testing by 'exclusion' (not eating the food at all for at least 3 weeks) the foods which appear most often on your list (in questions 1 to 6, and the ones underlined twice) are the ones to test first – one by one:

1. Decide which foods on your list are the ones you eat most often (say it happens to be bread). Your strategy is to test the effect of excluding wheat and other grains by leaving them out of your diet for at least 3 weeks (the grains are wheat, barley, rye, oats and millet).
2. You may not feel any benefit from this exclusion (if wheat or other grains have been causing allergic or intolerance reactions) for at least a week, and you may actually feel slightly unwell during that first week (caused by withdrawal symptoms).
3. If after a week your symptoms (whatever they are – fatigue, palpitations, skin reactions, breathing difficulty, muscle or joint ache, feelings of agitation, or whatever) are improving, you should maintain the exclusion for several weeks more, before reintroducing the excluded foods to challenge your body and see whether symptoms return. If the symptoms return after eating the foods for several days, at the same rate as you did before the exclusion period, you will have

© Harcourt Publishers Ltd 2002   Chaitow L, Bradley D, Gilbert C *Multidisciplinary Approaches to Breathing Pattern Disorders*. Churchill Livingstone, Edinburgh

shown that your body is better, for the time being at least, without the food you have identified.

4. Remove this food from your diet (in this case grains – or wheat if that is the only grain you tested) for at least 6 months before testing it again. By then you may have become desensitized to it and be able to tolerate it again.

5. If nothing was proved by the wheat/grain exclusion, similar elimination periods on a diet free of dairy produce, or fish, or citrus, or soya products, etc. can also be attempted – using your questionnaire results to guide you – always choosing the next most frequently listed food (or food family).

This method is often effective. Dairy products, for example, are among the commonest allergens in asthma and hay fever problems. A range of wheat-free and dairy-free foods are now available from health stores which makes such elimination far easier.

Rotation diet

There are other ways of reducing the stress of irritant foods, and one of these involves the use of a rotation diet, in which foods from any particular family of suspect foods (identified by the questionnaire you have completed) are eaten only once in 5 days or so.

This system is effective, especially if a detailed food and symptom diary is kept, in which all deviations from your normal state of health are noted down as are all foods eaten. Symptoms such as feelings of unusual fatigue, or irritability, or difficulty in concentrating, or muscular pains, or actual breathing difficulties, should be listed and given a daily 'score' out of (say) 3, where 0 = no problems and 3 = the worst it has ever been. Make sure to score each symptom each day to see how it varies, and to link this to when suspect foods are eaten (sometimes reaction to foods takes up to 12 hours to be noticed) (see symptom score sheet, p. 264).

If such a score sheet is kept and note is made of suspect foods, a link may be uncovered. By comparing the two lists (suspect foods and symptoms) it is often possible to note a pattern connecting particular foods and symptoms, at which time the exclusion pattern described above can be started.

Oligoantigenic diet

The oligoantigenic diet was developed at Great Ormond Street Hospital for Sick Children, London, and at Addenbrooke's Hospital, Cambridge, as a means of identifying foods which might be causing or aggravating the conditions of young patients.

Avoiding foods which may be provoking symptoms for not less than 5 days means that all traces of any of the food will have cleared the system and any symptoms caused by these should have vanished. Symptoms which remain are either caused by something else altogether (infection for example, or hormonal imbalance, or emotions) or by other foods or substances.

On reintroduction of foods in a carefully controlled sequence (the 'challenge') symptoms which reappear will have been shown to derive from a reaction to particular foods, which are then eliminated from the diet for at least 6 months.

There is some evidence to support the idea that those foods which have become a major part of human diet since Stone Age times – mainly grains (particularly wheat) of all sorts and dairy produce – are the foods which are most likely to provoke reactions. All modern processed foods involving any chemicals, colorings, flavorings, etc. are also suspect until proven safe.

The oligoantigenic diet is usually followed for 3 weeks while a careful check is kept on symptoms (pain, stiffness, mobility, etc.) If the symptoms improve or vanish, then one or more of the foods being avoided may be to blame. Identification and subsequent avoidance of the culprit food(s) depends upon the symptom returning upon the reintroduction (challenge) of the food.

The eating pattern listed below is a modified version of the hospital pattern. To try a modified oligoantigenic exclusion diet, evaluate the effect of following a pattern of eating in which the foods as listed below are included ('Allowed' on the list) or excluded ('Forbidden' on the list), for 3 weeks.

Fish
Allowed: white fish, oily fish
Forbidden: all smoked fish

Vegetables
None are forbidden: but people with bowel problems are asked to avoid beans, lentils, Brussels sprouts and cabbage

Fruit
Allowed: bananas, passion fruit, peeled pears, pomegranates, paw-paw (papaya), mango
Forbidden: all fruits except the six allowed ones

Cereals (and seeds, nuts)
Allowed: rice, sago, buckwheat, quinoa, sunflower seeds, pumpkin seeds, almonds
Forbidden: wheat, oats, rye, barley, corn, millet, sesame, all other nuts

Oils
Allowed: sunflower, safflower, linseed, olive
Forbidden: corn, soya, 'vegetable', nut (especially peanut)

Dairy
Allowed: none (rice milk may be used as a substitute)
Forbidden: cow's milk and all its products including yogurt, butter, most margarine, all goat, sheep **and soya** milk products, eggs

Drinks
Allowed: herbal teas such as camomile and peppermint
Forbidden: tea, coffee, fruit squashes, citrus drinks, apple juice, alcohol, tapwater, **carbonated drinks**

Miscellaneous
Allowed: sea salt
Forbidden: all yeast products, chocolate, preservatives, **all food additives**, herbs, spices, honey, **sugar of any sort**

If benefits are felt after this exclusion, a gradual introduction of <u>one food at a time</u>, leaving at least 4 days between each reintroduction, will allow you to identify those foods which should be left out altogether for at least 6 months – if symptoms reappear when they are reintroduced.

If a reaction occurs (symptoms return having eased or vanished during the 3-week exclusion trial), the offending food is eliminated for at least 6 months and a 5-day period of no further experimentation is followed (i.e. no further reintroduction of previously excluded foods to clear the body of all traces of the offending food), after which testing (challenge) can start again, one food at a time, involving anything you have previously been eating which was eliminated by the oligoantigenic diet.

⚠ When a food to which you are strongly allergic, and which you have been consuming regularly is stopped, you may experience 'withdrawal' symptoms for a week or so, including flu-like symptoms and mood swings, anxiety, restlessness, etc. This will pass after a few days. It can be a strong indication that whatever you have eliminated from the diet is at least partially responsible for a 'masked' allergy, which may be producing many of your symptoms.

© Harcourt Publishers Ltd 2002   Chaitow L, Bradley D, Gilbert C *Multidisciplinary Approaches to Breathing Pattern Disorders*. Churchill Livingstone, Edinburgh

POSITIONAL RELEASE SELF-HELP METHODS (FOR TIGHT, PAINFUL MUSCLES AND TRIGGER POINTS)

When we feel pain, the area which is troubled will usually have some degree of local muscle tension, even spasm, and there is probably a degree of local circulatory deficiency, with not enough oxygen getting to the troubled area and not enough of the normal waste products being removed.

Massage and stretching methods can often assist in helping these situations, even if only temporarily. However, massage is not always available, or it may be impractical if the region is out of reach and you are on your own.

If the pain problem is severe, stretching may help, but at times this may be too uncomfortable.

There is another way of easing tense, tight muscles, and improving local circulation, and it is called 'positional release technique' (PRT). In order to understand this method a brief explanation is needed.

It has been found in osteopathic medicine that almost all painful conditions relate in some way to areas which have been in some manner strained or stressed, either quickly in a sudden incident, or gradually over time because of habits of use, poor breathing habits, posture, etc. When these 'strains' – whether acute or chronic – develop, some tissues (muscles, fascia, ligaments, tendons, nerve fibers, etc.) may be stretched while others are in a contracted, or shortened state. It is not surprising that discomfort emerges out of such patterns, or that these tissues will be more likely to become painful when asked to do something out of the ordinary, such as lifting or stretching. The shortened structures will have lost their normal elasticity, at least partially. It is therefore not uncommon for strains to occur in tissues which are already chronically stressed in some way.

What has been found in PRT is that if the tissues which are short are gently eased to a position in which they are made *even shorter*, a degree of comfort or 'ease' is achieved which can remove pain from the area.

But how are we to know which direction is needed to move tissues which are very painful and tense?

There are some very simple rules and we can apply these to ourselves in an easy to apply 'experiment'.

PRT exercise

Sit in a chair, and with a finger search around in the muscles of the side of your neck, just behind your jaw, directly below your ear lobe. Most of us have painful muscles here. Find a place which is sensitive to pressure.

Press just hard enough to hurt a little, and grade this pain for yourself as a '10' (where 0 = no pain at all).

While still pressing the point, bend your neck forward – very slowly – so that your chin moves towards your chest. Keep deciding what the 'score' is in the painful point.

As soon as you feel it ease a little, start turning your head a little towards the side of the pain, until the pain drops some more.

By 'fine-tuning' your head position, with a little turning, or side-bending, or bending forward some more, you should be able to get the score close to '0'. When you find that position you have taken the pain point to its 'position of ease' and if you were to stay in that position (you don't have to keep pressing the point) for about half a minute, when you SLOWLY return to sitting up straight, the painful area should be less sensitive, and the area will have been flushed with fresh oxygenated blood.

If this were a really painful area, and not an 'experimental' one, the pain would ease over the next day or so, and the local tissues would become more relaxed.

You can do this to any pain point anywhere on the body, including a trigger point (see Ch. 6 and Fig. 10.6). It may not always cure the problem (sometimes it will), but it offers ease.

Rules for self-application of PRT

- Locate a painful point and press just hard enough to score '10'.
- If the point is on the front of the body, bend forward to ease it, and the further it is from

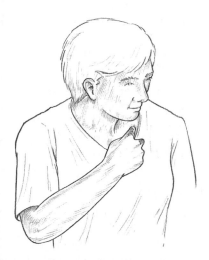

Figure 10.6 Strain/counterstrain self-treatment for second rib tender point. (Reproduced with kind permission from L. Chaitow 1996 Muscle energy techniques. Churchill Livingstone, Edinburgh.)

the midline of your body, the more you should ease yourself *toward* that side.

- If the point is on the back of the body, ease slightly backward until the 'score' drops a little, and then turn *away* from the side of the pain, and then 'fine-tune' to achieve ease.
- Hold the 'position of ease' for not less than 30 seconds and very slowly return to the neutral starting position.

- Make sure that no pain is being produced elsewhere when you are fine-tuning to find the position of ease.
- Do not treat more than 5 pain points on any one day as your body will need to adapt to these self-treatments.
- Expect improvement in function – ease of movement – fairly soon (minutes) after such self-treatment, but reduction in pain may take a day or so and you may actually feel a little stiff or achy in the previously painful area the next day. This will soon pass.
- If intercostal muscle tender points (the muscles between the ribs) are being self-treated, in order to ease feelings of tightness or discomfort in the chest, breathing should be felt to be easier, less constricted, after PRT self-treatment.
- Tender points to help release ribs are often found either very close to the sternum (breast bone), or between the ribs, either (for the upper ribs) in line with the nipple, or (for ribs lower than the 4th) in line with the front of the axilla (armpit).

If you follow these instructions carefully, creating no new pain when finding your positions of ease, and not pressing too hard, you cannot harm yourself and might release tense, tight and painful muscles.

MUSCLE ENERGY SELF-HELP METHODS (FOR TIGHT, PAINFUL MUSCLES AND TRIGGER POINTS)

When a muscle is contracted isometrically (which means contraction without any movement being allowed) for around 10 seconds, that muscle as well as the muscle(s) which performs the opposite action to it (called the antagonist(s)) will be far more relaxed than before the contraction, and can much more easily be stretched than previously. This is known as muscle energy technique (MET).

You can use MET to prepare a muscle for stretching if it feels tighter than it ought to, or before gently stretching it. It is also useful for self-treating muscles in which there are trigger points.

⚠ In this sort of exercise *light contractions only* are used, involving no more than a quarter of your available strength.

MET neck relaxation exercise

First phase of exercise

- Sit close to a table with your elbows on the table and rest your hands on each side of your face.
- Turn your head as far as you can comfortably turn it in one direction, say to the right, letting your hands move with your face, until you reach your pain free limit of rotation in that direction.
- Now use your left hand to resist as you try to turn your head back towards the left, using no more than a quarter of your strength and not allowing the head to actually move. Start the turn slowly, building up force which is matched by your resisting left hand.
- Hold this push – with no movement at all taking place – for about 7–10 seconds, and

then slowly stop trying to turn your head left.
- Now turn your head round to the right as far as is comfortable.

You should find that you can turn a good deal further than the first time you tried, before the contraction. You have been using MET to achieve what is called *post isometric relaxation* in tight muscles which were restricting you.

Second phase of exercise

- Both your hands should still be on the side of your face.
- Now use your right hand to resist your attempt to turn (using only 25% of strength again) even further to the right, starting slowly, and maintaining the turn and the resistance for a full 7–10 seconds.
- When your effort slowly stops, see if you can now go even further to the right than after your first two efforts. You have been using MET to achieve a different sort of release called *reciprocal inhibition*.

You have now used MET in two ways, using the muscles which need releasing and then using their antagonists. Both methods work to release tightness for about 20 seconds, which allows you the chance to stretch tight muscles after the contraction.

MET contractions are working with normal nerve pathways to achieve a release of undesirable excessive tightness in muscles.

You can use MET by contracting whatever part of your body is tight or needs stretching, and especially any muscle which houses a trigger point.

Always contract lightly, hold for 10 seconds, then stretch painlessly using either the tight muscle itself or its antagonist.

WORKBOOK

Have your symptoms checked by your doctor before starting breathing retraining. Check again if symptoms continue to worry you.

Commit to regular practice.

Completing these charts is a graphic way of finding how your stress levels, sleep and symptom patterns interrelate with each other and with you.

Start with the 'Identification of Symptoms' chart. This gives you a picture of how you are on day 1, at the start of breathing retraining. At the beginning of week 2, check symptoms on that day. Repeat on day 1 of week 3.

You can then compare progress from one week to the next. *Try not to look at the chart in between times* – paper clip the page to the previous one.

Fill in the other charts daily for the next fortnight. See if you can identify any patterns.

You should get an idea of what triggers to look out for. Adapt your practice routines accordingly to abolish symptoms.

Identification of symptoms

Listed here are some typical HVS symptoms. You may have only a few of these symptoms while others have the lot.

Start this chart the day you start breathing retraining. Compare day 1 (week 1) and day 1 (week 2) and then day 1 (week 3).

Symptoms	Example	Week 1	Week 2	Week 3
Chest wall pain				
Physical tension	✓ ✓ ✓			
Tiredness	✓ ✓			
Visual disturbances				
Dizziness	✓			
Upset gut	✓			
Poor concentration	✓ ✓			
Faster or deeper breathing	✓ ✓ ✓			
Tight chest	✓ ✓			
Feeling revved up				
Tingling fingers				
Sighing/yawning	✓ ✓			
Tight jaw/throat	✓ ✓			
Headache				
Clammy/cold hands and feet	✓			
Erratic/faster heart beats	✓			
Others				

✓✓✓ = symptoms all day ✓✓ = some of the day ✓ = intermittent

Chaitow L, Bradley D, Gilbert C *Multidisciplinary Approaches to Breathing Pattern Disorders*. Churchill Livingstone, Edinburgh

Which situations trigger breathing discomfort?

Here are some situations that may trigger HVS.

Complete this chart, starting the day you begin breathing retraining, in the same way as the 'identification of symptoms' chart. Compare day 1 (week 1) with day 1 (week 2) and then day 1 (week 3).

Triggers	Example	Week 1	Week 2	Week 3
Driving				
Household chores				
Telephoning	✓✓			
High humidity				
Kissing/making love	✓			
Watching TV/cinema				
Talking	✓✓			
Meetings/interviews	✓✓✓			
Queues/crowds				
Exercise	✓✓			
Others				

✓✓✓ = always ✓✓ = often ✓ = sometimes

Stress and strain gauge

	Day 1			Day 2			Day 3			Day 4			Day 5			Day 6			Day 7			Day 8			Day 9			Day 10			Day 11			Day 12			Day 13			Day 14		
	am	pm	n	am	pm	n	am	pm	n	am	pm	n	am	pm	n	am	pm	n	am	pm	n	am	pm	n	am	pm	n	am	pm	n	am	pm	n	am	pm	n	am	pm	n	am	pm	n
10																																										
9																																										
8																																										
7																																										
6																																										
5																																										
4																																										
3																																										
2																																										
1																																										

Every morning, afternoon and bedtime rate your stress levels by putting a bold dot in the appropriate box.
At the end of two weeks join the dots.
Compare this chart with your 'Symptoms', 'Eating' and 'Sleep' results (see overleaf). Is there a pattern?

1 = calm
10 = highly stressed
am = morning
pm = afternoon
n = night

Chaitow L, Bradley D, Gilbert C *Multidisciplinary Approaches to Breathing Pattern Disorders*. Churchill Livingstone, Edinburgh

Symptoms

Breathing discomfort/sighing/air hunger

Day	1	2	3	4	5	6	7	8	9	10	11	12	13	14
Morning														
Afternoon														
Evening														
Night														

✓ = Yes, I am experiencing HVS symptoms.
○ = I have no HVS symptoms.

Eating

Day	1	2	3	4	5	6	7	8	9	10	11	12	13	14
Breakfast														
Lunch														
Dinner														

✓ = Yes   ♡ = On the run   ○ = Skipped $ = Upset gut

Sleep

Day	1	2	3	4	5	6	7	8	9	10	11	12	13	14
No. of hours														
No. of wakes														
Wake refreshed? (✓ or ○)														

Breathing retraining/'time out'/relaxing

Before you get out of bed, lie on your back and nose/abdominal breathe for a couple of minutes to establish your breathing pattern for the day.

   In bed at night, low, slow nose-breathe while lying on your side to get off to sleep.

For the next two weeks, schedule time in the morning and afternoon or evening for 10 minutes of relaxed abdominal nose-breathing while lying. Make it a priority.

Day	1	2	3	4	5	6	7	8	9	10	11	12	13	14
Waking														
Morning														
Afternoon														
Night														

Be honest!
✓ = Yes   ○ = Forgot/no time

Chaitow L, Bradley D, Gilbert C *Multidisciplinary Approaches to Breathing Pattern Disorders*. Churchill Livingstone, Edinburgh

NASAL WASH RECIPE

This recipe for a nasal wash is an easy, cheap and effective remedy. Salt is a preservative so it won't 'go off.'

   Dissolve 1/2 a teaspoon of rock or sea salt and 1/2 a teaspoon of bicarbonate of soda in 500 ml of hot boiled water.

Fill a cleaned recycled nasal spray bottle with the solution, discard the rest. Spray each nostril morning and evening for two to three days: spray until you feel it hit the back of your throat – with the spray bottle almost horizontal for maximum saturation. Aim the nozzle toward the outside corner of the eye of the nostril being sprayed. Sniff gently, hoick and spit. Spray as required.

Chaitow L, Bradley D, Gilbert C *Multidisciplinary Approaches to Breathing Pattern Disorders*. Churchill Livingstone, Edinburgh

ONE EXAMPLE OF A PSYCHOSOCIAL SCORE: HAD SCORE

This simply administered score measures both anxiety and depression levels. Patients fill in the questionnaire themselves. The therapist adds the figures of all the *odd* numbered questions, which reveals anxiety levels. The total of all the *even* numbered questions gives a depression score. Eleven and above on either or both indicates a positive score and help from a psychologist or counselor may be offered to patients who request further help.

Redone at a later date, this score is also useful as a marker of symptom improvement and gives positive feedback to the patient.

Feelings

This questionnaire is designed to help us know how you feel. Read each item and *UNDERLINE* the reply that comes closest to *how you have been feeling in the past week*. Don't take too long over your replies; your immediate reaction to each item will probably be more accurate than a long thought out response.

1	I feel tense or wound up.	Most of the time.	3
		A lot of the time.	2
		From time to time – occasionally.	1
		Not at all.	0
2	I still enjoy the things I used to enjoy.	Definitely as much.	0
		Not quite so much.	1
		Only a little.	2
		Hardly at all.	3
3	I get a frightened sort of feeling as if something awful is about to happen.	Very definitely and quite badly.	3
		Yes but not too badly.	2
		A little but it doesn't worry me.	1
		Not at all.	0
4	I can laugh and see the funny side of things.	As much as I always could.	0
		Not quite so much now.	1
		Definitely not so much now.	2
		Not at all.	3
5	Worrying thoughts go through my mind.	A great deal of the time.	3
		A lot of the time.	2
		From time to time but not too often.	1
		Only occasionally.	0
6	I feel cheerful.	Not at all.	3
		Not often.	2
		Sometimes.	1
		Most of the time.	0

© Harcourt Publishers Ltd 2002   Chaitow L, Bradley D, Gilbert C *Multidisciplinary Approaches to Breathing Pattern Disorders*. Churchill Livingstone, Edinburgh

7	I can sit at ease and feel relaxed.	Definitely. Usually. Not often. Not at all.	0 1 2 3
8	I feel as if I am slowed down in my thinking.	Nearly all the time. Very often. Sometimes. Not at all.	3 2 1 0
9	I get a sort of frightened feeling like 'butterflies' in the stomach.	Not at all. Occasionally. Quite often. Very often.	0 1 2 3
10	I have lost interest in my appearance.	Definitely. I don't take as much care as I should. I may not take as much care as I should. I take just as much care as ever.	3 2 1 0
11	I feel restless as if I have to be on the move.	Very much indeed. Quite a lot. Not very much. Not at all.	3 2 1 0
12	I look forward with enjoyment to things.	As much as I ever did. Rather less than I used to. Definitely less than I used to. Hardly at all.	0 1 2 3
13	I get sudden feelings of panic.	Very often indeed. Quite often. Not very often. Not at all.	3 2 1 0
14	I can enjoy a good book or radio or TV program.	Often. Sometimes. Not often.	0 1 2

Chaitow L, Bradley D, Gilbert C *Multidisciplinary Approaches to Breathing Pattern Disorders*. Churchill Livingstone, Edinburgh

PERSONAL MONTHLY SYMPTOM SCORE SHEET

NAME: _____   DATE: _____

SYMPTOM SCORING 0 = No Symptoms; 1 = Mild; 2 = Moderate; 3 = Severe

Fill in your scores at the end of the day.

SYMPTOMS DATE:																															
1																															
2																															
3																															
4																															
5																															
6																															
7																															
8																															
9																															
10																															
11																															
12																															
TOTAL SCORE:																															
WEIGHT:																															
COMMENTS:																															

HOW TO USE THE SYMPTOM SCORE SHEET:
List your key symptoms in the left-hand column. Each day, at the same time if possible, estimate a value for each symptom. Write the date in the appropriate box and score: 0 if there was no symptom; 1 if it was mild; 2 if it was moderate to severe; and 3 if it was as bad as you can imagine. The score sheet can be used for any modification but is ideal for dietary change. The weight box is optional and the 'comments' box at the bottom is for entering key words, such as 'Stopped wheat' or 'Period started' or 'Started taking X supplement or medication', or to note anything else that might reflect on the scores of the key symptoms. The total symptom score and the individual scores provide a record of change, or non-change, and can therefore be used to evaluate the efficacy of different strategies. The score sheet may, over a period of a month or two, show a pattern, and can be used specifically to monitor what happens to all or some symptoms when a particular intervention such as a food exclusion or a new medication is being evaluated.

Chaitow L, Bradley D, Gilbert C *Multidisciplinary Approaches to Breathing Pattern Disorders*. Churchill Livingstone, Edinburgh

CAFFEINE: THE FACTS

The immediate effects of caffeine

In small doses

- Increases metabolism
- Increases body temperature
- Acts as a diuretic
- Stimulates the secretion of gastric acid

In large doses

- Can produce headaches and jitters

Long-term effects of caffeine

- Consumption over 600 mg/day may cause insomnia, anxiety, depression, stomach upset

Caffeine as a behavioral stimulant

- 1–2 cups of coffee (i.e. 100–200 mg) causes increased arousal and alertness
- This is followed by a behavioral depression (i.e. a dip in performance)
- If you are unused to consuming caffeine, the stimulant effects may be very noticeable
- If your body is accustomed to large quantities of caffeine you may experience withdrawal effects if you stop consumption (tiredness, lack of energy, headaches)
- The brain becomes accustomed to a certain level of caffeine, consequently more and more is needed to prevent fatigue
- The effects of caffeine may last as long as 5–8 hours after ingestion

Caffeine and sleep

- Caffeine may improve a worker's performance but the long-lasting effects can impair sleep the following day
- Taken prior to sleep, caffeine usually:
  — delays sleep
  — shortens sleep
  — reduces the overall amount of REM sleep

Caffeine intake and recommendations

- Limit yourself to 300 mg per day
- Do not consume caffeine 4 hours prior to sleep
- Use caffeine strategically
- To reduce caffeine, mix decaffeinated coffee with your regular brew and reduce quantity by 1 cup every 3 or 4 days

© Harcourt Publishers Ltd 2002   Chaitow L, Bradley D, Gilbert C *Multidisciplinary Approaches to Breathing Pattern Disorders*. Churchill Livingstone, Edinburgh

PANIC ATTACKS (ACUTE ON CHRONIC HYPERVENTILATION)

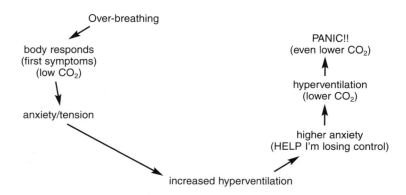

Panicky feelings signal that you have been overbreathing and exhaled too much carbon dioxide. Although these feelings are horrible, they are not dangerous, and will not cause harm. You can train yourself to control your breathing, and not allow your breathing to control you.

Accept the unpleasant symptoms for what they are – the consequence of overbreathing.

Ignore the urge to gasp. Softly breathe in through the nose, and out *slowly* through pursed lips, three times.

Now breathe slowly and gently, in and out through your nose, concentrating on the 'out' breath.

Restore a normal calm rhythmic breathing pattern.

Resting a relaxed hand on your stomach may help you focus.

Breathe the panic away. Congratulate yourself on your success.

From I. Rowbottom MCSP (1990) What is hyperventilation? City Hospital, Edinburgh (Modified 1998)

Chaitow L, Bradley D, Gilbert C *Multidisciplinary Approaches to Breathing Pattern Disorders*. Churchill Livingstone, Edinburgh

STRESS SCAN

Check for signs of tension in each area:

HEAD: Jaw, tongue, lips, eyes, forehead. Pressure, heat, or pulsations in head?
NECK: Braced? Out of balance?
SHOULDERS; *BACK*; *CHEST*: Rapid heart rate?
BREATHING: High? Stopped? Fast? Shallow? Uneven?
ABDOMEN: Tense muscles? Stomach discomfort?
HANDS: Cool? Moist?
OTHER AREAS: Legs, arms, feet, pelvic muscles, thighs.
THOUGHTS AND FEELINGS: Anger, fear, worry, guilt, impatience, insecurity, resentment.

Signs of effective relaxation:

- Muscles and joints looser
- Breathing fuller, slower, lower
- Heart rate slower, less noticeable
- Hands and feet warmer, drier
- Head cooler, less pressure
- Shoulders dropped to a natural position
- Jaw unclenched
- Thinking: better concentration, less pressured, more objective, broader perspective

    Chaitow L, Bradley D, Gilbert C *Multidisciplinary Approaches to Breathing Pattern Disorders*. Churchill Livingstone, Edinburgh

RECOMMENDATIONS FOR HYPERVENTILATION

Dr L. C. Lum served for many years as a chest physician at Papworth Hospital in Cambridge. He was very influential in bringing hyperventilation to the attention of the medical and psychological professions. The following pages contain two handouts that he provided for his patients.

     Chaitow L, Bradley D, Gilbert C *Multidisciplinary Approaches to Breathing Pattern Disorders*. Churchill Livingstone, Edinburgh

FACTORS INVOLVED IN HYPERVENTILATION

1. *Early history*. About 80% of hyperventilators give a history of poor bonding with one or other parent, often both. The remainder either have a family history of asthma, bronchitis or emphysema, or have clearly derived the habit of overbreathing from the parents. There is often a history of proneness to fainting in childhood, or of phobic tendencies. Often other members of the family have similar symptoms.

2. *Personality*. The usual personality is perfectionist, and often obsessional, while being basically insecure. I attribute this to the lack of parental bonding. Children need close ties with *both parents*.

3. *Onset on holiday*. It is very common for symptoms to start when on holiday after a period of stress. Hyperventilators seem to keep going while the pressure is on, and crack when it is relieved. (Weekends too are a favored time for symptoms to start.)

4. *Exacerbation of symptoms at rest*. There seems to be a failure of 'fine-tuning' of respiration, so that breathing changes do not follow accurately changes in activity. For example, in the evening, the breathing does not subside from the level appropriate to daytime activity, to the lower metabolic requirement of watching TV, or trying to go to sleep. A corollary to this is that the commonest situation for developing panic attacks is driving a car (maximum of stimulation combined with minimum of physical effort); next commonest are watching TV and in bed! There are probably physiological analogies with the holiday situation.

5. *Muscle pains*. These are very common, and most often affect the neck, shoulders and upper back. They were attributed to tetanic spasm in isolated muscle fibers as long ago as 1937, and I believe this to be correct, since one can usually locate tender trigger areas in these muscles. Similar tender nodules are usually present at the anterior edge of the parietal muscles when the patient complains of parietal or frontal headache, and at the insertion of the nuchal muscles into the occiput. Less commonly one finds general limb pains, particularly in the legs, associated with a tendency to spasm of whole muscle groups.

6. *Climate and weather*. Hyperventilation is exacerbated by hot (and particularly humid) weather – for the obvious reason of the importance of breathing in heat loss. The influence of hot, humid weather was well documented by American army doctors during the Second World War. Hypoxic stimulation at altitude is also important (the threshold seems to be about 5000 feet). Similarly, marked changes in barometric pressure as with the approach of frontal systems. The development of the painful muscular nodules of HV is probably how Farmer Giles predicts weather changes by his 'rheumaticks'. The turbulent weather in the UK at the end of 1987 provoked many exacerbations, and such severe panic attacks in some patients that I had to put them in hospital.

7. *Low blood sugar*. It is common for symptoms to occur or to get worse before lunch and in the late afternoon, since even a moderately low blood sugar can gravely exaggerate the symptoms of hyperventilation. The diet needs specific modification.

8. *Crying*. Hyperventilators often complain of emotional lability, and are prone to tears. In the laboratory after a session of breath testing, it was common for patients to begin crying, without knowing why. This is due to loss of cortical inhibition due to cerebral hypoxia.

9. *Menstruation*. Symptoms tend to be worse during the premenstrual week and the early days of the period. Progesterone, the hormone secreted by the ovaries after ovulation, is a strong respiratory stimulant, and can reduce carbon dioxide level of the blood by as much as 25%. Hence, any tendency to overbreathe is made worse during this time. Also the symptoms of premenstrual tension (PMT) – headache, tension, irritability, tendency to tears – are common in HV.

10. *Occupational hazards: the voice*. Singers, actors and wind instrumentalists are particularly vulnerable. It has terminated many operatic careers. One of the greatest dramatic sopranos of the 20th century, Rosa Ponselle, always suffered so severely with stage fright that she retired from opera at the height of her career. *Speech*.

Hyperventilators are usually animated, breathless talkers who try to get too many words on one breath. They must be taught to slow down, use shorter phrases, with a small sip of air between phrases, rather than a large gulp between long sentences.

11. *Allergy*. There is a high incidence of allergic phenomena – e.g. eczema, asthma, rhinitis and hay fever – in hyperventilation states. Hyperventilation causes certain blood cells to produce an excess of histamine, a substance which causes allergic reactions. (See also 'Hyperventilation syndromes: physiological considerations in clinical management. In: Timmons B H, Ley R (eds) 1994 Behavioral and psychological approaches to clinical management. Plenum, New York, pp 113–123.)

FAULTS IN HYPERVENTILATION AND CORRECTIVE EXERCISES

1. BREATHING TOO FAST (normal rate is 10–14 breaths per minute; hyperventilators are usually nearer 20, and often much higher)
2. IRREGULAR AMPLITUDE OF BREATHS
3. IRREGULAR RHYTHM
4. FREQUENT SIGHS OR YAWNS
5. HABITUAL SNIFFING AND COUGHING
6. FAST BREATHLESS TALKING

The above faults are all associated with excessive use of the upper thorax. Hyperventilators often do not use the diaphragm at all. Habitual diaphragmatic breathers do not suffer from chronic hyperventilation.

7. GENERAL TENSION OF THE WHOLE BODY

This shows up particularly in the muscles of the neck, just at the base of the skull, the shoulder muscles, and anywhere down the back on either side of the spinal processes. However, any muscles of the body or limbs may be affected. Chronic tension causes painful knots of muscle in spasm. Particularly liable to be affected are the locations listed above, muscles over the temples (which cause migraine-like headaches), muscles in the chest wall, particularly under the left breast or alongside the breast bone, around the shoulder, elbow and wrist joints. These are more common on the left side, but often affect the right side of the chest. However, virtually any muscle in the body may be affected. The usual result is an aching pain, sometimes stabbing. Occasionally a whole muscle may go into spasm, causing severe cramp-like pains.

Diaphragm exercises

NOTE: These exercises are designed to overcorrect the faults. The hyperventilator's respiratory center has become 'set' to keep the $PaCO_2$ at an abnormally low level; the very slow rate teaches the hyperventilator to resist the inspiratory drive.

Inhalation with the diaphragm *actively* pushes out the front wall of the abdomen. Exhalation is completely *passive*. The lung empties itself as a balloon does. NO exhalatory effort is required. One just relaxes, and lets the air fall out.

There must be no pause between inhalation and exhalation. As you begin to let the air come out, feel yourself relax, and continue to relax during the count before the next breath, resisting the desire to sneak in a small breath during this time. You should aim at getting the number of breaths down to between six and eight breaths a minute. Time yourself with a clock, and teach yourself how many counts it takes to achieve this. You may not be able to slow your breathing down this much at first. Eight is what you should aim for initially; eventually get down to six.

Practice sessions

You should do five or six sessions (minimum four), each lasting ten minutes, every day. These should be in the semi-recumbent position. You should not attempt to do anything else (e.g. watch TV, listen to music or the radio) during this time. It is helpful to do similar breathing before getting up and when settling down to sleep, but *do not count these as practice*; you don't learn much when you are half asleep.

Standing practice

Stand with the feet apart, weight more on one foot than the other (change the weight from time to time). Let the arms hang loosely across the front of the abdomen, with one hand loosely holding the other arm above the wrist, so that the forearms feel the movements of the abdominal wall. The shoulders should be down, and the whole attitude appear relaxed. You can do this for a few minutes at a time whenever the opportunity occurs, e.g. when shopping.

Periodic reminders

Develop the habit of paying attention to your breathing frequently (4–6 times an hour), by reminding yourself to take a couple of breaths with the diaphragm. Usually, this should be when you change from doing one thing to doing another (e.g. using the phone, in jobs around the house, in reading or writing, between paragraphs and pages).

Cultivate relaxation at all times

Watch your body language. Does your attitude reflect tension or relaxation? Most overbreathers are in a chronic state of tension which shows in the way they sit, stand, walk, hold a pen or drive a car – in fact their every attitude and movement.

Learn the relaxed way of sitting, standing and walking, and get the habit of asking yourself, 'What message is my body language sending out?' Whenever you change activity, action, or posture, your first thought must be to do it in a relaxed way.

Hyperventilators are invariably fast, breathless talkers. They put too much effort into voice, facial expression, and gesture. They speak in long sentences without pausing for breath and then have to take a gasp before the next sentence. Learn to break up your speech into small phrases of a few words each. Learn the trick of taking a short sip of air (with the diaphragm) after each short phrase. Talking on the telephone usually increases overbreathing. It is useful to make a tape of your voice on the telephone and in ordinary conversation round the house. This will help you to identify harmful mannerisms.

Walking rhythm

Hyperventilators' breathing is always fast and irregular. The rhythm of the feet provides a regular beat with which to coordinate your breathing. Walking at your normal pace, take two steps for breathing in, two for breathing out, and hold your breath for two steps. (This pause is shorter than the pause during practice, because walking requires twice as much air as sitting.) Do not worry about diaphragm breathing at first. First of all get the rhythm right. When you can do this easily, start to train yourself to breathe with the diaphragm while walking. It is difficult to learn two things at the same time.

Walking to eliminate body tension

The natural rhythm of the body requires that, as one leg goes forward, the opposite arm should swing forward. A limber, relaxed gait requires that the shoulder should also swing forward with the arm. This is known as 'contrary body movement' in dancing. What happens to the back muscles is that, as one shoulder is pulled forward by the muscles on one half of the back, the same muscles on the opposite side must relax (this is a physiological law). Consequently, during walking the back muscles alternately contract and relax, instead of being tense all the time. When you have mastered this method of walking you will soon find that the painful nodules in the back and neck disappear.

Try to walk as if you were pleased with yourself. Remember that body language is a two-way affair: if you make yourself move as if you were relaxed and pleased with yourself, you will begin to feel that way.

 Chaitow L, Bradley D, Gilbert C *Multidisciplinary Approaches to Breathing Pattern Disorders*. Churchill Livingstone, Edinburgh

Index

Page numbers in **bold** indicate figures and tables.

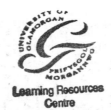